Springer Series on
LIFE STYLES AND ISSUES IN AGING

Series Editor: Bernard D. Starr, PhD
Marymount Manhattan College
New York, NY

Advisory Board: Robert C. Atchley, PhD; M. Powell Lawton, PhD;
Marjorie Cantor, PhD (Hon);
Harvey L. Sterns, PhD

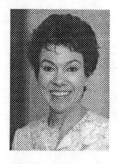 **Carole Cox, Ph.D.,** is Associate Professor at the Graduate School of Social Service, Fordham University. Her previous gerontological work and research have focused in the areas of caregiving, ethnicity, and service utilization, including international comparisons of programs. Dr. Cox is the author of numerous book chapters and articles dealing with various aspects of the issues confronting older persons and their families. Her previous books include *Home Care: An International Perspective* (co-author, Abraham Monk), published by Auburn House, *The Frail Elderly: Problems, Needs and Community Responses*, Auburn House, and *Ethnicity and Social Work Practice* (co-author, Paul Ephross), published by Oxford University Press. Her interest in custodial grandparents and the particular problems they face stems from her personal involvement with these grandparents both in grandparent groups and in the community.

To Grandmother's House We Go and Stay

Perspectives on Custodial Grandparents

Carole B. Cox, PhD
Editor

 **Springer Series on
Lifestyles and Issues in Aging**

Copyright © 2000 by Springer Publishing Company, Inc.

Springer Publishing Company, Inc.
536 Broadway
New York, NY 10012-3955

Cover design by James Scotto-Lavino
Acquisitions Editor: Bill Tucker
Production Editor: Jeanne Libby

00 01 02 03 / 5 4 3 2 1

Library of Congress Cataloging-in-Publication Data

To grandmother's house we go and stay: perspectives on custodial grandparents /
    Carole B. Cox, editor.
        p.   cm. — (Springer series on life styles and issues in aging)
    Includes bibliographical references and index.
    ISBN 0-8261-1286-2
    1. Grandparents as parents.   2. Grandparent and child.   3. Child rearing.
    I. Cox, Carole B.   II. Series.
    HQ759.9.T615   1999 2000
    306.874'5—dc21

                                                                99-15737
                                                                CIP

This book is dedicated to my grandparents and to all the grandparents who inspire, give shape to, and link the generations.

Contents

Contributors

Sandra Barnhill, JD
Executive Director
Aid to Children of Imprisoned
  Mothers
Atlanta, GA

Jacquelin Berman, PhD
Director of Research
New York City Department of the
  Aging
New York, NY

Lisette Resto Brooks, CSW
Director
Community School Program/PS5
New York, NY

Diane R. Brown, PhD
Professor and Director
Urban Health Program
Wayne State University
College of Urban, Labor, and
  Management Affairs
Detroit, MI

Patricia Brownell, PhD
Assistant Professor
Graduate School of Social Service
Fordham University
New York, NY

Carol S. Cohen, DSW
Assistant Professor
Graduate School of Social Service
Fordham University
New York, NY

Carole B. Cox, MSW, PhD
Associate Professor
Graduate School of Social Service
Fordham University
New York, NY

Paula Dressel, PhD
Senior Fellow
Anna E. Casey Foundation
Baltimore, MD

Diane Driver, PhD
Academic Coordinator
Center on Aging
University of California
Berkeley, CA

Du Feng, PhD
Assistant Professor
Department of Human
  Development and Family Studies
Texas Tech University
Lubbock, TX

Margaret M. Flynt, JD
Director, Elderly Project
Volunteers of Legal Services
New York, NY

Roseanne Giarrusso, PhD
Research Assistant
Professor of Gerontology
Andrus Gerontology Center
University of Southern California
Los Angeles, CA

Martha Johns, MSW
Senior Project Associate
National Resource Center for
  Permanency Planning
Hunter College
School of Social Work
New York, NY

Daphne Joslin, PhD
Associate Professor
Department of Community Health
William Patterson College
Wayne, NJ

Joan Mars, PhD
Assistant Professor
Department of Public Affairs
University of Wisconsin
Oshkosh, WI

Jonathan Marx, PhD
Associate Professor
Department of Sociology
Winthrop University
Rock Hill, SC

Meredith Minkler, Dr. PH
Professor of Health and Social
  Behavior
School of Public Health
University of California
Berkeley, CA

Faith Mullen, JD
Senior Policy Analyst
Public Policy Institute
American Association of Retired
  Persons
Washington, DC

Carol M. Musil, PhD, RN
Assistant Professor of Nursing
Bolton School of Nursing
Case Western Reserve University
Cleveland, OH

John Mutikani, MSN, RN
Bolton School of Nursing
Case Western Reserve University
Cleveland, OH

Melinda Perez-Porter, JD
Director, Grandparent Caregiver
  Law Center
Brookdale Center on Aging
Hunter College
New York, NY

Jeff Porterfield, PhD
Associate Professor
Department of Sociology and
  Criminal Justice
Clark Atlanta University
Atlanta, GA

Rolanda Pyle, MSW
Director, Grandparent Resource
  Center
New York City Department of the
  Aging
New York, NY

Kathleen M. Roe, DrPH, MPH
Professor of Community Health
  Education
Department of Health Science
San Jose State University
San Jose, CA

Susan Schrader, BSN, RN
Bolton School of Nursing
Case Western Reserve University
Cleveland, OH

Merril Silverstein, PhD
Hanson Family Assistant Professor
  of Gerontology and Sociology
Andrus Gerontology Center
University of Southern California
Los Angeles, CA

Nina M. Silverstein, PhD
Associate Professor
Gerontology Institute
University of Massachusetts
Boston, MA

Jennifer Crew Solomon, PhD
Associate Professor
Department of Sociology
Winthrop University
Rock Hill, SC

Esme Fuller Thomson, PhD
Anson Assistant Professor
Faculty of Social Work
University of Toronto
Toronto, Canada

Carmen Valcarcel, MA
Mental Health Clinician
Community School Program/PS5
New York, NY

Laila Vehvilainen, MPH
Gerontology Institute
University of Massachusetts
Boston, MA

Preface

This book addresses a growing phenomenon in American society, that of grandparents assuming responsibility for raising their grandchildren. Grandparents have always played important roles in the lives of grandchildren, but throughout the country more and more are finding that, because of the incapacity of their own children, they are assuming the roles of parents. The many factors contributing to this phenomenon and the impact that they have on grandparents, their grandchildren, and society itself are examined in the following chapters.

The 18 chapters address the varied spheres and dimensions of the grandparent-grandchild relationship as well as the policies and services, both existing and needed, which can strengthen it. The overall intention of this book is to underscore the issues faced by these grandparents. The diverse backgrounds and areas of specialization of the authors, which include lawyers, nurses, social workers, psychologists, sociologists, and public health professionals, give a unique breadth to the book. Their expertise is used to explore topics ranging from social and psychological concerns to diversity to policy issues and community programs and services.

Uniting the perspectives of this group of experts is a shared concern for the development of policies and interventions to support grandparent caregivers. As the book examines the many facets of these grandparent's lives, from these many perspectives, it will, I hope, lead to actions that realize these goals.

Throughout the book, it is apparent that grandparents, often in the face of tremendous odds and obstacles, are performing heroic tasks as they assume responsibility for their grandchildren. These grandparents underscore the continuing importance of family and responsibility. They demonstrate that "it doesn't take a village to raise a child"; it really takes a grand-mother!

Finally, I would like to add my own appreciation to a particular group of grandparents, the Grandparent Empowerment Movement (GEM) of the Harlem Interfaith Counseling Center. I have had the opportunity both to work with and to learn from these very special grandparents. In particular, I would like to thank Gwendolyn Florant, facilitator of the group and director of the Center, for her vision and enthusiasm and Celestine Grant, chairperson of GEM, a grandmother, a community activist, and a very wise woman, for her ceaseless energy and commitment. My special appreciation is given to the New York Community Trust for its understanding and support of my own and other projects designed to empower and address the needs of grandparent caregivers.

CAROLE COX
January, 1999

SECTION I

Setting the Stage

Chapter 1

Why Grandchildren Are Going to and Staying at Grandmother's House and What Happens When They Get There

Carole B. Cox

In response to shifts and changes in the structure of families and in response to changing social conditions, the role of grandparents in American society is being redefined. Increasingly, grandparents, rather than playing peripheral roles in the lives of their grandchildren, are becoming responsible for raising them.

Between the years 1980 to 1990, the number of children in the United States living with their grandparents or other relatives increased by 44%, and in a third of these homes, no parent was present (Saluter, 1992). In 1997, 3.7 million grandparents were raising their grandchildren, and most, 2.3 million, were grandmothers (Lugaila, 1998). The prevalence of grandparent-headed households is not evenly distributed among the population. It is most likely to occur among African-Americans, where 13.5% of all children are being raised by grandparents in comparison with 6.5% of Hispanics and 4.1% of White non-Hispanic children. Compared with other households, grandmothers raising grandchildren are more likely to be poor, more likely to be receiving public assistance, and less likely to have health insurance (Casper & Bryson, 1998).

The dramatic increase in grandparent-headed households has been attributed to many factors including parental substance abuse (Kelley, 1993; Minkler et al., 1992), AIDS (Joslin & Brouard, 1995), incarceration (Dressel & Barnhill, 1994), homicide (Kelley & Yonker, 1997), and mental illness (Dowdell, 1995; Kelley, 1993). Most grandparents heading these new households never anticipated becoming parents again. In most instances, they are thrust into the role as a result of the loss or incapacity of their own child.

The needs and problems encountered by these grandparents are not going unnoticed. Articles on grandparent caregivers continue to occur in the press as well as in feature stories on both local and national television stations and radio. Both the U.S. House of Representatives (1992) and the U.S. Senate (1992) have held hearings on the issue of grandparents raising grandchildren. In the past few years, a plethora of sites on the World Wide Web devoted to grandparents raising grandchildren has also developed. These sites offer support, "chat rooms," resources, and education. Underlying these sites is a common recognition of the needs of grandparents for assistance, information, and support.

Further underscoring the extent of this growing phenomenon is the attention that was paid to these grandparents at the 1995 White House Conference on Aging. For the first time, a specific session was devoted to the concerns of grandparents raising grandchildren with the objective of bringing these concerns to the attention of policy makers. Among the resolutions passed were the need to establish comprehensive programs for grandparents, financial, social and legal supports, removing barriers to public programs, development of supportive services, the need for legal surrogate decision-making authority, and the promotion of intergenerational programs to strengthen the family unit headed by the grandparent.

However, it is important to note that, to date, there is no comprehensive policy or program designed to meet the needs of custodial grandparents. Any efforts to meet the objectives have primarily been made at the state and local levels. In addition, private foundations and community agencies have assumed increasingly actives roles in meeting the needs of both grandparents and their grandchildren. As programs continue to develop throughout the country, there is a pressing need for information that can assist in their development. It is hoped that chapters in this book, through their in-depth examination of status, issues, and concerns of grandparents raising grandchildren, will contribute to the growth of programs sensitive to the needs of this population. In addition, chapters on policies and services affecting these grandparents present information, which is critical for professionals seeking to work with and to advocate for these grandparents.

Grandparents in American Society

As a prelude to understanding the current position of many American grandparents, an examination of their traditional positions in American society may be helpful. For the most part, grandparents have acted as adjuncts to the parents, available for assistance, but not responsible for actual child rearing.

Gratton and Haber (1996) tracing the role of grandparents through the advent of Social Security find that until the mid-19th century, they were viewed as figures of authority dependent on their means for economic and social control. By the early 20th century, as a result of economic changes, the status of older persons and thus of grandparents had declined, and grandparents were often perceived as a threat or burden rather than a resource. Following the depression and the advent of Social Security, grandparents, no longer a fiscal threat to families, assumed the role of companions and friends to grandchildren. As will be described throughout this book, new social forces are, for many, transforming this role of companion into that of parent.

Grandparents have also been described according to their styles of grandparenting (Neugarten & Weinstein, 1964), levels of activity in the role (Cherlin & Furstenberg, 1985), and according to others' expectations of their behavior. Grandparents may be expected to act as a type of "safety valve" that can be called upon to provide immediate assistance during a family crisis, such as divorce or unemployment (Cherlin & Furstenberg, 1986). Grandparents may also be expected to act as primary sources for instilling moral beliefs and values in children (Roberto & Stroes, 1992). Overall, the most important function expected of grandparents has simply been to "be there" and to help maintain a sense of family identity and continuity (Bengston, 1985).

This discussion of the roles that grandparents have traditionally assumed underscores the extent to which the role is shaped by individual personalities and interests and the expectations of others. Indeed, because of the absence of any prescribed functions associated with being a "grandparent," the role has been termed a "roleless role" (Troll, 1983). Moreover, any norms for behaviors that do exist tend to be more in terms of what grandparents should not do, how they should not interfere, rather than what they should do and how they should be (Johnson, 1983; Kornhaber & Woodward, 1981).

Given this paucity of positive expectations and functions, it is no wonder that grandparents raising grandchildren are often confused and unsure about their roles. Their roles as adjuncts to parents are in themselves vague, and there is a definite lack of guidelines for them when they assume the parenting role. This very ambiguity implies that these grandparents are largely responsible for shaping and giving meaning to this new identity, defining it according to their own personalities, resources, and values.

At the same time, as the role of parenting grandparent becomes increasingly prevalent, it is likely to assume the qualities of other normative social roles. As specific behaviors and patterns of interaction become expected and shared, they will strongly influence the ways in which the new grandparent role is enacted. Consequently, as with other social roles, grandparents raising grandchildren will find that they must fulfill certain obligations and actions meaning that they are no longer trapped in a "roleless role."

Theoretical Perspectives Related to Understanding the Parenting Grandparent

---

Role Theory

Many of the issues faced by parenting grandparents may be attributed to role uncertainty and ambiguity; thus, in attempting to understand the situations encountered by many grandparents, it may be helpful to briefly examine role theory. As discussed earlier, roles involve specific expected behaviors, and these behaviors form the basis for social interactions.

Persons learn how to perform their social roles through several processes. Anticipatory socialization refers to the process of learning what is expected in a role before assuming it (Sarbin & Allen, 1968). As an example, middle school students often attend a high school orientation before beginning the new school while expectant parents may attend parenting classes before the birth of their first child. Each of these strategies assist in preparing persons for new and unknown roles; helping them to learn correct patterns of behaviors and actions that can ease the transition. Unfortunately, these types of preparation are seldom available to grandparents who often enter the new role because of a family crisis or loss. Few anticipate or prepare for parenting their grandchildren.

Satisfactory role performance also depends on having the ability and motivation to meet the role's requirements (Brim, 1968). Waking during the night to care for infants and dealing with the rebelliousness of adolescents demands an energy level and physical status which many grandparents do not have. Poor health and chronic conditions, which afflict many older persons, can seriously impede their ability to carry out the new role effectively.

Motivation toward accepting the parenting role may also be lacking. Many grandparents are not eager to accept responsibility for their grandchildren and may do so as a result of coercion by other family members, the judicial system, or out of a sense of loyalty and responsibility. For some, the new responsibility may mean that they must give up work to provide care, whereas others find they have little or no time for their usual activities or friends.

An important factor in learning and accepting new roles is the presence of social supports. These supports are those with whom one interacts and confides and who are critical for providing necessary reinforcement and encouragement. Their relationships and assistance are important in helping grandparents to both define and accept the new roles. Many grandparents assuming the responsibility of raising their grandchildren are without these supports. In fact, by assuming the parenting role, established support networks may be disrupted. Developing new support systems, which can offer advice, teach skills, and provide emotional sustenance can be a critical factor in their well-being and successful role enactment.

In the course of aging, persons typically relinquish some roles and take on new ones (Riley et al., 1969). This role transition is easier if the individual understands and accepts the requirements associated with the new role and sees it as having certain esteem and status. The transition is difficult if the relinquished role is being replaced by one of less value. Continuity theory (Neugarten, Havighurst, & Tobin, 1968) further postulates that individuals strive to maintain psychological continuity as they age by substituting similar roles for lost ones. This type of continuity becomes important for maintaining self-esteem and life satisfaction with individuals seeking to retain those roles with which they most closely identified (Atchley, 1989).

Many grandparents who become parents again may perceive it as a positive transition as they gain a new important role. Moreover, those who most closely identified with the parent role and who received much satisfaction with it may enjoy the opportunity to enact it again with their grandchildren. Conversely, those who perceive the role as a loss, whether of status or freedom, are likely to find the transition stressful. Indeed, for some grandparents, the role may compensate for other losses, whereas for others, it may precipitate loss as it means that more valued roles must be forsaken.

Developmental Stages

Several theories related to adjustment and aging may also help in understanding the issues and stresses which may be encountered by grandparents raising grandchildren. According to developmental stage theorists, development through life occurs sequentially as persons move through predetermined stages closely tied to chronological age. Although there is more fluidity now regarding the timing of marriage, education, childbirth, and retirement, the parenting role is generally determined by choice and is associated with the early and middle stages of life. (Dannefer, 1984; Rindfuss, Swicegood & Rosenfeld, 1987) rather than the latter stages.

Erikson (1963) described the stages of late adulthood as periods of searching for meaning to one's life with the major task that of achieving a sense of integrity and wisdom. Rather than a period of activity, it is a time of integration. Havighurst (1972) identified the major tasks of later life as adjusting to limitations and losses including reduced income, strength, and health.

Levinson's model discusses three stages in adult life (Levinson et al., 1978) separated by transitional periods during which new life structures are created as individuals give up the past and move toward the future. During these transitions, particularly beginning at midlife, individuals must become sensitive to changes within themselves so that they may respond appropriately to the changing environment. For older persons, this involves increasing awareness of limitations so that they can make appropriate adjustments in their lifestyles.

All of these life-stage perspectives view the latter periods as ones of greater introspection, with persons seeking a sense of meaning to what has already occurred rather than taking on new challenges. The later stages are associated with a propensity to constrict one's life rather than expand, as adaptations to limitations become dominant preoccupations.

According to the developmental perspectives, grandparents raising grandchildren are psychologically and socially vulnerable as they are not complying with the expected tasks of later life. For grandparents who begin raising their grandchildren at midlife, their own transitions and quests for personal meaning are thwarted by new child-rearing responsibilities. For older grandparents, child rearing offers little time for reflection on the meaning of one's own life. In fact, one's own sense of wisdom may be continually provoked by the challenges incumbent within the new role.

Conversely, to the extent that grandparents effectively adjust to the demands of parenting, they challenge the theories themselves. By effectively assuming the parenting role, they give evidence that adult development does not occur in a linear process with one stage preceding another. Instead, a cyclical pattern, which gives persons the opportunity to repeat an earlier stage, may be most conducive to late-life integrity and fulfillment. For grandparents, having the opportunity to repeat an earlier stage with new experiences, skills, and learning may mean a "second chance," to more effectively enact the parent role, consequently enhancing feelings of self-esteem and control.

Other theoretical perspectives, such as exchange theory, age stratification, feminist theory, and family systems theories may also help in interpreting the experiences of grandparent caregivers. The use of these theories is critical for both guiding research and integrating the findings into a meaningful context. As theories assist in explaining and predicting the responses of grandparent caregivers, they provide the frameworks for developing interventions appropriate to the needs of grandparent caregivers.

Issues Confronting Grandparents

As can be seen in the preceding discussion and as will be discussed throughout this book, grandparents raising grandchildren are at risk for many problems, including social isolation, psychological and emotional stress, and financial strain. A lack of preparation for the role coupled with scarce resources to meet the new demands and responsibilities compound their difficulties in adjustment. Often, they find themselves attempting to adjust to the new situation while confronting the grief associated with the loss of their child. For many, poverty, little access to resources, and poor health further aggravate there coping efforts. The characteristics of a national sample of custodial grandparents described in the following chapter by Minkler, Fuller-Thompson, and Driver underscore the prevalence of these factors, which are subsequently referred to throughout the book.

The issue of health, as discussed in the chapter by Marx and Solomon, is a complex one. Although custodial grandparents report poorer health than noncustodial grandparents, these differences must be examined in conjunction with variables, such as marital status, income, supports, number and ages of the grandchildren, and race. Such understanding is essential for the development of appropriate policies and programs for both grandparents and grandchildren.

Accepting the reality that one's own child is not able to parent is for many an additional stress, which can undermine any feelings of competency in the grandparent role. For many, the communities in which they live are a constant source of anxiety. Worries about gangs, drugs, and violence that may tempt or affect their grandchildren and learning how to contend with these influences are major concerns. For those whose own children succumbed to these threats, these worries can be overwhelming.

Grandparents may also find themselves in conflict with their own children over either custody or parental involvement with the grandchildren. In situations where grandparents have been given custody because of neglect or abuse, they may find they are continually challenged by parents who see their rights having been usurped against their will. Grandparents often experience conflicting emotions and loyalties as they balance the desires of their children with the best interests of their grandchildren (Kelley & Damato, 1995). In situations where parents have been abusive, the grandparents may decide to forbid their contact with the children, while at the same time, struggling to not speak negatively about them to the grandchildren. Being able to cope effectively with the stresses involved in parenting is a major challenge. The chapter by Musil, Schrader, and Mutikani examines varying coping strategies used by grandparents as they attempt to meet these challenges.

Raising grandchildren may also be very rewarding. Many find enormous gratification in the parenting role; as discussed in the chapter by Giarrusso, Silverstein, and Du Feng, raising grandchildren offers both psychological costs and benefits, providing a "mixed bag" of stress and rewards. Understanding the response of grandparents to the situation necessitates special attention to the circumstances under which the grandparents obtained the grandchildren and their values and attitudes toward family responsibility.

Among the rewards that grandchildren may offer are a renewed purpose and excitement to life as well as new patterns for social interaction. Although there may be less time for leisure activities, there are also new opportunities for involvement. Grandchildren can also relieve isolation and loneliness that threaten many older persons. Although their social life may become constricted, many grandparents find that having someone in the home to care for compensates for other losses.

Any consideration of the roles and needs of grandparents must also examine the needs of the grandchildren they are raising, as they are caring for children who have, for whatever reason, lost their own parents. This loss impacts on the relationship between grandparent and grandchild, even among those for whom the relationship began almost at the child's birth. For all children, there is a need to know and understand the reasons why they are not being raised by their own parents. The needs and issues confronting these children and the ways they impact on the grandparents are discussed throughout the book.

Those children who have lived with their parents and developed a relationship with them, regardless of its nature or quality, are vulnerable to feeling abandoned. Grandchildren who have entered their grandparent's home after experiencing parental drug abuse, neglect, illness, or death are at particular risk for psychological and behavioral problems.

Even in the most ideal situation, insecurity and fear can lead to acting-out behaviors as grandchildren seek to determine the structure of the new household. Many of the grandchildren coming to live with their grandparents have lived in homes with no or very few restrictions. Consequently, attempts to control their behaviors may be met with rebellion. Learning to trust or feel secure in the new environment is difficult. Feelings of insecurity may be exacerbated by their fears about grandparents' health and continued ability to care for them.

The special needs of these children would be taxing for the most able parent. For grandparents, these needs can be overpowering. In addition to dealing with normal problems associated with the varied stages of child rearing, many grandparents must also learn to cope with hostility and aggressive behavior. Abuse against grandparents is an issue that is beginning to be explored as more and more cases become reported. As discussed in the chapter by Brownell and Berman, many factors, particularly associted with adolescence, make grandparents vulnerable to abuse.

Diversity in Grandparent Situations and Roles

Grandparents assume the role of parent as a result of diverse circumstances. One of the major contributors to the role has been HIV/AIDS, which is explored in depth in the chapter by Joslin. Although the impact of the disease is felt primarily among the younger population, it has concomitantly affected older persons as they become caregivers. Not only do they provide care to their ailing children; they frequently assume responsibility for raising their grandchildren. Developing programs and services that address the multiple and complex needs of these grandparents are a major concern.

Particular difficulties confront grandparents raising grandchildren of incarcerated parents. Incarceration is stigmatizing and traumatic for grandparents and grandchildren with grandparents in need of both resources and social services. However, obtaining such assistance can be frustrating with grandparents often having to make enormous sacrifices to meet the needs of their grandchildren. The chapter by Porterfield, Dressel, and Barnhill examines the circumstances affecting these grandparents while also offering suggestions for both policy and service reform.

The importance of cultural and ethnic values in defining the role of grandparents cannot be ignored. Common to other social roles, that of grandparent is similarly affected by norms and traditions. Among many ethnic groups in which strong intergenerational relations and supportive family environments have remained intact, the role of the grandparent has remained clearly defined (Baressi, 1987).

However, as younger generations assimilate into American society, the position and status of grandparents often becomes tenuous and impaired (Van Tran, 1988). To maintain relationships, older persons may be forced to accommodate to the needs of their family, even to the extent that their own concerns are ignored (Detzner, 1996). Consequently, many grandparents, even within diverse ethnic families, are raising grandchildren because of cultural and social necessities rather than personal choice. Thus, any assumption regarding the ethnic grandparent's willingness and eagerness to accept the parenting role should be made with caution. Indeed, as ethnic grandparents have themselves assimilated to the dominant society, they may experience strong reservations about their obligation to begin raising children again.

Two of the groups with the highest rates of custodial grandparenthood are African Americans and Latinos. A series of focus groups conducted with grandparents from both populations found each feeling strained in attempting to meet the demands of the grandchildren, many of whom had emotional problems (AARP, 1997). Both voiced two major concerns: their own physical and psychological limitations and finances. Moreover, their stress was often heightened by friction with their own child and by fears that the grandchild could be returned to an unsafe home. With both groups living on modest incomes, often close to the poverty line, worries about expenses associated with raising children were constant.

The histories and cultures of both African Americans and Latinos in the United States have contributed to both groups' preference for familial assistance in times of need. Distrust and suspicion of the greater society and its programs, negative experiences with these programs, and problems of accessibility and language are among the many factors affecting their use of programs and services. Consequently, it is not surprising that when parents are incapacitated or absent grandparents are the favored source of assistance.

African-American grandparents have often acted as surrogate parents to the grandchildren particularly in periods of social and economic upheaval when there was an overwhelming need for them to keep the family intact. Following the Civil War, grandmothers were frequently called on to raise the grandchildren as the children searched for work (Jackson, 1986) or migrated to urban areas in the North and West (Burton & Dilworth-Anderson, 1991). From the early 19th century until the mid-1960s, it was common for the black grandmother to accept and raise both her own grandchildren as well as more extended kin and orphans with no place else to live (Jones, 1973).

However, surrogate parenting, although a common historical tradition, should not be perceived as normative in today's society (Burton & Dilworth-Anderson, 1991). As with other grandparents raising their grandchildren, most African-American custodial grandparents had neither anticipated nor prepared for the situation. The chapter by Brown and Mars on the experiences of a sample of African-American grandparents raising grandchildren illustrates how family bonds continue to influence grandparents' acceptance of the parenting role. At the same time, the role remains stressful with grandparents in need of supports and resources.

Latino culture is often characterized through a commitment to the value of familism, which places the needs of the family above those of the individual. Marin (1989) defines familism as a sense of duty to provide emotional and material support to members of the extended family with relatives the more reliable preferred helpers. The value emphasizes the importance of children and the elderly and the strong obligation to help each as needed.

The elderly typically assist their children through child care. Economic uncertainty and poverty accentuates this involvement as grandparents act as a critical resource to families, which may allow parents to work. In fact, the role of child care provider may be the one role occupied by older people that increases in importance when Hispanic families immigrate to the United States (Gelfand, 1989). Consequently, assuming the parental role when children are absent or incapacitated may be perceived as simply extending traditional norms and patterns.

However, similar to African-American grandparents, the task of raising grandchildren is a challenging one to Latino grandparents. As discussed in the chapter by Cox, Brooks, and Valcarcel, traditional values, limited resources, and social institutions impact on their caregiving roles and ability.

Policy Issues

The many issues faced by grandparents raising grandchildren testify to a need for specific policies to support them. However, as discussed earlier, there is not yet any comprehensive federal policy or program that addresses the issues these older persons confront.

At the same time, some immediate policy issues affecting the relationship of the grandparent to the grandchild and to the children have begun to be addressed. Adoption, guardianship, kinship care, or foster care are strategies and means of legalizing the relationship of the grandparent to the grandchild. The chapter by Perez-Porter and Flint describes the legal mechanisms available to grandparents raising grandchildren. Types of legal arrangements vary by state, and it is essential that advocates are knowledgeable about the options available to grandparents in the state in which they live.

Kinship foster care is particularly relevant to grandparents as in most states nonrelative foster parents receive higher benefits than relatives. The underlying assumption seems to be that relatives, including grandparents, can assume the responsibility for caring for the children without experiencing it as a burden and that additional financial resources are not necessary. But, as has been discussed earlier, finances are one of the primary concerns of custodial grandparents, many of whom live below or near the poverty line.

Most states must assume legal custody of the child before the grandparent can become a foster parent. In addition, becoming a foster parent entails investigation, background checks, and often special classes. Grandparents who are unfamiliar with the legal and service systems, who are anxious about their own status in America, whose education and English are limited, or who have chronic health problems are frequently unwilling to go through the foster parent process. Consequently, they remain ineligible for payments that can help in support of the child.

Permanency planning for children living with grandparents remains an illusive goal. The needs and concerns of these grandparents do not generally fit with the demands and interests of child welfare systems. The chapter by Johns examines the growth of permanency planning movement and its relationship to grandparent caregivers while highlighting both the strengths and weaknesses of the policy. Meeting the needs of relative caregivers through a formal system designed for nonrelatives and trying to assure stability for children in a safe environment remains a formidable challenge.

Welfare reform, which occurred with passage of the Personal Responsibility and Work Opportunities Act of 1996, may have particularly onerous effects on grandparents seeking public benefits. The Temporary Assistance to Needy Families (TANF) emphasizes personal responsibility and self-sufficiency as well as the role of the biological parents in raising children.

Mullen's chapter addresses the benefits available under the Act and the ways in which they apply to custodial grandparents. Although the impact of this legislation on grandparent caregivers is not yet known and may vary with the ways in which states allocate funds and interpret eligibility requirements, several parts of the legislation have the potential to negatively impact grandparents. Particularly troubling parts of the TANF legislation, include the 5-year cap placed on benefits, the work requirement, and the cap on the level of benefits that denies any increase in cash assistance for children born after the family has applied for benefits. In addition, legal immigrants, depending on their date of arrival in the United States, may be denied benefits under TANF, creating additional risks for many grandparents.

Another area of concern under the TANF legislation, relevant to grandparents, is the penalties that may be imposed on families if children have excessive absences from school. The behavioral and learning problems that may afflict many of the grandchildren place grandparents at risk of being penalized. Even a temporary stop in assistance can be devastating to poor families and may indeed cause some to reconsider their decision to raise their grandchildren (Kelly, Yorker, & Whitley, 1997).

In addition to welfare benefits, both Medicaid and food stamps have also been affected by welfare reform. Although grandparents may not be eligible for TANF benefits, their grandchildren may remain eligible for Medicaid. Unfortunately, many do not enroll when they do not receive cash assistance. Changes in the definition of disability for children make it more difficult for grandchildren with many disorders to obtain Medicaid benefits. This places an additional burden on grandparents as many of the grand-children they are raising have been severely traumatized and are in need of extensive care.

Nutrition is also affected by welfare reform, and thus the ability of grandparents to provide healthy meals for their grandchildren may be restricted. Reductions in the Food Stamp program and changes in the ways in which income is assessed in determining eligibility will mean fewer resources for many grandparent headed households. Food stamps for legal immigrants have been eliminated, meaning that many grandparents will no longer be entitled to the benefit.

Supports and Services

The pressing emotional, psychological, social, and economic concerns affecting grandparents and their grandchildren indicate the need for myriad interventions. Support groups have played a dominant role in meeting the needs of many grandparents.

Support groups combat isolation and provide grandparents with the opportunity to learn from each other. They offer an arena in which persons can feel secure in expressing their concerns and problems. As discussed earlier, social supports can be critical factors in learning new roles, and consequently, these groups may be influential in this process. Cohen and Pyle discuss the nature and characteristics of grandparent support groups as well as their structure. The chapter offers examples of various types of groups, including respite programs for grandparents as well as suggestions for group development.

In addressing the needs of grandparents, it is easy to overlook their unique strengths. The chapter by Cox on empowerment for grandparents raising grandchildren illustrates how empowerment training can build on these strengths, increasing the grandparents' skill while enabling them to become community resources reaching out to other grandparents in need of support and information. Using a model and curriculum designed specifically for them, the grandparents are empowered to become their own advocates.

An area of concern to grandparents which is often overlooked are the schools which their grandchildren attend. Learning how to interact with these systems whose structure and curriculum vary distinctly from the schools that they attended can be difficult. These difficulties are compounded by the fact that often the grandchildren are at high risk for developmental delays and behavioral problems requiring special programs.

Silverstein and Vehvilainen describe grandparent interactions with school, ranging from administrative to interpersonal, faced by a sample of grandparents in Massachusetts. The authors present specific strategies, which may assist schools in meeting the needs of both grandparents and their grandchildren.

The burgeoning phenomenon of grandparents raising grandchildren has not occurred in a vacuum. The last 10 years has witnessed the emergence of support groups, resource centers, on-line chat rooms, and even video conferences addressing issues confronting grandparents. Roe's chapter traces the evolution of these programs and community interventions while providing suggestions for their continued development.

The issues involved with grandparents raising grandchildren are vast, ranging from emotional and psychological concerns to areas of social and public policy. In the following chapters, the authors share their expertise in an effort to present a comprehensive discussion of the many issues confronting these grandparents. Clearly, as this population continues to grow, there is a pressing need to learn from their experiences and research.

References

Atchley, R. (1989). A continuity theory of normal aging, *The Gerontologist, 99,* 183–190.

Bengston, V. (1985). Diversity and symbol in grandparent roles. In V. Bengston & J. Roberton (Eds.), *Grandparenthood.* Beverly Hills: Sage.

Brim, O. (1956). Socialization through the life cycle. In C. Gordon & K. Gergen (Eds.), *The self in social interaction.* New York: Dryden Press.

Burton, L. M. (1992). Black grandparents rearing children of drug-addicted parents: Stressor, outcomes, and social service needs. *The Gerontologist, 32,* 744–751.

Cherlin, A., & Furstenberg, F. (1985). Styles and strategies of grandparenthood. In V. Bengston & J. Robertson (Eds.), *Grandparenthood* (pp. 97–116). Beverly Hills: Sage.

Cherlin, A., & Furstenberg, F. (1986). Grandparents and family crisis. *Generations, 10,* 26–28.

Dannefer, D. (1984). Adult development and social theory. *American Sociological Review, 49,* 100–116.

Detzner, D. (1996). No place without a home; Southeast Asian grandparents in refugee families. *Generations, 20,* 45–48.

Dowdell, E. B. (1995). Caregiver burden: Grandmothers raising their high risk grandchildren. *Journal of Psychological Nursing and Mental Health Services, 33,* 3–8.

Dressel, P. L., & Barnhill, S. K. (1994). Reframing gerontological thought and practice: The case of grandmothers with daughters in prison. *The Gerontologist, 34,* 685–691.

Erikson, E. (1963). *Childhood and Society,* 2nd ed. New York: Norton.

Gelfand, D. (1989). Immigration, aging, and intergenerational relationships. *The Gerontologist, 29,* 366–372.

Jackson, J. (1986). Black grandparents: Who needs them? In R. Staples (Ed.), *The Black family: Essays and studies.* Belmont, CA: Wadsworth.

Jendrek, M. (1994). Grandparents who parent their grandchildren: Circumstances and decisions. *The Gerontologist, 34,* 206–216.

Johnson, C. (1983). A cultural analysis of the grandmother. *Research on Aging, 5,* 547–567.

Jones, F. (1973). The lofty role of the black grandmother. *Crises, 80,* 19–21.

Joslin, D., & Brouard, A. (1995) The prevalence of grandmothers as primary caregivers in a poor pediatric population. *Journal of Community Health, 20,* 383–400.

Kelly, S. J. (1993). Caregiver stress in grandparents raising grandchildren. *Image, Journal of Nursing Scholarship, 25,* 331–337.

Kelly, S. J., & Danato, E. G.(1995). Grandparents as primary caregivers. *Maternal and Child Nursing, 20,* 326–332.

Kornhaber, A., & Woodward, K. (1981). *Grandparents/grandchildren: The vital connection.* Garden City: Anchor Press/ Doubleday.

Levinson, D. J., Darrow, C. N., Klein, E. B., Levinson, M. H., & McGee, B. (1978). *The seasons of a man's life.* New York: Knopf.

Marin, G. (1989) Hispanic culture: Implications for AIDS prevention. In J. Boswell, R. Hexter, & J. Reinisch (Eds.), *Sexuality and disease: Metaphors, perceptions and behavior in AIDS era.* New York: Oxford University Press.

Minkler, M., Roe, K. M., & Price, M. (1992). The physical and emotional health of grandmothers raising grandchildren in the crak cocaine epidemic. *The Gerontologist, 32,* 752–761.

Neugarten, B. L., Moore, J. W., & Lowe, J. C. (1965). Age norms, age constraints, and adult socialization. *American Journal of Sociology, 70,* 710–717.

Nobles, W. (1974). African root and American fruit. *Journal of Social and Behavioral Sciences, 20,* 52–64.

Riley, M., Foner, A., Hess, B., & Toby, M. (1969). Socialization for the middle and later years. In D. A. Goslin (Ed.), *Handbook of socialization theory and research.* Chicago: Rand McNally.

Rindfuss, R. R., Swicegood, C. G., & Rosenfeld, R. A. (1987). Disorder in the life course: How common and does it matter? *American Sociological Review, 52,* 785–801.

Roberto, K., & Stroes, J. (1992). Grandchildren and grandparents: Roles, influences, and relationships. *International Journal of Aging and Human Development, 34,* 227–239.

Sabogal, F., Marin, G., Otero-Sabogal, R., Marin, B., & Perez-Stable, E. (1987). Hispanic familism and acculturation: What changes and what doesn't. *Hispanic Journal of Behavioral Sciences, 9,* 397–412.

Sarbin, T., & Allen, V. (1968). Role theory. In G. Lindzey & E. Aronson (Eds.), *The handbook of social psychology* (Vol. 1, pp. 488–567). Reading, MA: Addison-Wesley.

Strom, R., Collingsworth, P., Strom, S., & Griswold, D. (1993). Strengths and needs of black grandparents. *International Journal of Aging and Human Development, 36,* 255–268.

Tate, N. (1983). The black aging experience. In R. H. McNeely & J. L. Cohen (Eds.), *Aging in minority groups.* Beverly Hills: Sage.

Troll, L. (1983). Grandparents: The family watchdogs. In T. Brubaker (Ed.), *Family relationships in later life* (pp. 63–74). Beverly Hills: Sage.

Van Tran, T. (1988). In C. H. Mindel, R. W. Haberstein, & R. Wright Jr. (Eds.), *Ethnic families in America: Patterns and variations.* New York: Elsevier.

Chapter 2

A Profile of Grandparents Raising Grandchildren in the United States

Esme Fuller Thomson, Meredith Minkler, and Diane Driver

A much-discussed finding of the 1990 Census was the dramatic 44% increase over the preceding decade in the number of children living with grandparents or other relatives. Five percent of all American children were living with grandparents or other relatives by 1990, and in an estimated one third of these homes, neither parent was present (Saluter, 1992), often making the grandparent the sole or primary caregiver. Substance abuse, teen pregnancy, AIDS, incarceration, emotional problems, and parental

The authors gratefully acknowledge the Commonwealth Fund for its support of this research. The Commonwealth Fund is a New York City–based national foundation that undertakes independent research on health and social issues. From Minkler, M., & Fuller Thompson, E., & Diane Driver, *A profile of grandparents raising grandchildren in the United States. The Gerontologist,* 37, 1997. Adapted with permission of the Gerontological Society of America, 1030 15th Street NW, Suite 350, Washington DC 20005, via the Copyright Clearance Center, Inc.

death are among the factors that have been found to contribute to this phenomenon (Brouard & Joslin, 1995; Burton, 1992; Dressel & Barnhill, 1994; Feig, 1990; Jendrek, 1994; Minkler & Roe, 1993).

The early to mid-1990s saw increasing research attention to the phenomenon of grandparent caregiving (Burton, 1992; Dowdell, 1995; Dressel & Barnhill, 1995; Jendrek, 1994; Joslin & Brouard, 1995; Minkler & Roe, 1993; Shor & Hayslip, 1994). Although these studies provided much useful information, including initial explorations of the special problems and challenges faced by grandparents raising children of imprisoned mothers (Dressel & Barnhill, 1994) and of drug-involved parents (Burton, 1992; Minkler & Roe, 1993), most of the research to date has been based on small nonrandom samples in particular geographic areas. The findings of these studies, consequently, cannot be generalized to the growing population of custodial grandparents nationally.

An important recent exception is Chalfie's (1994) national look at grandparents raising grandchildren in skipped-generation households—those comprising grandparents and their grandchildren with neither of the child's parents present. Using previously unpublished data from the March 1992 Current Population Survey and conducted for the American Association of Retired Persons (AARP), the study provides important information about the minority subset of grandparent caregivers who reside in two generation households. However, 1990 census figures suggest that two-thirds of children living with grandparents live in homes in which at least one parent also is present (Saluter, 1992). Consequently, Chalfie's study does not provide nationally representative data on the broader population of grandparents who are raising their grandchildren. In addition, the latter study is solely concerned with bivariate analyses. Multivariate analyses are needed to clarify which characteristics are related to grandparent caregiving independently of other variables and which are primarily spurious.

The current research attempts to fill these gaps by developing a national profile of grandparent caregivers in the United States, including both skipped-generation households and those comprising three or more generations. Both bivariate and multivariate analyses were conducted to establish this comprehensive profile. The study, supported by the Commonwealth Fund, uses the second wave of data from the National Survey of Families and Households, collected from 1992 to 1994.

Following a brief look at the study's conceptual framework and its research design and methods, this chapter will present initial findings concerning the prevalence and lifetime incidence of grandparent caregiving in the United States and a demographic profile of the subgroup we have labeled America's "grandparent caregivers of the 1990s." Implications of our findings for future research, policy, and practice then will be discussed, with particular attention to their salience in light of recent national-level policy developments.

Conceptual Framework

As Bengston et al. (1995) have noted, contrary to popular notions of the American family in decline, a wealth of research evidence suggests that intergenerational solidarity and strong intergenerational bonds remain the rule rather than the exception in American family life (Bengston & Silverstein, 1993; Rossi & Rossi, 1990). The large number of grandparents who are involved in extensive caregiving for their grandchildren represent a graphic example of the strength of intergenerational bonds, and conceptualizations of solidarity between generations form an overarching conceptual framework for this study. In particular, the research is grounded in notions of functional solidarity, as witnessed in the level of assistance provided to grandchildren.

Studies of grandparents as surrogate parents to their grandchildren often have been framed in terms of "time disordered roles" (Selzer, 1976) and the stresses and disjunctures that may occur when heavy child care responsibilities are perceived as "off time" in the life cycle (Burton & Dilworth-Anderson, 1991; Dowdell, 1995; Jendrek, 1994). Although the increasing fluidity of the postmodern life course has called into question the notion of rigid age stages and age appropriate roles, a more general sense of certain events being "off time," and hence potentially more stressful, has conceptual relevance for the present research. This chapter provides a first step in exploring the impact of the off-time role by developing a profile of individuals who become custodial grandparents. These findings will provide a context for researchers to investigate the nature and significance of this impact in future studies.

Methodology

As noted earlier, data for this study come from a large longitudinal data set, the National Survey of Families and Households (NSFH) of adult Americans. The NSFH was funded by the Center for Population Research of the National Institute of Child Health and Human Development. The survey was conducted by the Center for Demography and Ecology at the University of Wisconsin-Madison.

The most recent wave of the NSFH, conducted during 1992 to 1994, interviewed a probability sample of 10,008 respondents. All data are weighted to adjust for nonresponse and for oversampling of ethnic minorities, nontraditional families, and recently married people. This weighting represents a sample that is demographically representative of the coterminous United States. (For a more detailed summary of study design and questions, see Sweet et al., 1988.) Our study's subsample consists of the 3,477 respondents to the 1992 to 1994 NSFH who reported having one or more grandchildren.

Lifetime incidence of grandparent caregiving was determined through the proportion of grandparents who replied in the affirmative to the question, "For various reasons, grandparents sometimes take on the primary responsibility for raising a grandchild. Have you ever had the primary responsibility for any of your grandchildren for 6 months or more?" To determine the subsample of recent grandparent caregivers, those caregivers who had responded "yes" to the preceding question and who reported beginning or ending caregiving during the 1990s were selected. This resulted in 173 recent caregivers, representing 5% of the grandparents in the study. Using bivariate techniques, these recent caregivers were compared and contrasted with the noncaregiving grandparents with respect to their gender, marital status, family size, total number of grandchildren, number of coresident children, experience of a child's death in the last five years, race, education, urban/rural status, age and family income. These variables were then included in a logistic regression predicting caregiver status to untangle the relative importance of each of these characteristics while controlling for other variables.

Results

Of the 3,477 grandparents in this study, 380 (10.9%) reported having had primary responsibility for raising a grandchild for a period of 6 months or more at some point in their life (see Table 2.1). In other words, more than 1 in 10 grandparents have raised a grandchild for at least 6 months. As indicated in Table 2.1, nearly half (44%) of the grandparents in our study who had been primary caregivers for a grandchild took over parenting responsibilities when their grandchild was still an infant. Close to three quarters (72%) began caregiving before the child turned five. Two thirds

(69%) of the grandparents were raising the child of a daughter, and one third (31%) were raising a son's child.

For many caregiving grandparents, this role did not represent a short-term commitment, and indeed more than half (56%) had given care for a period of at least three years. In fact, one in five grandparent caregivers took care of a grandchild for 10 or more years.

Table 2.2 provides a profile of the 173 grandparents who reported that they had raised a grandchild for at least six months during the 1990s and contrasts it with a profile of non–caregiving grandparents. As Table 2.2 suggests, slightly more than half (54%) of custodial grandparents in the United States were married. More than three quarters (77%) of all caregiving grandparents were women. Most (62%) were non-Hispanic White, with more than a quarter African American (27%), 10% Hispanic, and 1% classified as another race or ethnicity. Custodial grandparents had a mean age of 59.4 years. Almost three quarters (74%) of recent custodial grandparents lived in urban areas during the baseline year of 1987–1988. More than half (57%) of caregivers had completed high school.

Caregiving grandparents had lower mean incomes ($31,643 vs. $37,814, $p<.05$) and median incomes ($22,176 vs. $29,000). If fact, caregiving grandparents were 60% more likely than noncusdodial grandparents to report incomes below the poverty line (23% vs. 14%, $p<.01$). In 1992, the poverty line was a mere $9,395 for a couple and $14,228 for a family of four.

Custodial grandparents differed markedly from noncustodial grandparents on many demographic variables. Our findings indicate that custodial grandparents in the 1990s were significantly ($p<.01$) less likely to be married, to be non-Hispanic White, to be male, and to have completed high school. Furthermore, they were, on average, 3 years younger than non-caregiving grandparents ($p<.01$). Custodial grandparents did not differ significantly from their noncustodial peers with respect to 1987–88 urban/rural status but were significantly more likely to have lived in the South (42.5% vs. 34.8%, $p<.05$) during the first wave of interviews (1987/1988). The current region of residence is not yet available from the second wave of the NSFH.

To create a broader family context within which to understand the situation of grandparent caregivers better, data also were examined on total family size, number of and proximity to one's children and grandchildren, and parental bereavement within the last 5 years. Caregiving grandparents of the 1990s were significantly more likely to have more children (4.0 vs. 3.3) and more grandchildren (7.3 vs. 5.4) than noncaregiving grandparents

TABLE 2.1 Lifetime Incidence, Duration, and Nature of Custodial
Grandparenting in America

Variable	%
Lifetime incidence (n = 380)	
Percentage of grandparents having ever raised a grandchild for 6 months or more	10.9
Age of child when caregiving undertaken (n = 3 72)	
Under 1 year	43.5
1 through 4 years	28.4
5 to 10 years	15.7
Eleven years or more	12.4
Duration of primary caregiving (n = 286)	
Less than 1 year	16.9
1 to 2 years	26.8
3 to 4 years	15.4
5 to 9 years	21.1
Ten or more years	19.8

and also were more likely to have children in their immediate vicinity. More than half (52.8%) of the caregiving grandparents had one or more of their offspring in their home versus less than a third (30.4%) of the non-caregiving grandparents ($p<.001$). In addition, caregiving grandparents were slightly more likely than noncaregivers to have their noncoresident children residing within 20 miles (76% vs. 69%, $p<.05$).

A logistic regression was run to verify which factors help predict caregiving status in a multivariate analysis (see Table 2.3). In general, these findings supported the results of the bivariate analyses. The results shown in Table 2.3 indicate that the odds of being a caregiving grandparent were more than twice as high (odds ratio [OR]=2.18, $p<.001$) for females and for those who had experienced the death of a child in the previous 5 years [OR]=2.16, $p<.05$). African Americans had 83% higher odds of being grandparent caregivers than respondents from other races (OR=1.83, $p<.01$). For every decade of age, the odds of being a custodial grandparent decreased 25% ($p<.001$). There was a trend ($p<.10$) indicating that those with a high school diploma had somewhat lower odds of being a caregiver; however, this trend did not reach the level of significance it had

TABLE 2.2 Comparative Profile of Custodial Grandparents
vs. Noncustodial Grandparents of the 1990s

Variable	Noncaregiving Grandparents (n = 3304)	Grandparents (n = 173)
Marital status in 1993		
Widowed/divorced/separated/		
never married	32%	46%[a]
Married	68%	54%
Mean age in 1993	62.3 years	59.4 years[b]
Race		
Black	10%	27%[a]
White, non-Hispanic	84%	62%
Hispanic	6%q	10%
Other	0%	1%
Gender		
Male	44%	23%[a]
Female	56%	77%
Education level in 1993		
Grade 11 or less	29%	43%[a]
Grade 12 or higher	71%	57%
Geographic region in 1988		
South	34.8%	42.5%[c]
Elsewhere	65.2%	57.5%
Urban/rural status in 1988		
Nonstandard metropolitan area (rural)	27%	26%
Standard metropolitan areas (urban)	73%	74%
Income in 1993		
Mean income	$37,814	$31,643[c]
Median income	$29,000	$22,176
Families below poverty line	13.7%	22.9%[b]
Families above poverty line	86.3%	77.1%
Offspring		
Total number of children	3.25	3.94a
One or more coresident children	30.4%	52.8%a
One or more non-coresident children		
within 20 miles	69%	76%[c]
Total number of grandchildren	5.39	7.29a
Child died in past 5 years	2.7%	6.5%

p Values are based on the chi-squared statistic for proportions and t-test statistic for means:
[a] $p<.05$.
[b] $p<.01$.
[c] $p<.001$.

achieved in the bivariate analyses. Family size and structure also played a significant role. Although in contrast to the findings of the bivariate analyses, overall number of children was not significantly associated with caregiving status in the multivariate analysis, number of coresident children remained a significant factor. For every coresident child, the odds of being a grandparent caregiver increased 23%. Furthermore, the number of grandchildren was directly related to the odds of being a grandparent caregiver. The odds of reporting caregiving responsibilities were 8% higher (OR = 1.08, $p<.001$) per grandchild. Finally, in contrast to the cross-sectional findings, marital status, living in the South, and living below the poverty line no longer contributed significantly to the equation once included in a multivariate model. Urban/rural status did not contribute significantly to our understanding of caregiving status in either bivariate or multivariate equations.

Discussion

The findings of this study indicate that grandparent caregiving is not as rare a phenomenon as is commonly believed, and that it cuts across class, race, and gender lines. The facts that nearly three quarters of the custodial grandparents in this national study took in grandchildren when they were under age 5, and that more than half provided care for at least 3 years, suggests that for many, this role involves a long-term and labor-intensive commitment. Yet our knowledge of the real parameters of this experience remains fragmentary. A major limitation of the present study, for example, lay in the failure of the NSFH data set to include information on the number of grandchildren and other relatives for whom a grandparent had primary responsibility. Because earlier studies have suggested that most custodial grandparents were raising two or more of their grandchildren (Joslin & Brouard, 1995; Minkler & Roe, 1993), it is important to determine the proportion of grandparent caregivers nationally who are, in fact, raising multiple grandchildren. Further, national data are needed on the reasons why grandparents undertake primary responsibility for raising their grandchildren or other young relatives.

The finding that grandparents with coresident offspring are considerably more likely to be caregivers than those without children in the home lends support to our conviction that analyses, such as Chalfie's (1994), that are limited to skipped-generation households pose too narrow a definition of grandparent caregiver families. Further, this finding underscores the

TABLE 2.3 Logistic Regression of Custodial Grandparents
vs. Noncustodial Grandparents of the 1990s

Variable	Odds ratio	(95% Confidence interval)
Marital status in 1993 (married = 1)[a]	0.76	(0.53,1.10)
Age in 1993 (by decade)	0.75***	(0.63, 0.89)
Race (Black = 1)[b]	1.83**	(1.19, 2.81)
Gender (female = 1)	2.18***	(1.47, 3.22)
Education (high school graduate = 1)[c]	0.72+	(0.50, 1.03)
Geographic region in 1988 (South = 1)[d]	1.17	(0.84, 1.66)
Urban status in 1988 (Urban = 1)	0.99	(0.69, 1.44)
Poverty level (families below poverty line = 1)	1.08	(0.71, 1.65)
Total number of children	0.98	(0.88, 1.09)
Number of coresident children	1.23*	(1.02, 1.49)
Total number of grandchildren	1.08***	(1.03, 1.12)
Parental bereavement (child died in past five years = 1)	2.16*	(1.06, 4.38)

[a] Reference category includes all people not currently married—widowed, divorced, separated, never married.
[b] Reference category includes all non-Blacks.
[c] Reference category is 11 or fewer years of education.
[d] Reference category is all other areas of the United States.
+ $p < .10$.
* $p < .05$.
** $p < .01$.
*** $p < .001$.

importance of an ecological perspective that stresses the "double duties" many grandparent caregivers fulfill when they find themselves caring for their own children and one or more of their grandchildren. The ecological perspective further is supported by our findings that grandparent caregivers have significantly more grandchildren than noncaregivers as well as having more of their offspring living within 20 miles. Research is needed to determine the patterns of help and support received from and given to the additional proximate family members. In sum, far more information is needed about the entire caregiving picture of which caring for one's grandchildren may be only a part.

The importance of examining multiple bonds and relationships across generations is particularly well highlighted in the case of African Americans, who in our study had twice the odds of becoming caregiving grandparents. The overrepresentation of African Americans among grandparent caregivers reflects, in part, a long tradition of caregiving across generations in Black families that has its roots in West African culture (Sudarkasa, 1981; Wilson, 1989). But as Burton and Dilworth-Anderson (1991) suggest, the experience of many of today's African-American grandmothers, who assume the role of caregiver as a result of a daughter's drug addiction, incarceration, teen pregnancy, or incapacitation resulting from AIDS, may be very different from that of their foremothers and forefathers who took on a caregiving role under far different sociohistorical circumstances. Further studies of the meaning and significance of grandparent caregiving for different racial and ethnic groups, and in different situational contexts, are needed to flesh out our understanding of this phenomenon and its contemporary manifestations.

The significantly greater tendency of females than males in this study to be primary caregivers for their grandchildren is, of course, in keeping with the pronounced sexual division of labor around family caregiving of all types (Abel, 1991; Brody, 1985). It should be noted, however, that although most grandparent caregivers in this study were female, close to a quarter were grandfathers, whose roles in grandparenting have been almost totally ignored in the extant studies (see Thomas, 1990, 1994, for, important recent exceptions). As Bengston et al. (1995) have noted, this neglect stems in part from "methodological individualism" through which single family members, typically women caregivers, or dyads (caregiver and care recipient), are focused upon and the roles of secondary caregivers or other family members largely ignored. Increased research attention to the roles and circumstances of grandfathers who are primary or secondary caregivers for their grandchildren, and a focus beyond individuals to the broader family as the unit of analysis should be undertaken to enrich our understanding of the complexity of care relationships in surrogate parent households. Similarly, more research should be directed to the many grandparent caregivers who are unmarried, and for whom the challenge of "unplanned parenthood" in middle or late life may also entail greater financial vulnerability and the lack of respite that might have been provided by a spouse.

An important finding of this study was that four variables which were signficant in bivariate relationships were not found to be significant in the subsequent multivariate analysis. Neither marital status, living under the poverty line, living in the South nor number of children provided a unique contribution to our understanding of custodial grandparenting when these factors were included in multivariate equations. In other words, the connection between these variables and caregiving status in the bivariate analysis may have been primarily spurious. Living below the poverty line, for example, is related to marital status, age, gender, education, and being African American. It appears to be these other variables—rather than poverty itself—which have the direct relationship with caregiving status. Such findings clearly underscore the need for further research using multivariate analyses.

Panel studies using multivariate techniques also are needed to follow up on earlier cross sectional studies indicating an association between grandparent caregiving and depression (Minkler et al., 1992); changes in self-rated health and health behaviors (Burton, 1992; Minkler et al., 1992); isolation from friends (Burton, 1992; Shor & Hayslip, 1994) ; lowered satisfaction with the grandparent role (Shor & Hayslip, 1994); and severe economic hardship (Minkler & Roe, 1993).

In addition to offering a number of promising avenues for further research, the results of our research have implications for current policy and practice. Although living below the poverty line did not contribute signficantly to the odds of being a grandparent caregiver in our multivariate analysis, for example, it is important, from a policy perspective, to underscore our finding that almost a quarter of grandparents raising grandchildren were living below the poverty threshold. Although 28% of grandparents in skipped-generation families receive Aid to Families with Dependent Children (AFDC) (Chalfie, 1994), the low level of benefits received, the stigmatizing nature of the program, and eligibility problems faced by many grandparent applicants make this a less than adequate option.

Our findings concerning the large proportion of grandparent caregivers who are below poverty line appear to support the the need for more widely available "kinship care" programs through which low-income custodial grandparents in some states receive the more generous and less stigmatizing payments available to foster care parents (Takas, 1992). Futher, our findings suggests that the recently signed Welfare Reform Act (which places a lifetime limit of 5 years on AFDC and imposes a mandatory work requirement after 2 years) may not bode well for the "economic health" of many intergenerational households headed by grandparents.

In addition to underscoring the 1995 White House Conference on Aging's call for stepped-up, rather than cut-back, financial assistance to grandparent caregivers, our findings on the prevalence and intensity of care provision suggest the importance of other types of supportive programs and policies as well. The American Association for Retired Person's (AARP's) Grandparent Information Center has identified more than 400 support groups for grandparent caregivers around the United States (Woodworth, 1996), in addition to several more comprehensive programs that include counseling, respite, tutoring for children in the care of their grandparents, and other services (Dressel & Barnhill, 1994; Miller, 1991; Minkler et al., 1993). Yet many of these programs are short lived, and almost no evaluative studies have been conducted to determine their efficacy.

Evaluative research on a variety of interventions to assist grandparent caregivers is needed, as is increased education of health and social service providers about the needs and concerns of grandparent caregivers and the children in their care. A combination of carefully focused research and appropriate policy and practice measures in short is recommended in recognition of the vital role that grandparent caregivers are playing in raising some of the nation's most vulnerable children.

References

Abel, E. K. (1991). *Who cares for the elderly? Public policy and the experiences of adult daughters.* Philadelphia: Temple University Press.

Aldous, J. (1995). New views of grandparents in intergenerational context. *Journal of Family Issues, 16,* 104–122.

Bengston, V., Rosenthal, C., & Burton, L. (1995). Paradoxes of families and aging. In R. H. Binstock & L. K. George (Eds.), *Handbook of aging and the social sciences* (4th ed., pp. 253–282). San Diego: Academic Press.

Bengtson, V. L., & Silverstein, M. (1993). Families, aging, and social changes: Seven agendas for 21st century researchers. In B. Maddox, & M. P. Lawton (Eds.), *Kinship, aging, and social change: Annual review of gerontology and geriatrics* (Vol. 13, pp. 15–38). New York: Springer.

Brody, E. M. (1985). Parent care as a normative family stress. *The Gerontologist, 25,* 19–28.

Burton, L. (1992). Black grandmothers rearing children of drug-addicted parents: Stressors, outcomes and social service needs. *The Gerontologist, 32,* 744–751.

Burton, L. M., & Dilworth-Anderson, P. (1991). The intergenerational roles of aged Black Americans. *Marriage and Family Review, 16,* 311–330.

Chalfie, D. (1994). *Going it alone: A closer look at grandparents parenting grandchildren.* Washington DC: American Association of Retired Persons.

Cherlin, A. J., & Furstenberg, F. F., Jr. (1986). *The new American grandparent: A place in the family, a life apart.* New York: Basic Books.

Dowdell, E. B. (1995). Caregiver burden: Grandparents raising their high risk children. *Journal of Psychosocial Nursing, 33,* 27–30.

Dressel, P., & Barnhill, S. (1994). Reframing gerontological thought and practice: The case of grandmothers with daughters in prison. *The Gerontologist, 34,* 685–690.

Feig, L. (1990, January 29). *Drug exposed infants and children: Service needs and policy questions.* Washington, DC: Department of Health and Human Services.

Flaherty, M. J. (1988). Seven caring functions of black grandmothers in adolescent mothering. *Maternal Child Nursing Journal, 17,* 191–207.

Jendrek, M. P. (1994). Grandparents who parent their grandchildren: Circumstances and decisions. *The Gerontologist, 34,* 206–216.

Joslin, D., & Brouard, A. (1995). The prevalence of grandmothers as primary caregivers in a poor pediatric population. *Journal of Community Health, 20,* 383–401.

Kornhaber, A. (1985). Grandparenthood and the "new social contract." In V. Bengston & J. F. Robertson (Eds.), *Grandparenthood* (pp. 159–172). Beverly Hills: Sage.

Miller, D. (1991, November 24). The "grandparents who care" support project of San Francisco. Paper presented at the annual meeting of the Gerontological Society of America, San Francisco.

Minkler, M., Roe, K. M., & Price, M. (1992). Physical and emotional health of grandmothers raising grandchildren in the crack cocaine epidemic. *The Gerontologist, 32,* 752–761.

Minkler, M., & Roe, K. M. (1993). *Grandmothers as caregivers: Raising children of the crack cocaine epidemic.* Newbury Park, CA: Sage.

Minkler, M., et al. (1993). Community interventions to support grandparent caregivers. *The Gerontologist, 33,* 807–811.

Roe, K. M., Minkler, M., & Barnwell, R. S. (1994). The assumption of caregiving: Grandmothers raising the children of the crack cocaine epidemic. *Qualitative Health Research, 4,* 281–303.

Roe, K. M., Minkler, M., & Saunders, F. F. (1995). Combining research, advocacy and education: The methods of the grandparent caregiver study. *Health Education Quarterly, 22,* 458–475.

Roe, K. M., Minkler, M., Thompson, G., & Saunders, F. F. (1996). Health of grandmothers raising children of the crack cocaine epidemic. *Medical Care, 34,* 1072–1089

Rossi, A., & Rossi, P. (1990). *Of human bonding: Parent-child relations across the life course.* New York: Aldine de Gruyter.

Saluter, A. F. (1992). Marital status and living arrangements: March 1991. *Current population reports* (Series P-20, No. 461). Washington, DC: U.S. Government Printing Office.

Selzer, M. (1976). Suggestions for the examination of time-disordered relationships. In J. F. Gubrium (Ed.), *Time, roles and self in old age* (pp. 111–125). New York: Human Sciences Press.

Shor, R. J., & Hayslip, B. (1994). Custodial grandparenting: Implications for children's development. In A. Godfried & A. Godfried (Eds.), *Redefining families: Implications for children's development.* New York: Plenum.

Sudarkasa, N. (1981). Interpreting the African heritage in Afro-American family organization. In H. P. McAdoo (Ed.), *Black families* (pp. 37–53). Beverly Hills: Sage.

Sweet, J., Bumpass, L., & Call, V. (1988). *The design and content of the national survey of families and households* (NSFH Working Paper No. 1). Madison: Center for Demography and Ecology, University of Wisconsin.

Takas, M. (1992). *Kinship care: Developing a safe and effective framework for protective placement of children with relatives.* Washington, DC: American Bar Association Center on Children and the Law.

Thomas, J. L. (1990). The grandparent role: A double bind. *International Journal of Aging and Human Development, 31,* 169–171.

Thomas, J. L. (1994). Older men as fathers and grandfathers. In E. H. Thompson, Jr. (Ed.), *Older men's lives* (Vol. 6, pp. 197–217). Thousand Oaks, CA: Sage.

Troll, L. (1983). Grandparents: The family watchdogs. In T. H. Brubaker (Ed.), *Family relationships in later life.* Beverly Hills: Sage.

Wilson, M. N. (1989). Child development in the context of the black extended family. *American Psychologist, 44,* 380–385.

The Status of Grandparents

Chapter 3

Physical Health of Custodial Grandparents

Jonathan Marx and
Jennifer Crew Solomon

Physical health is an important factor in determining quality of life and longevity. A person's health impacts his or her ability to carry out basic daily activities, such as bathing, dressing, and eating. It also influences social interaction as well as opportunities for employment and thus financial security. What is the health status of custodial grandparents? Does assuming responsibility for raising grandchildren affect their health? If so, how? For example, does being an important part of a grandchild's life enhance the health of custodial grandparents, or does the added responsibility of caregiving tax their health? In this chapter, we discuss the health status of custodial grandparents and make comparisons with people of similar ages. We then profile custodial grandparents and discuss major factors influencing their health and health care needs. We conclude by offering recommendations for policies and services to assist grandparent-grandchild families.

Concept of Health

To discuss the physical health of custodial grandparents, we must first clarify the concept of health. In everyday conversation, we often speak of health in dichotomous terms. A person is in good health or experiencing poor health—someone is either sick or well. This way of talking about health conceptualizes it as the presence or absence of disability or disease. Atchley (1997), however, suggests that it is more useful to think of health as a continuum with excellent health at one end and poor health at the other. Points along the continuum from excellent to poor health may be characterized as "social, physical, and mental well-being, absence of disease or impairment, presence of health condition, restriction of activity, mild disability, severe disability, and extreme frailty" (p. 86).

Although the focus of this chapter is the physical health of custodial grandparents, social, mental, and physical well-being are intertwined, and their reciprocal cause-and-effect relationships are not easily disentangled. For example, the existence of a network of friends or family members who can provide emotional support, personal assistance, and information (i.e., social support) has been shown to influence both mortality and morbidity (see Uchino, Cacioppo, & Kiecolt-Glaser, 1996, for a review of the literature). However, poor health may limit a person's ability to engage in interaction with others and thus acquire social support. Similarly, considerable research evidence connects stress with depressed immune function (see Herbert & Cohen, 1993, for a meta-analytic review of the research), but being ill also produces stress.

Health status is influenced by both nature and nurture. People inherit tendencies or vulnerabilities to some diseases, for example, diabetes and certain types of cancer. Conversely, lifestyle choices related to smoking, eating, and exercise also impact health. Atchley (1997) suggests that chance plays a part in determining health status. That is, people do not always know that the consequences of their actions, such as job choices, may jeopardize their health.

Health can be viewed as a continuum of conditions from excellent health to poor health and extreme frailty. A person's health status is related to social and mental factors as well as genetics, lifestyle, and luck.

Overview of Health Status: People 40+

As a basis for understanding the health status of grandparents and appraising the impact of raising grandchildren on grandparents' health, we will examine the health of relevant age groups in the population according to types of conditions as measured by various health indicators.

Types of Health Conditions

Health conditions can be categorized as acute or chronic. Designation of a condition as acute or chronic is based on the length of time the condition is expected to last—not its seriousness or likelihood of causing death. Acute conditions are short term and temporary (e.g., pneumonia, the common cold). In general, the number of acute conditions decreases with age, for example, people ages 18 to 24 average 1.7 acute conditions per year, whereas the 45 and older age group average 1.1 acute conditions per year (Atchley, 1997).

Chronic conditions are long term and range in severity from dermatitis to heart disease. Although some conditions may require special rehabilitation or extended care, many chronic conditions are not disabling. For example, people adapt and learn to live with the effects of arthritis and hypertension, two of the most common chronic conditions of middle-aged and older people.

Measuring Health Status

Research on health status employs a variety of measures—prevalence rates, number of medical conditions, functional ability, and self-assessed health status. Prevalence rates indicate how common a certain condition is among various groups of people. Younger people and thus younger grandparents (45–64 years) have much lower rates of hypertension, diabetes, arthritis, and heart disease than older people/grandparents (65+ years) (Adams & Marano, 1995). Moreover, race and social class are associated with variations in health within age groups. Hypertension, arthritis, and diabetes are more common among older (65+ years) Blacks than Whites, and heart disease is more common among Whites than Blacks: 339.3 and 200.9 per thousand older people, respectively (Adams & Marano, 1995). However, in all age groups, Blacks are more likely than Whites to die from heart disease (Becker, 1993). Hispanics have lower death rates from heart disease and cancer than either older Whites or Blacks (National Center for Health Statistics, 1991).

People in lower social classes are more vulnerable than people in upper classes to all of these illnesses. Variation by gender is also evident with women suffering more than men from hypertension and arthritis.

Conversely, men are more vulnerable than women to heart disease (Adams & Marano, 1995). In general, women experience higher rates of acute diseases, short-term disabilities, and nonfatal chronic diseases, such as arthritis, and men have more injuries and higher rates of life-threatening chronic diseases, such as heart disease and emphysema (Verbrugge, 1985).

A second measure of health status is the number of different chronic medical conditions reported by people in different age and gender categories. In a 1989 study by Verbrugge, Lepkowski, and Imanaka using National Health Interview Survey (NHIS) data found that 60% of those 55+ year reported more than one chronic condition—an average 2.6 chronic conditions per person 55 and older. Older women report more chronic conditions than do older men (Herzog, 1989).

Functional ability is another important indicator of health status. This measure examines the degree of limitation people have in carrying out basic daily activities (e.g., walking, bathing, dressing, and personal hygiene), instrumental activities (e.g., household maintenance, managing finances, and shopping), and work roles. According to LaPlante and Miller (1992), 6% of the 55 to 64 age group have difficulty with basic life activities, 11.8% of the 65 to 74 age group, 26.5% of the 75 to 84 age group, and 57.6% of the 85+ age group. Considering gender and racial differences and controlling for age distributions, 13.9% of men and 14.6% of women report some degree of activity limitation (NCHS, 1992). Blacks, on average, report more activity limitations than whites (Clark & Maddox, 1992; NCHS, 1992). Older Hispanics (65+) report higher rates of needing assistance with ADLs than do similarly aged whites (U.S. Bureau of the Census, 1990). Within the category of Hispanics, Puerto Rican, Cuban, and Mexican Americans have poorer health and than white Americans with Puerto Ricans being the least healthy. People with lower incomes also generally report more acute conditions and more restricted days than those with higher incomes (U.S. Department of Health and Human Services, 1991).

Having people rate their own health is an additional approach to determining health status. People are asked to rate their own health as either "excellent, very good, good, fair, or poor." The results of previous research indicate that self-assessed health is strongly related to other more objective measures of health status such as physical exams and physician ratings and may quite accurately reflect a person's ability to perform daily activities (Atchley, 1997).

In general, self-ratings of health as fair to poor increase with age for both African Americans and European Americans. According to the National Health Interview Survey (1990), 6% of people aged 25-44 reported their health as fair to poor along with 16% of the 45 to 64 age group, and 28% of the 65+ age group. It should be noted that the majority of respondents in every age group, including the oldest, rated their health as good to excellent.

Other factors besides age are also associated with self-assessments of health. Race and income are two of the most consistent factors. African Americans are more likely at every age to rate their health as fair or poor than are European Americans.

Income is also an important correlate of self-rated health status. More than 52% of people in families with incomes of $50,000 a year or more rated their health as excellent, but only 28% of people in families with incomes less than $14,000 rated their health as excellent, (U.S. Department of Health & Human Services, 1991b). Among older people, only 10% of those 65+ years with incomes less than $10,0000 rated their health as excellent compared with 26% of those with incomes more than $25,000 (AARP, 1991). The impact of the combination of race and poverty status is clearly highlighted in such areas as poor inner-city neighborhoods where older Hispanics and African Americans are more likely to report fair or poor health status as well as greater functional disability than older Whites (Cantor & Mayer, 1976). Moreover, people living at or below poverty level develop poor health at younger ages than people with higher incomes (Butler & Newacheck, 1981).

The health of grandparents should parallel the health status of the general population as indicated by prevalence rates, number of chronic conditions, functional ability, and self-ratings. Thus, as we look more closely at grandparents and custodial grandparents in particular, we would expect to find that White grandparents have better health than Black grandparents, grandmothers have more nonfatal chronic conditions than grandfathers, and that higher social classes have better health than lower.

As people (grandparents) age, it appears that chronic conditions and functional disability increase. Self-ratings of health, however, remain relatively high despite the prevalence of chronic and potentially disabling conditions. Some scholars suggest that people's expectations and basis of comparison change as they age (Cockerham, 1998) or that the slow development of many chronic conditions allows people to adjust and cope with physical limitations in ways that do not limit their ability to perform their regular activities (Atchley, 1997).

As we proceed in our discussion of grandparents' health, focusing on custodial grandparents, we must remain attuned to the previously discussed factors (e.g., poverty, race, gender, and age) associated with health status in general to understand the impact of caring for grandchildren on the physical well-being of grandparents.

Caregiving Grandparents-Factors Influencing Health

Although the word "grandparent" may conjure up images of people older than 65 years with gray hair and glasses, grandparents vary considerably in terms of age. It is common to become a grandparent in the middle 40s; however, grandparents can be "30 or 110 years old" (Pruchno & Johnson, 1995, p. 65). Therefore, to assess the health and health care needs of custodial grandparents, we will first compare custodial grandparents with noncustodial grandparents and then consider variation in health among custodial grandparents considering age, household composition, and financial well-being.

Using the Health and Retirement Study (HRS), Wave 1 (1995), we compared demographic and physical health characteristics of custodial ($N = $ 123) and noncustodial grandparents ($N = 1152$). The HRS uses a national probability sample of U.S. households with an oversample of Blacks, Hispanics, and residents of Florida. The average age for both custodial and noncustodial grandparents in the study was 55 years. A larger proportion of custodial grandparents (47.2%) compared with noncustodial grandparents (23.7%) were African American. The mean level of education was 10.7 years for custodial and 11.7 years for noncustodial. A larger percentage of noncustodial (59.9%) than custodial (41.5%) were married. Although 57.6% of noncustodial grandparents indicated they were somewhat or very satisfied with their financial situation, only 39% of custodial grandparents were similarly satisfied. The breakdown on satisfaction with financial status within the custodial/noncustodial categories by racial groups was as follows: White custodial grandparents 41.9% dissatisfied, noncustodial 24.4%; Black custodial grandparents 51.7% dissatisfied, noncustodial 45.4%; Hispanics custodial grandparents 50% dissatisfied, noncustodial 27.2%. Furthermore, custodial grandparents (44.7%) are more than 80% more likely to report fair to poor physical health than noncustodial grandparents (24.3%). In addition, a larger percentage (21.2%) of custodial than noncustodial (13.9%) grandparents reported a decline in their physical health in the last year. Interestingly, a higher percentage (20.3%) of custodial versus noncustodial (17.5%) also reported an improvement in health during this period. Although these findings are purely descriptive, the results of this research indicate that the health of custodial grandparents differs from that of noncustodial grandparents and thus deserves special attention. It also suggests influences on their health, such as financial well-being and marital status and highlights the importance of examining subcultural differences.

The following review of the literature illustrates the current knowledge base on the health of custodial grandparents. As you will see, some research findings indicate that caregiving may have negative health consequences for custodial grandparents; however, other evidence suggests possible positive health outcomes.

The results of several studies describe the health of custodial grandparents as poor. For example, studies of African-American grandmothers and great-grandmothers raising children as a result of parental drug addiction (Burton, 1992; Minkler & Roe, 1993; Minkler, Roe, & Price, 1992; Smith, 1994) indicate that some grandmothers experience disability and increased illness. In addition, clinicians have noted depression and insomnia, hypertension, and back and stomach problems among grandparent caregivers (Miller, 1991). A little more than one third of respondents in the Minkler, Roe, and Price (1992) study of 71 African-American grandmothers and great-grandmothers indicated that their health had worsened since beginning caregiving. Many of the grandmothers whose health worsened attributed the change in their health status to caregiving. For example, caregiving responsibilities made them miss medical appointments or dealing with the stress motivated them to drink and smoke more. Furthermore, Minkler, Roe, and Price (1992, 1993) found that grandmothers may de-emphasize or downplay their health problems to protect grandchildren. Thus, grandmothers may have severer health limitations than current studies indicate.

However, in the same study, nearly half of the grandparents indicated no change in their health and about one fifth reported improved health. Moreover, about one quarter of those who reported better health also attributed the improvement to lifestyle changes because of caregiving (e.g., increased exercise with grandchildren, quitting smoking). Giarusso, Wang, and Silverstein (1996) used the University of Southern California Longitudinal Study of Generations to compare the physical well-being of coparenting grandparents (at least one parent present), parenting grandparents (no parent present), and a control group of grandparents who had not parented or coparented grandchildren. Health status was measured using a 4-point scale ("excellent, good, fair, or poor") to answer the following question: "Compared with other people your own age, how would you rate your overall physical health at the present time?" Overall, the study found that caregiving negatively affected few grandparents. The coparenting group were the youngest but reported the poorest physical well-being. The control group of nonparenting grandparents had the best health. The parenting group was in the middle, having better health than the coparenting grandparents and poorer health than the control group; however, the differences between the parenting group and the other groups were not statistically significant. Similarly, there was no difference between the health of grandmothers and grandfathers. Moreover, measures taken 3 years later revealed no significant deterioration in parenting grandparents' physical well-being. It should be noted, however, that most (72%) of the grandparent households in this study had incomes above the national median income, and 90% were above the poverty line. Once again, we see a connection between financial well-being and health status.

Results from analysis of the Health and Retirement Survey (HRS), Wave 1, 1995 provide additional insights into the physical health and other characteristics of custodial grandparents. Of the 123 grandparents in the study, 35% were White, 47.2% Black, and 13.8% Hispanic. In all racial categories, most were women (only two men). Most Whites and Hispanics were married: 62% and 64.7%, respectively. However, only 22.4% of Blacks were married. Average age differences were slight—55 years for Whites, 55.7 years for Blacks, and 53.7 years for Hispanics. Education levels were similar for Whites (11.5 years) and Blacks (11 years); however, Hispanics were much lower at 7.5 years. Using a 5-item (poor, fair, good, very good, excellent) self-reported health measure, 39.6% of Whites indicated their health was fair to poor, 50% of Blacks, and 47% of Hispanics. Comparing their health now to 1 year ago, most stated that their health status was the same: 60.5% of Whites, 55.2% of Blacks, and 64.7% of Hispanics. However, 18.6% of White respondents, 24.1% of Blacks, and 17.7% of Hispanics reported that their health was somewhat or much worse than a year ago.

Caring for a grandchild can in and of itself influence grandparents health, but other factors, such as household composition, financial well-being, and characteristics of the grandchild, may also influence the health of custodial grandparents. Research by Solomon and Marx (forthcoming,1999) examined the coexisting factors of household composition, poverty status, and characteristics of the grandchild in studying the health status of women 40 years old and older living in four different types of households: (a) single custodial grandmothers, (b) married custodial grandmothers living with a spouse, (c) women living alone, and (d) women living with only a spouse. Health status was measured using four different indicators: self-rated health, number of health conditions, activity limitations related to normal daily activities, and restricted activities of more than half a day in the last 2 weeks because of illness or injury.

In terms of all health indicators examined, women with husbands and no dependents in the household were consistently the healthiest compared with women in the other three household categories. Most of these women indicated strong health status and fewer reported restricted days, health conditions, or activity limitations. Women as part of a married couple raising a grandchild had better health than women in any other family structure except the previously discussed women living only with their husbands. Compared with either women alone or single custodial grandmothers, more women in this category had no restricted days, health conditions, or activity limitations. There were, however, slightly more who indicated weak health status compared with both married women no dependents and women alone.

Comparing women living alone to single and married custodial grandmothers, we found that they were more likely to have restricted days than custodial grandmothers with husbands. Moreover, women living alone scored higher on the overall self-reported rating of health status than custodial grandmothers whether the woman was married and living with a spouse or living with only the grandchild. Health conditions and activity limitations were also more prevalent in the women living alone than any other group except grandmothers alone raising grandchildren.

Women alone raising grandchildren had the poorest health relative to women in the other three types of households. More single custodial grandmothers viewed themselves as being in poor health, as restricted in their daily activities in the last 2 weeks, and limited because of an impairment or health problem. They were also more likely to report health conditions.

The finding that married custodial grandmothers have much better health than single custodial grandmothers seems to indicate that other factors besides the presence or absence of grandchildren in the household are associated with grandparent health status. For example, it was mentioned earlier that financial status is strongly correlated with health status. It is, therefore, not surprising that grandmothers alone raising grandchildren were both less healthy and more likely to live below the official poverty line than women living in the other types of households. Nearly half of the grandmothers alone raising grandchildren reported weak health status and activity limitations. Forty-seven percent also had incomes below the poverty index. In contrast, 72% of married custodial grandmothers reported good to excellent health, and only 18.4% had incomes below the poverty index. Moreover, living with an income below the poverty index was also associated with married custodial grandmothers reporting more restricted days, and activity limitations as well as being less likely to evaluate themselves as having good health.

The finding that women living alone had better health than single women living with grandchildren suggests that the characteristics of the grandchild (e.g., the age of the grandchild, the grandchild's behavior in school, and the number of grandchildren in the household) may influence the health of custodial grandmothers. Grandmothers raising grandchildren alone seemed to have increased health risks when raising older children. Single custodial grandmothers were less likely to describe their health as good and more likely to have recently restricted their activities for health reasons. In addition, having more than one child living in the household increased the likelihood that a single custodial grandmothers was limited in everyday activities and living with the grandchild since birth also reduced the odds of grandmothers reporting good health status. In contrast, younger grandchildren and grandchildren who are well behaved in school had positive influences on grandmother's health. The likelihood of married custodial grandmothers reporting good health was increased when the health status of the grandchild was strong; however, the impact of the grandchild's health on the single custodial grandmother's health was not statistically significant.

As our earlier review of the literature on factors associated with health status indicated, older people generally have poorer health than younger people. The average age for women in the study was married custodial grandmothers, 55.2 years; married women living with spouse only, 60.4 years; women living alone, 68.3 years; and single custodial grandmothers, 59 years. We found that older women were more likely to report restricted activities in the last two weeks but less likely to have health conditions. Among the single custodial grandmothers, older women were less likely to report good health status and to have no activity limitations. Age did not differentiate among the married custodial grandmothers.

The results of this study strongly suggest that health differences exist not just between custodial and noncustodial grandparents. It is not simply the presence of and responsibility for grandchildren that influences the health of custodial grandparents. Marital and financial status, as well as characteristics of the grandchild also influence the physical well-being of custodial grandparents.

Summary and Explanations

We will now review what we know from research evidence about the health of custodial grandparents. First, the research findings indicate that custodial grandparents health is generally worse than that of noncustodial grandparents. However, within the category of custodial grandparents, we found variations in health status between single and married grandparents. Single custodial grandmothers are more likely to have health problems than do their married counterparts. At least some of the difference between married and single custodial grandmothers can be understood by considering differences in financial status and the impact of living at or below the official poverty level. A lack of money makes access to medical care, a safe living environment, and good nutrition more difficult to acquire.

Marital status itself, however, may have a positive influence on grandmothers' health because of the presence of a spouse who can provide social, emotional, and physical support. For example, when one partner becomes ill, the other can take care of the partner by offering physical and emotional assistance to speed recovery (Ross, Mirowsky, & Goldstein, 1991). Not only do single custodial grandmothers lack social support from a spouse, but they may also be cut off from other sources of support, such as friends, because of time constraints imposed by caregiving responsibilities. Moreover, single custodial grandparents may find that their lives as surrogate parents to young children alienates them from their age peers whose children are grown and out of the home. At the same time, age differences may be an obstacle in developing support systems with younger parents raising their own children. Custodial grandparents also report being limited in their other social roles including decreased contact with family and lowered marital quality, leading to divorce (Jendrek, 1994; Minkler, Roe, & Robertson-Beckley, 1994; Shore & Hayslip, 1994). Furthermore, the health of divorced or widowed women may suffer as a result of the stresses associated with the consequences of divorce and bereavement.

Adverse health conditions of many custodial grandparents may also be related to factors associated with the grandchildren, such as the compounding of stresses from having the child for an extended period. The probability of single grandmothers reporting good health status was lowered more than 50% when children lived with them since birth. Thirty-nine percent of married grandmothers and 41% of unmarried grandmothers in our study had grandchildren living with them since birth. Moreover, assuming responsibility for the care of a grandchild at birth may be the culmination of traumatic and stress producing events, such as the death of the child's parents or parental drug addition and emotional problems.

Shore and Hayslip (1994) suggest that for grandparents who do not have legal guardianship, there is also insecurity concerning when one of the child's parents might return to reclaim the child, particularly when the parent has a drug or mental problem that may present a danger to the grandchild's well-being. In addition, Jendrek (1996) found that custodial grandparents reported less time to get things done, less time with spouse and contact with friends, less privacy, and increases in worrying and physical tiredness. Therefore, the ill health of grandmother with older grandchildren may reflect the compounding of stresses from having the grandchild for a long time as well as not knowing how much longer the child will be with them.

Research evidence also suggests that the number and ages of grandchildren as well as their behavior in school impact grandparent health. Both the responsibility for more than one grandchild and raising older grandchildren are negatively related to grandparents' good health. Taking on the responsibility for two or more children is likely to mean more financial strain, more stress, and more time in child care activities. Older children, especially teenagers, can be difficult and harder to please than younger children who enjoy being played with and cuddled (Cherlin & Furstenburg, 1986). Children who are well behaved in school are certainly much easier and less stressful to deal with than troublemakers. Moreover, good behavior in school may be an indication of good behavior at home. It seems reasonable, therefore, that being obedient at school would have a positive effect on grandparents' physical well-being.

Finally, racial differences were also noted in several studies. For instance, Minkler, Roe, and Price (1992, 1993) and Smith (1994) focused on the poor health of African-American custodial grandmothers. Similarly, most of the single custodial grandmothers discussed earlier whose health was poor were Black. Our research also indicated that married custodial black grandmothers' health was worse than married custodial white grandmothers' health.

Considerations and Limitations

We must now consider the following limitations of the current research: (a) the adequacy of the measures of health status and other variables, (b) the subjects of the research, and (c) the ability to identify the determinants of health status. At the beginning of the chapter, we discussed various measures of health status. Several studies (Anderson, Mullner, & Cornelius, 1987; Gibson, 1991) report race differences in the self-reported health of Black and White Americans on subjective and objective measures of health. Some studies report similar biases in self-ratings using the subjective indicator of health for Blacks and Whites (Blazer & Houpt, 1979), others find that this measure over estimates poor health among Blacks (Ferraro, 1987; Maddox, 1962), and still others that it underestimates poor health (Cockerham, Sharp, & Wilcox; Linn, Hunter, & Linn, 1980).

There may also be problems of interpretation and possible self-report bias. For example, health measures used in the study included global self-rated health that correlates well with objective health indicators and physician ratings (Ferraro, 1980; Kaplan & Comacho, 1983). However, grandparents may either consciously or unconsciously report their health as better than it actually is for fear of losing custody of grandchildren who may be sent to foster care.

Low socioeconomic status is consistently associated with poor health. We, therefore, need more precise measures of financial well-being and a better understanding of the mechanisms by which it affects health status. Incomes below the official poverty line are associated with a lowered quality of physical health; however, at what point does not having enough money begin to impact a person's health, and how does low socioeconomic statue (SES) "cause" poor health? Furthermore, how does poor health impact financial status in terms of occupational opportunities, education, and income level? Are low SES and poor health reciprocally related in a self-perpetuating cycle? And if so, how can the cycle be halted? Does disease and disability result not only from the lack of proper nutrition and access to health services but also from increased stress, low self-esteem, and social isolation?

If, for example, low SES operates through stress and low self-esteem and social isolation to produce illness, can social support play a mediating role in buffering the negative health aspects of low SES and perhaps bringing an end to the cycle? If so, what type of social support is most beneficial (e.g., emotional, functional, support from neighbors, friends, or family)? The results of a metaanalysis by Uchino, Cacioppo, and Kiecolt-Glaser (1996) provide encouraging evidence for the possibility that certain types of social support, particularly from family, may have beneficial effects on the cardiovascular, endocrine, and immune systems. Because all of these systems show declines in function as people age, older grandparents would particularly benefit from this effect of social support.

Second, the subjects of research on custodial grandparents have primarily been White and Black women. Few studies have included Hispanics or other minorities. Thus, we know much less about surrogate parenting among those populations in general and about the health of the grandparents in particular.

Furthermore, although the chapter is on the health of custodial grandparents and the word "grandparent" has often been used, we have really been talking about grandmothers. Research has focused almost exclusively on the health of custodial grandmothers. One explanation for the lack of information on custodial grandfathers is that the current research reflects the reality that most single custodial grandparents are women and thus most of the research has focused on them. Fewer studies have included married custodial grandparents. Giarrusso, Wang, and Silverstein (1996) included grandfathers as part of the custodial grandparents in their study but did not compare their health to that of the grandmothers, probably because of the small number of grandfathers in the sample. The fact is we simply do not know much about the health of custodial grandfathers— single or married. This deficit needs to be addressed not only because of the need to know the health status of grandfathers and how it may be affected by caregiving for grandchildren but also to more fully understand the factors related to grandmother's health. For example, grandmothers may be taking care of health care needs of grandfathers while at the same time caring for small children. Conversely, a healthy grandfather can provide child care assistance as well as social and physical support for the grandmother. A question that might be asked is just who is taking care of whom? Grandchildren may, in fact, find themselves in the role of caregiver because of their grandparents' ill health.

Finally, longitudinal research is necessary to evaluate the causal impact of various factors influencing custodial grandparents' health. For example, Minkler, Roe, and Price (1992) suggest that health status may be a basis for choosing grandparents as surrogate parents. Conversely, the health status of some grandparents could have been worse before taking on the surrogate parenting of grandchildren. Grandparents report changing their health habits and lifestyle (e.g., quit smoking) because of caring for grandchildren (Minkler, Roe, & Price, 1992).

At the beginning of this chapter, we suggested that health be viewed not in dichotomous terms, such as sick or well, but as a continuum from excellent health and the absence of disease or impairment to poor health and extreme disability. People whose health status falls between the extremes of excellent and poor health experience the presence of a health condition or disease, activity restriction as a result of the condition, mild disability, and severe disability. This continuum is not necessarily unidirectional. Over their lifetimes, people move back and forth along the continuum. For example, a person may get the flu and move from excellent health to a health condition, which restricts activity and back to excellent health again. Unfortunately, the health trajectory of some people is one of a continuing lifetime decline in the quality of physical health perhaps because of genetic factors, lifestyle choices, or social class inequities. All custodial grandparents are at some point along this continuum of health. The evidence from current research seems to indicate that many custodial grandparents, particularly single custodial grandmothers, are at the end of the continuum characterized by poor health. As people age, they are more likely to move in a unidirectional way toward the extreme disability end of the continuum. Thus, to recommend policies and services to assist grandparent-grandchild families and improve the health of custodial grandparents, it is important to know whether the poor health of custodial grandparents who are in their 50s or 60s is the result of recent events or part of a lifetime pattern of decline.

Policy Implications

Current knowledge of the health status of custodial grandparents suggests a two-pronged approach for addressing the needs of custodial grandparents. First, policies and resources need to be developed that broadly address the needs shared by most custodial grandparents, such as legal assistance/advice, access to medical care for themselves and their grandchildren, and social support. For example, the AARP Grandparent Information Center serves as a clearinghouse for medical and legal advice and provides information on forming support groups.

Second, programs are needed that address the special situations of subcategories of custodial grandparents. Single grandparents and those living near or below the official poverty line require different programs of assistance than do married and more financially stable grandparents. For example, Minkler and Roe (1993) found that about a third of the grandmothers in their study continued to work outside the home. These grandmothers need help with child care to continue working. Some grandmothers are already caring for other family members—their own children, parents, or other relatives. These women would benefit from practical assistance as well as relief from the stresses of caregiving.

Programs and services designed to improve the health status of custodial grandparents must consider whether poor health is caused by factors associated with caregiving or existed before assuming the responsibility for raising grandchildren. For example, if the time constraints of surrogate parenting have resulted in custodial grandparents missing medical appointments and simply having less time to take care of themselves, then programs that offer respite or child day care options might be helpful. Conversely, although custodial grandparents who have long-term chronic illnesses, such as diabetes, might also benefit from respite services, their health care needs are much more complex. Continuing reliable access to good medical care is a critical component of any program designed to help custodial grandparents with debilitating chronic illnesses maintain a level of functioning that allows them to carry out the responsibilities associated with parenting their grandchildren. Access to good health care, however, is usually costly.

Thus, the necessity for some type of financial assistance for poverty-level custodial grandparents is obvious. However, it is difficult to discuss new policy issues falling under the heading of "welfare," given today's political climate, which produced the recent welfare reform legislation. It remains to be seen how new limits on lifetime eligibility for receiving AFDC affects low-income grandparents raising grandchildren. The current welfare reform legislation that emphasizes a welfare-to-work approach assumes that most, if not all, welfare recipients are young, healthy, and able to work. The fact that most single custodial grandparents are in their mid-50s or older and have health problems that may limit their ability to work does not bode well for the possibility that these already impoverished families will be able to elevate their financial standing and thus avoid continuing negative health outcomes associated with poverty, such as the lack of adequate nutrition and limited access to medical care.

Although creating new programs specifically for custodial grandparents may be difficult, existing programs could be expanded or modified to address some of the needs. Foster care programs should remove bureaucratic barriers to allow family members to become foster parents. In addition, programs that target older people do not affect only older people but often benefit younger people as well. Social Security pensions and Supplemental Security Insurance (SSI) may be a major source of income for grandparents parenting their grandchildren. Consequently, addressing the needs of grandparent/grandchild families does not necessarily mean creating new programs specifically designed for grandparent-headed families. Expanding or maintaining existing programs to support grandparent-grandchild families could result in improved health status for custodial grandparents. It is hoped that future research will provide additional information on the complex influences (e.g., physical, social, psychological, and financial) on the health of these grandparents. This knowledge can then be used to guide the creation and implementation of policies and services specifically designed to foster good health among custodial grandparents.

References

Adams, P. F., & Marano, M. A. (1995). National Center for Health Statistics. *Vital Health Statistics, 10,* 83–84.

American Association of Retired Persons (1991). *A profile of older Americans 1990.* Washington, DC: Author.

Anderson, R. M., Mullner, R. M., & Cornelius, L. J. (1987). Black-white differences in health status: Methods or substance? *The Milbank Quarterly, 65,* 72–99.

Atchley, (1997). *Social forces and aging: An introduction to social gerontology* (7th Ed.). Belmont, CA: Wadsworth.

Becker, L. B., Han, B. H., Meyer, P. M., Wright, F. A., Rhodes, K. V., Smth, D. W., Barrett, J., & the Chicago Project. (1993). Racial differences in the incidence of cardiac arrest and subsequent survival. *New England Journal of Medicine, 329,* 600–606.

Blazer, D. G., & Houpt, J. L. (1979). Perception of poor health in the healthy older adult. *Journal of the American Geriatric Society, 27,* 330–334.

Burton, L. M. (1992). Black grandparents rearing grandchildren of drug-addicted parents: Stressors, outcomes, and social service needs. *The Gerontologist, 32,* 744–751.

Cherlin, A. J., & Furstenberg, F. F. (1986). *The new American grandparent.* New York: Basic Books.

Cockerham, W. C., Sharp, K., & Wilcox, J. A. (1983). Aging and perceived health status. *Journal of Gerontology, 38,* 349–355.

Ferraro, K. F. (1980). Self rating of health among the old and the old old. *Journal of Health and Social Behavior, 21,* 377.

Ferraro, K. F. (1987). Double jeopardy to health for black older adults? *Journal of Gerontology, 42,* 528–533.

Gibson, R. C. (1991). Race and the self-reported health of elderly persons. *Journal of Gerontology, 46*(Suppl.), S235–242.

Herbert, T. B., & Cohen, S. (1993). Depression and immunity: A meta-analytic review. *Psychological Bulletin, 113,* 472–486.

Jendrek, M. P. (1996). Grandparents who parent their grandchildren: Effects on lifestyle. In J. Quadagno & D. Street (Eds.), *Aging for the twenty-first cen-*

tury: Readings in social gerontology (pp. 286–305). New York: St. Martins Press.

Kaplan, G. A. & Comacho, T. C. (1983). Perceived health and mortality: A nine-year follow-up of the human population laboratory cohort. *American Journal of Epidemiology, 117,* 292–304.

Maddox, G. L. (1962). Some correlates of differences in self-assessment of health status among the elderly. *Journal of Gerontology, 17,* 180–185.

Miller, D. (1991). The "Grandparents Who Care" support project of San Francisco. Paper presented at the annual meeting of the Gerontological Society of America, San Francisco.

Minkler, M. (1994). Grandparents as parents: The American experience. *Ageing International, 1,* 24–28.

Minkler, M., & Roe, K. M. (1993). *Grandmothers as caregivers: raising children of the crack cocaine epidemic.* Newberry Park, CA: Sage.

Minkler, M., Roe, K. M., & Price, M. (1992). The physical and emotional health of grandmothers raising grandchildren in the crack cocaine epidemic. *The Gerontologist, 32,* 752–761.

Minkler, M., Roe, K. M., & Roberton-Beckley, R. (1994). Raising grandchildren from crack-cocaine households: Effects on family and friendship ties of African-American women. *American Journal of Orthopsychiatry, 64,* 20–29.

National Center for Health Statistics. (1991). Current estimates from the National Health Interview Survey, 1990 (Vital and Health Statistics, Series 10, No. 181). Washington, DC: U.S. Government Printing Office.

Pruchno, R. A., & Johnson, K. W. (1996). Research on grandparenting: Current studies and future needs. *Generations, 20,* 65–70.

Ross, C. E., Mirowsky, J., & Goldstein, K. (1991). The impact of family on health: The decade in review. In A. Booth (Ed.), *Contemporary families: Looking forward, looking back.* Minneapolis: National Council on Family Relations.

Shore, J. R., & Hayslip, B., Jr. (1994). Custodial grandparenting: Implications for children's development. In A. E. Gottfried & A. W. Gottfried (Eds.), *Redefining families: Implications for children's development.* New York: Plenum.

Smith, A. (1994). African-American grandmothers' war against the crack cocaine epidemic. *Arete, 19,* 22–36.

Solomon, J. C. & Marx, J. (1995). "To grandmother's house we go": Health and school adjustment of children raised solely by grandparents. *The Gerontologist, 35,* 386–394.

Uchino, B. N., Cacioppo, J. T., & Kiecolt-Glaser, J. K. (1996). The relationship between social support and physiological processes: A review with emphasis on underlying mechanisms and implications for health. *Psychological Bulletin, 119,* 488–531.

U.S. Bureau of Census. (1990). *The need for personal assistance with everyday activities: Recipients and caregivers.* (Current Population Reports, Series, P-70, No. 19). Washington, DC: U.S. Government Printing Office.

U.S. Department of Health & Human Services. (1991a). *Current Estimates from the National Health Interview Survey, 1990.* Washington, DC: Author.

U.S. Department of Health & Human Services. (1991b). *Healthy People 2000: National health promotion and disease prevention activities.* Washington, DC: Author.

Verbrugge, L. M. (1984). Longer life but worsening health? Trends in health and mortality of middle-aged and older persons. *Milbank Memorial Fund Quarterly, 62,* 475–519.

Chapter 4

Social Support, Stress, and Special Coping Tasks of Grandmother Caregivers

Carol M. Musil, Susan Schrader, and John Mutikani

Although there has been increased understanding regarding the stresses of grandmother caregivers, the issues of social support and coping have received far less consideration. This chapter examines three interrelated factors that are central to the well-being of grandmother caregivers: the stresses, social supports, coping tasks, and strategies required to rear grandchildren effectively.

Stress

From a theoretical perspective, stress derives from environmental, social, or internal demands that may tax an individual's usual responses or that require an individual to adjust patterns of behavior (Holmes & Rahe, 1967; Lazarus & Folkman, 1984; Thoits, 1995). The stressors encountered by grandmother caregivers include not only discrete life events but also ongoing, daily strains related to the context of caregiving, including their family situations, and their psychosocial and physical health.

The Context of Caregiving

The context of the caregiving situation is a defining feature of the stress experienced by grandmother caregivers. When grandmothers begin rearing grandchildren, the family structure is reconfigured (Goodman & Silverstein, 1997). Often, as in cases of substance abuse, the grandparent-adult child relationship has been previously marked by discord. New conflicts, both intrapersonal and interpersonal, may arise, particularly if the grandparent must choose between the needs of the (adult) child and the needs of the grandchild. In many instances, the grandmother must seek legal action against her adult child to limit abusive or disruptive behavior or to secure an endangered or neglected grandchild (Kelley, Yorker, & Whitley, 1997).

Even after the grandparent assumes caregiving, the parent is rarely entirely separated from the family structure. In these situations, when the parent is not estranged, there is a structural role reversal in which the grandparent assumes the daily parenting for the grandchild, and the (adult) child has occasional, grandparent-like visits with limited responsibility (Goodman & Silverstein, 1997; Kelley, Yorker, & Whitley, 1997).

Drug abuse, death, mental illness, and incarceration in the parental generation are among the most recognized, but not the only, reasons that grandmothers assume the primary caregiving role. Many grandmothers assume legal responsibility for the grandchild until a young teenage parent is recognized by the state as a legal guardian, usually at age 18. Although most of these grandmothers will play a supportive or supplemental role in rearing their grandchild(ren), some grandmothers will assume a relatively greater proportion of the caretaking because the teen parent is unable to provide adequate care to the child. In other instances, the grandmother may choose not to limit her caregiving to a supplemental role, particularly if she did not have an opportunity to rear her own children (Burton, 1996).

The high rate of teen pregnancy has contributed to a number of young grandmothers who may have had their children reared, in part or in whole, by their own mothers (Burton, 1996). Odulana, Camblin, and White (1996) describe the "parental replacement model" of grandmother involvement with their teenage daughters' children. In these situations, grandmothers take over the child-rearing activities and often assume financial responsibility for the teen child and grandchild, whereas the teen mother may develop a more sibling-like relationship with her own child. Many strains occur in these intergenerational households associated with early mothering and grandmothering, and in some instances, the development of independent maternal caretaking skills in the young mother may be inhibited (Chase-Lansdale, Brooks-Gunn & Zamsky, 1994; Odulana, Camblin, & White, 1996).

The degree of choice that a woman has in undertaking the custodial role is not well understood. In some households, grandmothers elect to be caregivers and may even assume the child-rearing function for several children from multiple families (Burton, 1992). Sands and Goldberg-Glen (1998) noted that many of their subjects were never without children in their home and suggest that some grandmothers self-select into the caregiver role. They reported that 40% of the caregiver grandmothers in their study, both African American and White, felt that they had a choice about whether or not to assume caregiving and believed that if something happened to them, another family member, generally female, likely would be available. Conversely, many grandmothers anecdotally report that they assumed responsibility for their grandchildren as the alternative of having them placed in the home of a stranger, an unacceptable option.

Parenting Role

Assuming the role of parent is stressful for many grandmothers (Burton, 1992). Several researchers have found that grandmother caregivers are likely to report greater parenting stress than mothers (Kelley, 1993; Musil, 1998a; Musil, Youngblut, & Ahn, 1998). Cultural norms and values have changed greatly since grandmothers reared their own children, and they may have difficulty advising and disciplining their grandchild, particularly when the situations confronting the child are outside the grandparent's experience (Boksay, 1998). Some feel inadequate to the task, because of perceptions (either their own or others) that they may have failed to rear their own children successfully. These perceptions can in themselves be stressful as they begin to doubt their adequacy in the parenting role.

Creating a family and home environment that accommodates the unique needs of children is challenging. Although having more grandchildren in the home may be associated with somewhat greater stress (Musil, 1998a), the ages and special needs of the grandchildren determine, to a large extent, the nature of child-rearing stresses (Kelley, 1993). For example, in grandparent homes with infants and small children, structuring a child-proof and safe environment, perhaps after years of living without children, is a priority. Young children tax the physical reserves of the grandparents, whereas the school, sports, and recreational activities of elementary and middle school children present problems related to scheduling and over-involvement that are different from when grandparents reared their own children. For those rearing adolescents, issues related to independence intensify, along with grandparent concerns about the child's exposure to drugs, alcohol, and sexual situations. Teenagers pose a number of challenges including career planning, dating, birth control issues, driving, and the ever-present penchant for risk taking. Although there are many programs for families with children in the middle school years and younger, few programs are targeted to the needs of teens and preteens, a deficiency noted by some grandmother caregivers with children in this age group.

If the grandchild has special needs because of HIV infection or developmental disabilities resulting from prenatal drug exposure or fetal alcohol syndrome, child rearing is likely to be even more demanding. Children with attention deficit disorders, behavior problems or developmental disabilities require specialized health care, including medication, psychological or behavioral interventions, and sometimes even residential treatment programs. Grandchildren who were abused or neglected usually require individual or family counseling.

Educating grandchildren and becoming involved in school and other activities necessary for the child's growth and well-being can be daunting. The educational environment, including expectations for caregiver involvement, has changed dramatically over recent years (Rothenberg, 1997). In addition, grandparent-grandchild relationship requirements vary among school districts, and some schools may be less prepared to recognize or help meet the special needs of the family. Although some require a formal legal relationship, such as guardianship, before a grandparent may make educational decisions for their grandchild, others recognize informal authority (Rothenberg, 1997). When coupled with other developmental or family problems, tailoring an adequate educational experience for grandchildren is often difficult.

Financial and Employment Issues

The financial burden of rearing another generation of children is consistently cited as the major source of stress by grandparent caregivers (Burton, 1992; Kelley, Yorker, & Whitley,1997; Simon-Rusinowitz, Krach, Marks, Piktalis, & Wilson, 1996). Many caregivers are on fixed incomes, and 39% have annual family incomes of $20,000 or less (AARP, 1994). Often, grandparents do not seek government assistance even when warranted for fear of exposing the situation and losing the grandchild or due to the complexity of eligibility requirements, which may include time limits, work requirements, and legal relationships (Kleiner, Hertzog, & Targ, 1998; Towle, 1997). Others may not be eligible for age-related Social Security benefits for themselves as they did not pay into the system (Kelley, Yorker, & Whitley, 1997).

Employment issues arise as many grandmothers find it necessary to give up or reduce participation in the job market when they begin rearing their grandchildren (Odulana, Camblin & White, 1996; Simon-Rusinowitz, Krach, Marks, Piktalis, & Wilson, 1996). Balancing work and the daily tasks of child rearing is challenging for parents as well as grandparent caregivers under the best of circumstances. For grandmother caregivers, coping with the two responsiblities, particularly if the child has special needs or if the grandparent has additional caregiving responsibilities to other family members, can be very taxing (Minkler, Roe, & Price, 1992). However, despite complications from employment, employed grandmother caregivers reported less parenting stress and less ill health than nonemployed grandmothers (Minkler, Roe, & Price, 1992; Musil, Youngblut & Ahn, 1998; Sands & Goldberg-Glen, 1998). This may be due to the support and personal rewards received from their work and the work setting.

The environment in which the grandmothers must care for their grandchildren is a significant component of the caregiving situation. Neighborhood problems related to crime, drug trafficking, and safety contribute to chronic strain, especially in the inner city (Burton, 1992). Violence in the school setting adds to difficulties grandchildren must face, particularly if they have had limited experience with positive interpersonal relationships or if the stresses in the home contribute to poor peer relationships.

Psychosocial and Physical Health Stresses

Grandmother caregivers report several psychological stresses related to their role as caregivers. A major source of stress is the very reason that the adult child is unable to rear his or her own offspring. Death, incarceration, drug use, or HIV infection in the adult child has likely led to many legal and interpersonal problems preceding the grandmother's assumption of consistent and primary caregiving responsibilities. Thus, these grandmothers deal with complex family situations about which they often have ambivalent feelings, especially toward their own children. Trying to manage both the situations and concurrent emotions are stressful, especially when there is no anticipated resolution.

The overall picture of the lives of grandmother caregivers is not entirely clear. Several studies suggest that grandmother caregivers experience worse mental health and more depression than other women (Kelley, 1993; Musil, 1998a). However, these studies did not use comparisons with matched samples of noncaregiving grandmothers. At the same time, there has been little consideration of whether the role of grandmother caregiver promotes the same type of social integration and life satisfaction for women that occurs with other types of caregiving (Moen, Robison, & Dempster-McClain, 1995; Pearson, Hunter, Ensingmer, & Kellam, 1990).

Grandmother caregivers are likely to report stress-related emotional disturbances, such as frustration, fear, anxiety, and anger (Odulana, Camblin, & White, 1996). Minkler, Roe, and Price (1992) indicated that many reported a decline in their emotional health because they began caregiving, in part owing to watching the deterioration of their adult child from drug use. Although those same grandmothers appraised their overall emotional health as good or excellent, most reported some loneliness and depression sometime during the week. Other evidence suggests that many grandmothers have led difficult lives before their role as caregivers, experiencing more depression and worse health before assuming that role (Minkler, Fuller-Thompson, Miller, & Driver, 1997; Strawbridge, Wallhagen, Shema, & Kaplan, 1997).

Regardless of whether a pattern exists of prior ongoing stress, grandmothers also experience new emotional stresses resulting from their caregiving role. The job of parenting a grandchild drives the grandparent into unexpected personal transitions while possibly removing or distancing her from usual activities and sources of support. The consequences of these transitions, perhaps as much as the actual parenting activities, may contribute to psychological stress in the grandmother.

Despite their own child's inability to fulfill parental caretaking responsibilities, many grandparents continue to regard their (adult) child as good and caring (Jendrek, 1994), and isolate such problems as drug abuse and incarceration from their overall appraisal of that child. Other grandmothers are less willing to defend their own children's behavior and live with mixed feelings of regret and hope, underscoring the complicated feelings that many grandmother caregivers have about their families. Closeness between the grandmother caregiver and her own child (as well as grandmother closeness with the grandchild) has been found to be positively related to life satisfaction and less negative affect in the grandmother (Goodman & Silverstein; 1997)

The physical health of the grandmothers can be a source and consequence of stress. Many grandparent caregivers are older than 55 years (Burton, 1992; Chalfie, 1994), corresponding with a time in which they are likely to experience the emergence of their own health problems. Chronic conditions, such as heart disease, arthritis, or diabetes, become more prominent, with an increased risk among Blacks, adding to the burden of rearing a grandchild (Minkler, Roe, & Price, 1992; National Center for Health Statistics, 1990). Regardless of their health status, grandmothers often report feeling emotionally depleted and physically exhausted as a result of parenting their grandchildren, which is unrelated to their baseline health (Kleiner, Hertzog, & Targ, 1998; Towle, 1997). According to one grandmother, "There are parts of my old life that I miss, and there are times that both my husband and I are so tired we don't think we'll make it through the day" (Musil, 1997). Such age-related declines in energy can have subtle effects on the type of involvement grandmothers have with their grandchildren, although the cumulative effects of such daily interaction patterns on many aspects of the family system are unknown.

Additional stress stems from the grandmothers' own developmental tasks of late adulthood or emerging old age. Dealing with menopause, coming to terms with one's own life's worth, and making decisions about work and retirement are complicated by the prospect of caregiving responsibilities that may extend for many years. For many grandmothers, this simultaneous juggling of personal developmental tasks, along with those of their grandchildren, often occurs within the context of poverty (Chase-Lansdale, Brooks-Gunn, & Zamsky, 1994).

Social Support

Social support—the network of supports that provides informational, emotional, and tangible assistance—is vital to the health of grandparent caregivers. Support includes informal support provided by family, friends, church organizations, and others, whereas formal support, such as informational support, group support, financial assistance, and respite care, is rendered by professionals and social systems. Social support consistently has been associated with less distress in several stressful situations (see Thoits, 1995, for a review; Turner & Marino, 1994). Theoretical models have been applied to the relationship of social support to mental health outcomes of many types of caregivers (Kahana & Young, 1990; Li, Seltzer, & Greenberg, 1997; Pruchno, Peters, & Burant, 1995) but have been virtually unexamined in samples of grandmother caregivers.

Informal Support

Informal social support comes from the immediate and extended family, friends, and the church, among others, and includes both emotional support and tangible/instrumental aid. Grandmother caregivers are often at increased risk to experience social isolation and lack of support (Kelley, 1993). For example, grandmothers with primary responsibility for rearing their grandchildren reported less subjective and instrumental support than grandmothers with only supplemental responsibility for child rearing (Musil, 1998a).

At the same time, the benefits of informal supports shown in other caregivers of the elderly, (Li, Seltzer, & Greenberg, 1997; Schultz & Williamson, 1991) may be the same for grandmother caregivers. Appraisals of greater subjective, emotional support, such as feeling understood by family and friends, and instrumental support, such as being able to count on others in times of specific need, have been associated with less depression in grandmother caregivers (Musil & Ahn, 1997).

Although, to date, there is little research about informal support among grandmother caregivers, feeling a genuine concern from others and safety when venting feelings are likely to be essential aspects of support (Rose, 1997). However, locating such support may be difficult. Many grandmother caregivers isolate themselves from their peers because of embarrassment, restricted ability to participate in social events because of financial or time constraints, or fear of being criticized for their adult child's behavior (Ginchild-Abeje & Perez-Porter, 1997; Kelley, 1993). Others are unable to draw such acceptance from their personal networks but find that formal support group participation is helpful.

Grandmothers with a spouse or a partner may report less parenting stress, because of immediate support, than those without a companion (Musil, 1998b). Commenting on the support she received from her spouse, one grandmother said, "My husband, who had taken early retirement just before our assuming responsibility for the children, provides as much care as I do." However, about one third of grandmother caregivers are not currently married and find themselves with little or no support in caring for their grandchildren (AARP, 1994).

When looking at support provided by the family, important cultural factors may contribute to grandmothers' perceptions of their caregiving obligations and expectations for others' assistance. For example, there is a fairly consistent agreement that child rearing is viewed, to some extent, as a shared responsibility among African-American families (Chase-Lansdale, Brooks-Gunn, & Zamsky, 1994; Odulana, Lantham, Camblin, & White, 1996). The resiliency of these networks, however, should not be readily assumed. Although some earlier studies suggest that older African Americans generally belong to extended family networks with considerable intergenerational support (Taylor, Chatters, Tucker, & Lewis, 1990), Burton (1992) found that few Black grandmothers with such kinship ties received consistent economic and social support from their networks. Although those with a larger social network may have a correspondingly greater reservoir of support in times of need, they also have the potential of being called to provide assistance.

Other work has focused less directly on grandmother caregivers but points to a beginning understanding about cultural influences on the grandmother role including racial and geographic considerations. For example, in a comparison of Black and White grandmothers in a rural area, including those with no caretaking responsibilities, Kivett (1993) found both differences and similarities between and within racial groups. Although there were many racial similarities about the dimensions of the grandmother role, different patterns of grandmother-grandchild exchanges were identified (Kivett, 1993). In the Older Native Women's Health Project (1995), changes in aboriginal society and family structure have caused many women to express concern about their children and grandchildren and the grandmother's role in the family.

A strong belief and trust in God has been identified as a source of personal strength and support for many persons including caregivers (Picot, Debanne, Namazi, & Wykle, 1997; Taylor, 1985). The social networks found in the church may offer a safe source of peer support. Many grandmothers in Musil's (1997) study noted that they used faith in God and prayer to find strength to continue caregiving.

Formal Support

Formal support to grandmothers rearing grandchildren includes a range of services, although the most well known are support groups. Support groups are quite diverse, serving a variety of purposes. Although Vardi and Buchholz (1994) describe a support group process that is primarily psychotherapeutic in nature, other groups focus more on the social or educational aspects of support. An important secondary function of grandmother support groups is that they may serve as a base for organizing and mobilizing participants to become politically active in the issues facing grandparent/kin caregivers. Such activities foster community awareness and contribute to the reform of social policy, while channeling the energy of interested parties in external, goal-oriented projects. Support groups and their many considerations are presented in detail elsewhere in this book.

An underused source of formal support for grandmother caregivers is the computer. Hundreds of web sites are now available that provide information and assistance. Some of the sites provide information on various topics including support for women at midlife, questions of seeking legal custody, and guides for grandmother caregivers. Bulletin boards are available where grandparents may ask questions and interact with other grandparents and professionals. Other sites provide pertinent legislative information at the federal, state and local levels. Information on education, product safety, and referral sources for mental health problems for both the grandparent and the grandchild are also available.

Coping

Coping generally refers to coping strategies: behavioral or cognitive attempts to manage demands perceived as taxing or exceeding one's resources (Lazarus & Folkman, 1984). The stress and coping literature suggests that although coping is situational, an individual may tend to use particular coping strategies across situations (Lazarus & Folkman, 1984; Thoits, 1995). There has been only minimal account of how grandmother caregivers cope with the issues they encounter.

There is a growing base of literature that describes why grandmothers become involved in caretaking (Burton, 1992; Kelley, 1993; Minkler, Roe, & Price, 1992; Musil, 1998a). Less has been written describing the process of becoming a grandmother caregiver and considerably less describes how the family adapts to the initial and ongoing tasks and emotional demands of caregiving. Sands and Goldberg-Glen (1998) reported that the impetus for caregiving developed over time for roughly half the 123 families in their sample, that the onset was precipitous for 27%, and that a crisis within an ongoing situation prompted the decision for caregiving for the remaining grandparent families. Thus, it appears that for many grandmothers, the transition to caregiving was an evolutionary process, suggestive of an ongoing coping situation.

Health, Stress, Coping, and Social Support

Musil (1998a, 1998b) examined health, stress, coping, and social support in grandmothers who lived with their grandchildren and had either primary or supplemental responsibility for their care. Included in the sample were 58 women with primary responsibility for their grandchildren, most often because of the parents' drug abuse and related neglect of their children. Approximately two thirds of the primary caregivers were Black, and about 74% had legal custody of their grandchildren.

The study assessed coping with with the Ways of Coping Checklist (Lazarus & Folkman, 1984), using the three-factor structure of coping— coping actively, avoiding coping, and minimizing the situation— determined by Smyth and Yarandi (1996) from a sample of Black women. In active coping, the caregiver is involved in such activities as talking to someone or making plans of action and following them. Avoidance coping includes wishing the situation would change or attempting to avoid the situation. Minimizing includes efforts to reduce the weight or burden of caring by accepting the situation as it arises and by downplaying the problem.

The findings indicated that avoidant and minimization coping were related to greater depression, anxiety, and parenting stress but were unrelated to demographic factors, such as age of grandchildren and race or education of the grandmother (Musil & Ahn, 1997; Musil, 1998b). Relative stability in stress, coping, and support among grandmother caregivers over 10 months was found.

Many of the written comments of these grandmother amplify these findings (Musil, 1997). Those who used active coping involved themselves in communication and discussions with others about grandparent caregiving, sought possible solutions to specific problems, and may have participated in local or state efforts focused on kinship care issues. Many found direction by reading all they could get on child care or by attending seminars and workshops for grandmothers caring for grandchildren. Others commented on the importance of a sense of humor and the need to take things one day at a time. And, as noted earlier, employment, although not a coping strategy per se, was reported as providing both financial and other benefits and helped grandmothers to retain their identity (Musil, Youngblut, & Ahn, 1998). Finding ways to maintain individuality in the face of many responsibilities was acknowledged as an important challenge associated with caregiving.

In addition, grandmothers' comments (Musil, 1997) illustrated two important coping strategies: perceiving the caregiving role as rewarding and using prayer/spirituality. Being able to find meaning and purpose in the situation was reported to minimize the negative effects of caregiving for many of the grandmothers (Musil, 1997). A notable majority of the grandmothers who provided written comments expressed the rewards of providing such care. Despite the difficulty and burden in their role as the primary caregiver, many grandmothers remarked on their satisfaction in being active participants in the grandchild's care. The frustrations and demands of caregiving were counterbalanced by the rewards of caregiving such as personal growth. One grandmother commented, "I have learned more about looking at things in a different perspective, and I'm focusing on the important issues in my life. Through [her granddaughter's] presence I have discovered the joy of inner peace and genuine contentment."

Secondly, spirituality and prayer, especially in Black grandmothers, was viewed as a coping strategy for some women. For example, about 90% of Black grandmothers, compared with only 60% of White grandmothers, indicated that they used prayer as a coping strategy "often" or "a great deal" (Musil, 1997). These findings are consistent with those of other researchers (Chatters, Levin, & Taylor,1992; Taylor, 1986) who found that Blacks, especially women, were more likely to be religiously involved.

Based on the comments of the sample, spirituality appears to be a more critical coping strategy than is often recognized and needs to be incorporated in studies examining coping strategies of grandmother caregivers. About 10% of the sample provided additional comments indicating that the use of prayer, faith, and trust in God were coping strategies on which they relied (Musil, 1997). Several also noted that investigators seem to underestimate the importance of these strategies.

Religiosity, whether organized or nonorganized, may have important implications for health and well-being. Dimensions of religiosity, including prayer, self-rated religiosity, and church attendance, have been related to the perceived rewards of caregivers of the elderly, especially among Black caregivers (Picot et al.,1997). However, only organizational religiosity have been associated with better health (Levin, Chatters, & Taylor,1995).

Conclusion

Grandmothers assume the caretaking role for various reasons with drug abuse in the (adult) child one of the most common. Stress in grandmothers varies according to the initial reason for caregiving, the age and number of grandchildren, the grandmother's health, and socioeconomic factors.

Supports that can help in coping with this stress have received little attention by researchers. However, preliminary evidence suggests that support is particularly beneficial in reducing depression and promoting well-being. Sprituality may play a prominent role in helping grandmothers to cope with the stress of the overall family situation. Further research is essential to understand the relationships among stress, coping, and support in caregiver grandmothers. It is through such studies that more effective strategies to support the efforts of grandparent caregivers and their families can be made.

References

American Association of Retired Persons (1994, September). AARP grandparent information center. Washington, DC: Author.

Boksay, I. (1998). *Grandparents face unusual problems in raising their grandchildren*. The Shawnee News-Star, (on-line): http://www.newsstar.com/stories/011598/lfe_gparent.html.

Burton, L. M. (1992). Black grandparents rearing children of drug-addicted parents: Stress, outcomes, and social service needs. *The Gerontologist, 32*, 744–751.

Chalfie, D. (1994). *Going it alone: A closer look at grandparents parenting grandchildren*. Washington, DC: American Association of Retired Persons.

Chase-Lansdale, P. L., Brooks-Gunn, J., & Zamsky, E. S. (1994). Young African American multigenerational families in poverty: Quality of mothering and grandmothering. *Child Development, 65*, 373–93.

Chatters, L. M., Levin, J. S., & Taylor, R. J. Antecedents and dimensions of religious involvement among older black adults. *The Journal of Gerontology: Social Sciences, 47* (Suppl.), S269–S278.

Ginchild-Abeje, R., & Perez-Porter, M. (1997). In conversation with . . . Dr. Lenora Poe, author of *Black grandparents as parents*. *Grandparent caregivers: A national guide (on-line)*: http://www.igc.org/justice/cjc/lspc/manual/foster.html.

Goodman, C. C., & Silverstein, M. (1997, November). *Grandparents who parent intergenerational triads and well being*. Paper presented at the meeting of the Gerontological Society of America, Cincinnati.

Holmes, T. H., & Rahe, R. H. (1967). The social readjustment rating scale. *Journal of Psychosomatic Research, 11*, 213–218.

Jendrek, M. (1994). Grandparents who parent their grandchildren: Circumstances and decisions. *The Gerontologist, 34*, 206–216.

Kahana, E., & Young, R. (1990). Clarifying the caregiving paradigm: Challenges for the future. In D. E. Biegel & A. Blum (Eds.), *Aging and caregiving: Theory, research, and policy* (pp. 76–97). Newbury Park, CA: Sage.

Kelley, S. J. (1993). Caregiver stress in grandparents raising grandchildren. *Image*, *25*, 331–337.

Kelley, S. J., Yorker, B. C., & Whitley, D. (1997). To grandmother's house we go . . . and stay: Children raised in intergenerational families. *Journal of Gerontological Nursing, 23*, 12–20.

Kerns, R., & Turk, D. (1985). Behavioral Medicine and the family: Historical perspectives and future directions. In D. C. Turk & R. D. Kerns (Eds.), *Health, illness, and families: A lifespan perspective.* New York: Wiley.

Kleiner, H. S., Hertzog, J., & Targ, D. B. (1998). Background information for educators. *Grandparents acting as parents* (online): http://www.nnfr.org/nnfr/igen/gaap.html.

Lazarus, R., & Folkman, S. (1984). *Stress, appraisal and coping.* New York: Springer.

Leventhal, H., Leventhal, E., Turk, D. C., & Kerns, R. D. (Eds.). (1985). *Health, illness, and families: A life span perspective.* New York: Wiley.

Levin, J. S., Chatters, L. M., & Taylor, R. J. (1995). Religious effects on health status and life satisfaction among black Americans. *Journal of Gerontology, 50B* (Suppl.), S154–S163.

Li, L. W., Seltzer, M. M., & Greenberg, J. S. (1997). Social support and depressive symptoms: Differential patterns in wife and daughter caregivers. *Journal of Gerontology, 52* (Suppl.), S200–S211.

Minkler, M., Fuller-Thompson, E., Miller, D., & Driver, D. (1997). Depression in grandparents raising grandchildren: Results of a national longitudinal study. *Archives of Family Medicine, 6*, 445–452.

Minkler, M., Roe, K., & Price, M. (1992). The physical and emotional health of grandmothers raising grandchildren in the crack cocaine epidemic. *The Gerontologist, 32*, 752–761.

Moen, P., Robison, J., & Dempster-McClain, D. (1995). Caregiving and women's well-being: A life course approach. *Journal of Health and Social Behavior, 36*, 259–273.

Musil, C. M. (1997). *Psychosocial and self-assessed health of grandmothers giving care to grandchildren: A descriptive study.* Unpublished data.

Musil, C. M. (1998a). Health, stress, coping, and social support in grandmother caregivers. *Health Care for Women International, 19*, 101–114.

Musil, C. M. (1998b). *Health of grandmothers as caregivers: A 10 month follow-up.* Submitted for publication.

Musil, C. M., & Ahn, S. (1997, November). *Grandmothers raising grandchildren: Is support linked to depression?* Paper presented at the meeting of the Gerontological Society of America, Cincinnati.

Musil, C. M., Youngblut, J. M., & Ahn, S. (1998, March). *Parenting stress: A comparison of grandmother caretakers and mothers.* Paper presented at the meeting of the Midwest Nursing Research Society of America, Columbus.

National Center for Health Statistics (1990). The health of black and white Americans, 1985–1987. *National Health Interview Survey* (Series 10, No.171). Washington DC: US Government Printing Office.

Odulana, J. A., Camblin, L. D., & White, P. (1996). Cultural roles and health status of contemporary African American young grandmothers. *The Journal of Multicultural Nursing and Health, 2,* 28–35.

Pearson, J. L., Hunter, A. G., Ensminger, M. E., & Kellam, S. G. (1990). Black grandmothers in multigenerational households: Diversity in family structure and parenting involvement in the Woodlawn Community. *Child Development, 61,* 434–442.

Picot, S., Debanne, S., Namazi, K., & Wykle, M. (1997). Religiosity and perceived rewards of black and white caregivers. *The Gerontologist, 37,* 89–101.

Pruchno, R. A., Burant, C. J., & Peters, N. D. (1995). Typologies of caregiving families: Family congruence and individual well-being. *The Gerontologist, 37,* 137–167.

Rose, L. E. (1997). Caring for caregivers: perceptions of social support. *Journal of Psychological Nursing, 35,* 17–24.

Rothenberg, D. (1997). Grandparents as parents: A primer for schools. *KidSource* (online): wysiwyg://60/http://www.kidsource/content2/grandparents.3.html.

Sands, R. G., & Goldberg-Glen, R. S. (1998). The impact of employment and serious illness on grandmothers who are raising their grandchildren. *Journal of Women & Aging, 10,* 41–58.

Simon-Rusinowitz, L., Krach, C. A., Marks, L. N., Piktalis, D., & Wilson, L. B. (1996). Grandparents in the workplace: The effects of economic and labor trends. *Generations, 20,* 41–43.

Smyth, K., & Yarandi, H. (1996). Factor analysis of the Ways of Coping Questionnaire for African American women. *Nursing Research, 45,* 25–29.

Strawbridge, W., Wallhagen, M., Shema, S., & Kaplan, G. (1997). New burdens or more of the same? Comparing adult grandparent, spouse and adult-child caregivers. *The Gerontologist, 37,* 505–510.

Taylor, R. J. (1985). The extended family as a form of support to elderly blacks. *The Gerontologist, 25,* 488–489.

Taylor, R. J. (1986). Religious participation among elderly blacks. *The Gerontologist, 26,* 630–635.

Taylor, R. J., Chatters, L. M., Tucker, M. B., & Lewis, E. (1990). Development in research in black families: A decade review. *Journal of Marriage and the Family, 52,* 993–1014.

Thoits, P. A. (1995). Stress, coping and social support processes: Where are we? What next? *Journal of Health and Social Behavior,* Special Review, 53–79.

Towle, L. H. (1997). *Grandma, where's mommy? Carolina parent,* (on-line): http://family.disney.com/Categ...97_01/dony/dony199701_grandma.

Turner R. J., & Marino, F. (1994, September). Social support and social structure: A descriptive edipemiology. *Journal of Health and Social Behavior, 35,* 193–212.

Vardi, D., & Bucholz, E. (1994). Group psychotherapy with inner city grandmothers raising their grandchildren. *International Journal of Group Psychotherapy, 44,* 101–122.

Chapter 5

Psychological Costs and Benefits of Raising Grandchildren: Evidence From a National Survey of Grandparents

Roseann Giarrusso, Merril Silverstein, and Du Feng

As with other forms of caregiving, caregiving for grandchildren has been found to be stressful. Indeed, recent research suggests that caring for grandchildren may be even more stressful than caring for an elderly spouse or parent. According to Strawbridge, Wallhagen, Shema, and Kaplan (1997), grandparent caregiving usually occurs within the context of an already difficult life course. Thus, the psychological difficulties for grandparents, which often begin with the dysfunctional behavior of the

This research was supported by a grant from the American Association of Retired Persons.

adult child, are compounded with the assumption of full-time caregiving for grandchildren.

Yet, although some grandparents are likely to experience grave psychological distress from their caregiving activities, others are less affected and, in fact, may derive great psychological rewards from their caregiving duties. Thus, in order for service providers and policy makers to target support to caregiving grandparents better, a better understanding of the process and risk factors of psychological distress of caregiving is needed.

The study described in this chapter uses data from a recent (1997–98) nationally representative sample of grandparents in the United States to examine the psychological costs and benefits to grandparents of taking primary responsibility for the care of one or more of their grandchildren. Four research questions are addressed. First, what proportion of caregiving grandparents experience caregiving for their grandchild as stressful? What proportion experience it as rewarding? Second, what factors are associated with experiencing higher levels of stress or reward? Third, what is the balance between stress and reward, and, is this balance related to grandparents' overall psychological well-being? Fourth, does social support buffer the negative affect of stress on the psychological well-being of grandparents?

Is Caregiving for Grandchildren Stressful or Rewarding?

Research has begun to identify the burdens faced by grandparents who assume direct, full-time caregiving responsibilities for their grandchildren (e.g., Burton 1992; Chalfie 1994; Shore & Hayslip, 1994). Empirical evidence strongly suggests that grandparents who assume full-time caregiving responsibilities for their grandchildren experience high levels of stress. As discussed earlier in this book, their sources of stress are many and include economic difficulties; social isolation; grandchildren who have physical and psychological problems; adult children who are dysfunctional, sick, addicted, or incarcerated; conflict with spouses and friends; an overall lack of time (Dressel, 1994; Hirshorn, 1998; Roe, Minkler, Saunders, & Thomson, 1996; Jendrek, 1993, 1994; Minkler, Roe, & Price, 1992). Further, caregiving grandparents have little institutional support. They confront obstacles in obtaining such basics as public financial assistance, health insurance coverage, and housing and have difficulty in gaining legal rights to make decisions regarding the grandchild's education and medical care (Chalfie, 1994; Minkler & Roe, 1993; Minkler, Roe, & Price, 1992).

Thus, most research on caregiving grandparents has highlighted the negative impact that caregiving responsibilities have on these grandparents.

The a priori assumption of most studies on this subject is that caregiving for grandchildren produces stress and that this stress has negative consequences for grandparents' psychological well-being.

Conversely, an opposing perspective views the caregiving grandparent as deriving positive rewards from the experience as well as stress and distress. This idea has been touched upon in a few of the studies of grandparent caregiving (Giarrusso, Feng, Wang, & Silverstein, 1996; Hayslip, Shore, Henderson, & Lambert, 1998). These studies show that caregiving for a grandchild can be rewarding in several ways. First, caregiving for a grandchild can provide a meaningful new role for a grandparent, leading the grandparent to feel more useful and productive (Emick & Hayslip, 1996). Second, it can be intrinsically rewarding to care for a child (Giarrusso et al., 1996). Third, it can make the grandparent feel good that they are able to simultaneously help their child and grandchild (Burton, 1992).

What Factors Are Associated with Experiencing Caregiving as Stressful or Rewarding?

One possible reason that research has tended to focus on negative, as opposed to positive, aspects of caregiving may be because many of the early studies on this topic were based on clinical samples of distressed grandparent caregivers who sought support. However, contemporary studies using more representative samples of grandparents have also focused on the negative consequences of caregiving. For instance, Minkler, Fuller-Thomson, Miller, and Driver (1997) using, the NSFH, found that grandparents who had recently undertaken primary responsibility for the care of a grandchild were more than twice as likely than their noncaregiving counterparts to score above the traditional Center for Epidemologic Depression Scale threshold designating clinical depression.

Although it is vitally important to identify the factors that are associated with caregiving stress among grandparents, it is equally important to understand whether there are aspects of caregiving that are perceived as rewarding. Using a two-pronged strategy, examining both rewards and benefits, this study seeks to identify the demographic, social, and attitudinal factors that predispose grandparents to experience caregiving as more stressful as well as those factors that predispose grandparents to experience caregiving as more rewarding. In addition, we also investigate whether the rewards of caregiving act as a psychic resource that buffers the deleterious effects of stress on psychological health. Finally, we seek to discover whether having a supportive social network buffers the harmful effect of stress on grandparents' psychological well-being.

We complement the existing literature on the sources of stress and reward in grandparent caregiving by including as risk factors, in addition to sociodemographic characteristics, the orientations of grandparents to kinship norms, roles, and behavioral styles. One factor we examine that has not been examined in the current literature is the grandparent's level of normative solidarity and the degree to which it influences whether grandparents perceive caregiving for a grandchild as stressful or rewarding. Normative solidarity—the degree of filial obligation felt toward family members—is defined as one of the key bases of intergenerational solidarity and has been found to be a strong predictor of family interaction and function (Bengtson & Schrader, 1982). Thus, it is hypothesized that grandparents with a stronger sense of normative solidarity will experience caregiving as less stressful and more rewarding than those grandparents with a weaker sense of normative solidarity.

Another factor that may be related to the psychological stresses and rewards of caregiving for a grandchild is the adequacy with which grandparents feel they are performing their role. Identity theory (Stryker, 1987; Stryker & Serpe, 1982) suggests that people who feel that they adequately perform a particular social role are better able to meet the demands of that role, more likely to derive a sense of self-worth from it, and better equipped to manage the stresses associated with role conflict and role overload. Thus, grandparents who feel they are highly effective in performing their grandparent role may derive greater psychological benefits and fewer psychological costs from caregiving than those who feel they perform the role poorly.

A third factor that may influence the degree to which a grandparent perceives caregiving to be stressful and rewarding is the style of grandparenting that is engaged. The literature on grandparenting styles reveals a wide variety of ways that the grandparent role is enacted, ranging from surrogate parenthood to being virtual strangers to grandchildren. In their landmark study, Cherlin and Furstenberg (1988) identified five types of grandparenting styles based on the exchange of services with grandchildren, influence over grandchildren, and frequency contact with grandchildren. They labeled these types of involvement as follows: detached, passive, supportive, authoritative, and influential. More recently, Baydar and Brooks-Gunn (1998) outlined four types of grandmothers: homemaker, young and connected, remote, and frail. We speculate that caregiving grandparents who are "supportive" or "homemaker" types may find caregiving to be rewarding even if they are involuntarily thrust into the role.

Conversely, caregiving grandparents who are "detached" or "remote" in their orientation toward grandchildren may be at greater risk of experiencing the caregiving role as stressful.

Do the Rewards of Caregiving and Social Support Buffer the Effects of Stress on Grandparents' Psychological Well-Being?

A major goal of this chapter is to investigate the balance between the rewards and stresses experienced by grandparents who care for their grandchildren and to determine how this balance is related to grandparents' psychological well-being. Little research has investigated the compensatory interplay between the psychological costs and benefits of grandparent caregiving. We address the unanswered question of whether the rewards of caregiving can offset or minimize the harmful influence of caregiving stress on grandparents' psychological well-being.

Another goal of this chapter is to investigate whether social support moderates the strength with which caregiving stress contributes to psychological distress. In contrast to the previous discussion, there is quite a large body of literature demonstrating the capacity of social support to buffer the negative effect of caregiver stress on psychological well-being, (Pearlin, Lieberman, Menaghan, & Mullan, 1981; Pearlin & Schooler, 1978). Thus, we expect that the availability of social support among caregiving grandparents will attenuate the impact that caregiving stress has on their psychological well-being.

In summary, grandparents who encounter a variety of stressors in raising their grandchildren may still be able to successfully cope with these stresses and strains if they derive a sufficient amount of psychological rewards from caregiving, or if they receive adequate social support from others. If the psychological benefits of caregiving, or the importance of looking to others for support, can be highlighted for caregiving grandparents, they may be able to deal more effectively with the stressful circumstances with which they are presented.

Method

Sample

The present study is based on data from the Study of Intergenerational Linkages II, a 1997 national sample consisting of 2,000 individuals aged 18 and older, including an oversample of 500 grandparents. Respondents were randomly selected though random digit dialing procedures and surveyed over the telephone. A total of 940 self-identified grandparents were obtained by the sampling method. The operational sample consists of 162 respondents who identified themselves as grandparents and who reported ever having had primary responsibility for any of their grandchildren for a period of 6 months or more. About one quarter (24%) of these grandparents are currently caregiving. Among the three quarters who gave care in the past, 70% provided care within the last 10 years.

The average age of the caregiving grandparents is 63 years (SD = 9.56 years). Approximately three fourths of these grandparents are females (74%) and a quarter are males (26%). Thirty-nine percent of the sample reported that they had less than high school education, 37% of the respondents graduated from high school, 24% of the respondents had college or above education. A breakdown of the sample by race reveals that 78% are White, 13% are Black, and 6% belong to other racial groups.

Grandparents were raising between one and five grandchildren (with 104 respondents raising/raised one grandchild, 33 raised two grandchildren, and 25 raised three to five grandchildren). The average age of the youngest grandchild raised by the respondents is 4.20 years (SD = 5.49). The average number of years these grandparents took responsibility for raising their grandchildren is 5.95 years (SD = 5.50). About 50% of these grandparents (N = 79) reported that the parents of the grandchildren they took care of also lived with them.

Measures

Dependent Variables

Stress

Respondents were asked how stressful it was raising a grandchild, and responded to this question on a 5-point scale ranging from "not at all stressful" (1) to "extremely stressful" (5).

Reward

Similarly, respondents were asked how rewarding it was raising a grandchild, and responded on a 5-point scale ranging from "not at all rewarding" (1) to "extremely rewarding" (5).

Self-esteem

Four items were selected from the Rosenberg Self-Esteem Scale including items, such as: "On the whole, I am satisfied with myself," "I certainly feel useless at times," "I take a positive attitude toward myself," and "I wish I could have more respect for myself." Responses to these statements range from "strongly agree" (1) to "strongly disagree" (4). The positive items were reverse coded, and a scale score was computed as the total of the scores on the four items such that a high score indicates a higher level of self-esteem. The reliability of this short-version of the Rosenberg Self-Esteem Scale is .55 based on the current sample.

Independent Variables

Normative Solidarity

Normative solidarity was measured using a three-item scale. The items are "parents whose adult children have financial problems should assist them with housing costs," "parents should save money or property to leave as an inheritance for their children" and "parents should assist adult children with their child care if needed." Responses to these items were coded using a 5-point scale (1 = strongly disagree; 5 = strongly agree). A scale score was computed by averaging the three items, with a high score indicating a high level of normative solidarity. The mean level of normative solidarity for this sample was 3.61 (SD = 1.17).

Perceived Quality of Performance as a Grandparent

Scores of this variable reveal respondents' answers to the question: "How well do you perform your role as a grandparent these days?" on a 5-point scale ranging from poorly (1) to extremely well (5). The mean level of performance was 4.58 (SD = .76).

Degree of Involvement with Grandchildren

Respondents reported whether they shared certain activities (such as doing fun and recreational activities, baby-sitting, attending family gatherings together, attending religious activities or services together, and talking about personal concerns) with any of their grandchildren over the last year. Responses of "yes" were coded as 1 and "no" as 0. The scale score was calculated as the total number of "yes" answers to these items, where a higher score indicates a higher degree of involvement with grandchildren.

Grandparents' mean level of involvement was 4.26 (SD = .93).

Characteristics of Grandparents

Characteristics of the grandparents, such as age, gender, race, and highest achieved educational level, were measured. Because of the highly uneven distribution of race and education, these two variables were dichotomized. A dummy variable was created indicating whether the respondent was White, and another one indicating whether the respondent had any college education.

Characteristics of the Grandchild

The grandparents reported the age of the youngest grandchild being raised.

Social Support

Social support was operationally defined as the number of people in whom the grandparent felt that he or she could confide. The number of confidants grandparents reported ranged from 1 to 25, with a mean of 3.07 (SD = 3.15).

Results

The frequency distribution of the variable measuring "how stressful it is raising a grandchild?" shows that 30% of the grandparents in the current study thought that it was not at all stressful to raise a grandchild and that only 9% of the respondents thought that it was extremely stressful to raise a grandchild (see Figure 5.1). The frequency distribution of the variable measuring "how rewarding it is raising a grandchild" shows that most (81%) of these grandparents thought that it was extremely rewarding to raise a grandchild, and a very few (2%) thought it was not at all rewarding to raise a grandchild (see Figure 5.2).

Ordinary least squares multiple regression analysis was performed to examine which factors predict whether grandparents would perceive raising a grandchild as stressful. The independent variables include sociodemographic variables of age, gender, race, education of grandparents, and age of the youngest grandchild being raised as well as normative solidarity and performance and involvement as grandparents. The results indicate that normative solidarity of the grandparent is negatively related to grandparents' perception of raising a grandchild as a stressful experience, and that involvement as a grandparent is positively related to the stress resulting from grandparenting.

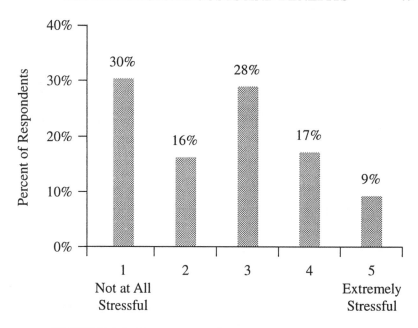

FIGURE 5.1 Extent to which grandparents thought it was stressful to raise a grandchild.

Because of the highly skewed distribution of grandparents' perception of raising grandchildren as a rewarding experience, this variable was dichotomized (1 = extremely rewarding, 0 = less than extremely rewarding). A logistic regression analysis was then conducted to examine the predictors of grandparents' perception of raising grandchildren as rewarding. The independent variables are the same as those included in the multiple regression. The results indicate that education of the grandparent, normative solidarity, age of the youngest grandchild raised, performance as a grandparent, and involvement as grandparent, are significant predictors of grandparents' perception of raising a grandchild as rewarding. Specifically, those grandparents with a college education, who are raising younger grandchildren, have stronger normative solidarity, better self-rated performance as a grandparent, and more involvement as a grandparent are more likely to perceive raising grandchildren as extremely rewarding.

As for the balance between stress and reward related to raising grandchildren, approximately more than half of the respondents (54%) thought that raising a grandchild was both stressful and rewarding, and approximately one fifth of the respondents (19%) thought that raising a grandchild

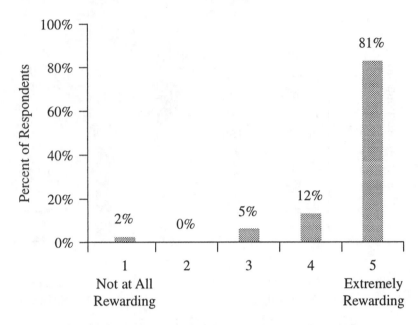

FIGURE 5.2 Extent to which grandparent thought it was rewarding to raise a grandchild.

was mostly stressful. Slightly more than a quarter of the respondents (27%) thought that raising a grandchild was mostly rewarding (see Figure 5.3).

In examining the effects of the balance of stress and rewards of caregiving on grandparents' psychological well-being, we compared mean self-esteem scores of grandparents across three groups: those who perceived raising a grandchild as "mostly rewarding," those who perceived raising a grandchild as "both rewarding and stressful," and those who perceived raising a grandchild as "mostly stressful." (These groups are formed by cross-classifying dummy variables for "stress" and "reward" to form one group that was relatively "concordant" on the measures and two groups that were relatively "discordant" on the measures in opposite directions.) For the dependent measure, self-esteem, to be relevant, we restrict this and the subsequent analysis to those respondents who were raising a grandchild at the time of data collection or had done so within the past 10 years. Results based on ANOVA reveal that the preceding three groups have significantly different means on self-esteem (F=2.988, df=111, p=.055). Figure 5.4 shows the group means. Post hoc comparisons indicate that the "mostly rewarding" grandparents have significantly higher self-esteem than the "mostly stressful" grandparents (*p*=.06).

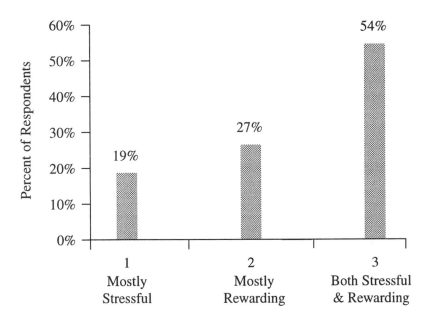

FIGURE 5.3 The balance between stress and reward.

We further examined potential for confidants to moderate the effect of stress on grandparents' self esteem. Using multiple regression, we regressed self-esteem on caregiving stress, the number of confidants, and the interaction between stress and the number of confidants. In brief, it was found that the number of people with whom subjects can share their private feelings and concerns interacts with caregiving stress in predicting grandparents' self-esteem. That is, the stress of caregiving more severely lowers self-esteem among grandparents with fewer confidants.

To test whether grandparents with more confidants are unaffected by the stress of caregiving, the sample was divided into two groups: those with two or less confidants and those with three or more confidants. As expected, the correlation between the stress and self-esteem of grandparents is significant for those respondents who have two or less confidants ($r = -28$, p = .03). The same correlation is not significant for those who have three or more confidants ($r = -18$, not significant). In other words, the number of confidants tends to suppress the harmful effects of caregiving stress on grandparents' self-esteem.

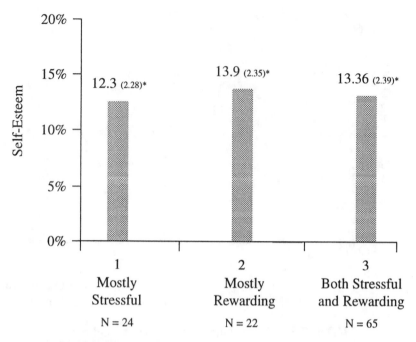

FIGURE 5.4 Mean level of self-esteem by balance between stress and reward.

Discussion

Full-time caregiving of grandchildren by grandparents is a growing national phenomenon. Although social scientists and policy makers are beginning to address the issues related to grandparent caregiving, the majority of research to date has been based on small, nonrepresentative samples. Only recently has research been done with nationally representative samples of grandparents in the United States (Baydar & Brooks-Gunn, 1998; Fuller-Thomson, Minkler, & Driver, 1997; Minkler, Fuller-Thomson, Miller, & Driver, 1997). The purpose of this chapter was to present findings from a recent (1997–98) nationally representative sample of grandparents to assess the psychological costs and benefits they may experience as a result of raising their grandchildren.

Surprisingly, only one quarter of our sample of grandparents found caregiving for grandchildren to be either "very" or "extremely" stressful. The rest of the grandparents found it to be little to somewhat stressful, with almost one third finding it to be "not at all" stressful. This lower than expected level of stress may be attributable to the greater diversity of grandparents available in a nationally representative sample compared with those recruited in opportunity or specialized samples of grandparents raising grandchildren. Previous studies using small, nonrepresentative samples have examined grandparent caregiving that generally resulted from tragic circumstances, such as drug abuse, incarceration, child neglect, and violent death of the parent generation. These studies underscored the stressful nature under which caregiving for grandchildren was assumed. These grandparents were often of low income and from neighborhoods that were under siege from drug dealing and violence. The stress of caregiving for grandchildren under these circumstances would likely be much greater than under circumstances that may have been brought about due to other less tragic circumstances and assumed by grandparents who were less economically deprived.

Another possibility is that when grandparents are asked directly, in a structured interview, how stressful it is for them to provide full-time care for grandchildren, they may feel the need to provide a socially acceptable answer. They may downplay the stress with which they deal to present their adult children (and by implication themselves) in a more favorable light to the researcher. Alternatively, grandparents may minimize or deny the stress that they experienced not just because they want to give a socially acceptable answer but because may not be able to admit, even to themselves, just how much of a toll caregiving for grandchildren is taking on them. Other researchers using qualitative methods indicated that grandparents often minimize the psychological and physical costs of caregiving to themselves because they were all that their grandchildren have left (Burton, 1992). Admitting that they are suffering opens up the possibility that they may have to give their grandchildren up to a dysfunctional parent or to social services.

When looking at the factors associated with experiencing caregiving for grandchildren as stressful, we see that there are no differences by the demographic characteristics of the grandparents: grandparents of all ages, genders, races, and levels of education report equal levels of stress. Thus, older grandparents did not seem to perceive caregiving for grandchildren to be any more stressful than did their younger caregiving counterparts. Although income is likely an important determinant of caregiving stress, this variable was not available in this data set for the time that caregiving occurred. However, education, which is correlated with income, was not found to make a difference. Nevertheless, future research should examine the influence of household income on whether caregiving for grandchildren is experienced as stressful.

Higher levels of normative solidarity were negatively associated with the perception of caregiving for grandchildren as stressful. Grandparents who had strong feelings of family obligation reported experiencing significantly less stress than grandparents who had weaker feelings of family obligation. Previous research has attributed the tendency of minority racial/ethnic groups (such as African Americans and Hispanics) to willingly take primary responsibility for the care of their grandchildren to cultural factors. However, this research suggests that feelings of stress may be more determined by general values toward family responsibility than by cultural-group membership per se. Thus, normative solidarity may be more important in the reduction of stress than racial/ethnic subcultures.

Another factor that was negatively associated with psychological stress was grandparents' general level of involvement with their grandchildren. Those grandparents who reported high levels of involvement also reported significantly lower levels of stress. One reason why involvement with grandchildren may lessen the experience of stress may be because it indicates a "good fit" between the desired role that the grandparent wants to play and the role they are called on to play. This suggests that if grandparents are forced to assume a different type of involvement than they desire (as a result of an action on the part of the adult child), they may find the caregiving of grandchildren to be more stressful. For example, if a grandparent, who would prefer to remain "detached" is involuntarily called on to assume primary responsibility for a grandchild, caregiving is likely to be stressful. Alternatively, when the types of involvement with the grandchild being raised include more volitional activities (e.g., fun and recreation), then the stresses of caregiving may be mitigated.

Another reason why increased general involvement with grandchildren may lead to lower levels of stress is because it may indicate the degree to which the grandparent is integrated within a larger social network—of church members, extended family, and community at large. This increased integration may help lessen grandparents' feelings of isolation that are often cited as a problem for caregiving grandparents (Emick & Hayslip, 1996).

Interestingly, the age of the youngest grandchild being raised did not influence the extent to which the grandparent caregiver experienced stress. Thus, raising a teenager was perceived as no more stressful by grandparent caregivers than raising a toddler. Unfortunately, this data set did not contain information on the gender or on other important characteristics of the grandchild, such as behavioral problems. Previous research has shown that raising grandsons and grandchildren with behavioral problems is more stressful than raising granddaughters and those without behavioral problems.

Turning to the degree to which the caregiving of grandchildren by grandparents was viewed as rewarding, the current study found that four of five grandparents described their caregiving responsibility to be "extremely rewarding," with only 2% describing it as "not at all rewarding." This finding is surprising and appears to be at odds with the dire tone of other research on caregiving grandparents. However, ours was the first nationally representative sample of grandparents that directly asked about the rewarding nature of their caregiving responsibilities. Other research has only indirectly touched on the psychological benefits that grandparents derive from their charges. Again, other studies have been largely based on caregivers who have been thrust into this responsibility because of tragic circumstances beyond their control. In a nationally representative sample, many of the caregivers may be facing very different sets of circumstances in providing care to their grandchildren.

Regarding the factors that were associated with experiencing caregiving as rewarding, no differences were found in the demographic characteristics of the grandparents. That is, grandparents of all ages, genders, and races found caregiving to be equally rewarding. However, education was positively associated with finding the experience of caregiving to be rewarding. Compared with grandparents with less than a college education, grandparents with at least some college found caregiving to be more rewarding. The reason why education influences the perception of reward may have important policy implications. More highly educated grandparents may find the caregiving experience to be more rewarding because they tend to be more knowledgeable about childhood development and thus are better able to choose mutually rewarding activities and better communicate with the child. Programs that educate grandparents on childhood development and other related information requisite to caring for a child may help to make their task more interesting and, therefore, more rewarding.

As was found with stress, normative solidarity was significantly related to the experience of psychological rewards for grandparents. The stronger a grandparents' feeling of family obligation, the more rewarding they found caregiving to be. Perhaps those who have high normative solidarity are more likely than those with low normative solidarity to perceive caregiving as an intrinsic part of their family role. Future research in this area should examine the reasons grandparents assumed primary responsibility for the care of their grandchild. For instance, if the reasons for caregiving resulted from circumstances beyond the control of the adult child, greater normative solidarity may result in the grandparent perceiving their role as more rewarding. However, it is unclear whether normative solidarity would serve the same function if the grandparent had to assume the caregiving role as a result of some dysfunction of the adult child, such as drug addiction or incarceration. In any event, it is likely that normative solidarity interacts with the reason for caregiving in its effect on the perception of rewards.

Although performance as a grandparent was not associated with the perception of caregiving as stressful, it was associated with the perception of caregiving as rewarding. Grandparents who felt they were performing their role well were more likely to find caregiving to be rewarding. In other words, a caregiving job felt to be well done may be it's own reward. Level of involvement as a grandparent was also positively associated with the perception of caregiving as rewarding. The more involved grandparent found caregiving to be more rewarding. Thus, the more fully grandparents embraced their role the more they derived psychological rewards from their caregiving.

Although age of the youngest child being cared for was not significantly related to the level of stress grandparents experienced, it was significantly related to the level of reward. Grandparents who were caring for younger grandchildren found the experience to be more rewarding than those who were caring for older grandchildren. This is consistent with other research that shows that although younger grandchildren may involve more physical labor, they also provide greater satisfaction. Younger children are more appreciative, loving, and less disrespectful and rebellious than are older children. Also, younger children have had less time to be negatively influenced by a dysfunctional parent.

Some grandparents in our sample had multiple grandchildren in their charge. This data set only allows us to identify the age of the youngest child and not the age of other grandchildren who may also be receiving care. Future research should address the psychological costs and benefits of each grandchild being cared for. One child may make caregiving rewarding, whereas others may make it stressful. This would be especially true if one of the grandchildren had special needs, as a result of, for example, being born drug addicted.

When considering the psychological costs and benefits of grandparent caregiving simultaneously, we found that more than half (54%) of the grandparents found the experience to be a "mixed bag" (i.e., they found it both stressful and rewarding). Twenty-seven percent found caregiving to be mostly rewarding, and only 19% found it to be mostly stressful. The important implication of this finding is that stress and reward in the caregiving experience are not mutually exclusive: Grandparents can find caregiving rewarding, even if they also find it stressful.

Another issue we addressed in this chapter is how the balance between stresses and rewards relates to grandparents' psychological well-being. Put another way, we ask whether rewards offset the harmful effects of stress on grandparents' psychological well-being. Our findings reveal that grandparents who found caregiving to be mostly rewarding had significantly higher levels of self-esteem than those who found it mostly stressful. However, those who found it both stressful *and* rewarding also had higher levels of self-esteem than those who found it mostly stressful, suggesting that the rewards of caregiving may overcome the power of stress to lower self-esteem; but the post hoc comparison fell short of statistical significance.

Another important question we addressed was whether social support buffers the effect of stress on grandparents' psychological well-being. Consistent with a large body of literature on social support, the current study found that social support buffers the negative effect of stress on grandparents' self-esteem. Grandparents who had more individuals in whom they could confide were better protected from the negative psychological effects of stress when compared with grandparents who had fewer confidants.

This finding has important implications for existing programs of support for grandparent caregivers. The current research suggests that support groups serve a needed function for grandparent caregivers. Even without providing economic resources to grandparents, programs that provide grandparents with social support through informal groups or through therapist-headed psychotherapy groups help to buffer the effect of stress on grandparents' self-esteem. Also, it suggests that when grandparents seek counseling for their grandchildren who have behavioral or emotional disorders, they should be encouraged to participate in some form of group counseling themselves.

A limitation of this study is that it is not longitudinal. Consequently, it is difficult to say anything about the causal sequencing of the factors considered in our analysis. An alternative explanation of the findings is that grandparents who have a high level of psychological well-being before assuming primary responsibility for the care of a grandchild are more capable of dealing with the stresses that caregiving may bring. Thus, those who are psychologically healthy may have better coping skills that help them lower their stress levels directly or allow them to appraise the caregiving experience as less stressful and more rewarding.

In conclusion, our findings point to some intriguing avenues for future research among grandparents who raise their grandchildren. Caregiving activities of grandparents are similar to most supportive family interactions in that they also can be characterized by a certain degree of ambivalence that lies at the intersection of coercion and choice (Luescher & Pillemer, 1998). Attention to only the stressful and obligatory nature of grandparent caregiving may mask the full social and psychological range of the experience and deny the underlying value and meaning that grandparents often attribute to this important societal role. We suggest that future studies more completely represent the complex, multidimensional, and often equivocal nature of caregiving when grandparents take on this unexpected responsibility.

References

Barnhill, S. (1996, Spring). Three generations at risk: Imprisoned women, their children, and grandmother caregivers. *Generations*, 39–40.

Baydar, N., & Brooks-Gunn, J. (1998). Profiles of grandmothers who help care for their grandchildren in the United States. *Family Relations, 47*, 385–393.

Bengtson, V. L., & Schrader, S. S. (1982). Parent-child relations. In D. Mangen & W. Peterson (Eds.), *Handbook of research instruments in social gerontology* (Vol. 2, pp. 115–185). Minneapolis: University of Minnesota Press.

Burton, L. M. (1992). Black grandparents rearing children of drug-addicted parents: Stressors, outcomes, and social service needs. *The Gerontologist, 32*, 744–751.

Chalfie, D. (1994) *Going it alone: A closer look at grandparents parenting grandchildren.* A Publication of the Women's Initiative. Washington, DC: American Association of Retired Persons.

Cherlin, A., & Furstenberg (1986). *The new American grandparent: A place in the family, a life apart.* New York: Basic Books.

Dressel, P. L., & Barnhill, S. K. (1994). Reframing gerontological thought and practice: The case of grandmothers with daughters in prison. *The Gerontologist, 34*, 685–691.

Emick, M. A., & Hayslip, B. (1996). Custodial grandparenting: New roles for middle-aged and older adults. *International Journal of Aging and Human Development, 43*, 135–154.

Fuller-Thomson, E., Minkler, M., & Driver D. (1997). A profile of grandparents raising grandchildren in the United States. *The Gerontologist, 37*, 406–411.

Giarrusso, R., Feng, D., Wang, Q., & Silverstein, M. (1996). Parenting and co-parenting of grandchildren: Effects on grandparents' well-being and family solidarity. *International Journal of Sociology and Social Policy, 16*, 124–154.

Goldberg-Glen, R., Sands, R. G., Cole, R. D., & Cristofalo, C. (1998). Multi-generational patterns and internal structures in families in which grandparents raise grandchildren. *Families in Society: The Journal of Contemporary Human Services, 79*, 477–489.

Hayslip, B., Shore, R. J., Henderson, C. E., & Lambert, P. L. (1998). Custodial grandparenting and the impact of grandchildren with problems on role satisfaction and role meaning. *Journal of Gerontology, 53B* (Suppl.), S164–S173.

Hirshorn, B. A., (1998). Grandparents as caregivers. In M. E. Szinovacz (Ed.), *Handbook on grandparenthood* (pp. 200–214). Westport, CT: Greenwood Press.

Jendrek, M. P. (1993). Grandparents who parent their grandchildren: Effects on lifestyle. *Journal of Marriage and the Family, 55*, 609–621.

Jendrek, M. P. (1994). Grandparents who parent their grandchildren: Circumstances and decisions. *The Gerontologist, 34*, 206–216.

Joslin, D., & Brouard, A. (1995). The prevalence of grandmothers as primary caregivers in a poor pediatric population. Journal of Community Health, 20, 383–401.

King, V., & Elder, G. H. (1998). Perceived self-efficacy and grandparenting. *Journal of Gerontology, 53B* (Suppl.), S249–S257.

Kivnick, H. Q. (1982). Grandparenthood: An overview of the meaning and mental health. *The Gerontologist, 22*, 59–66.

Luescher, K., & Pillemer, K. (1998). Intergenerational ambivalence: A new approach to the study of parent-child relations in later life. *Journal of Marriage and the Family, 60*, 413–425.

Minkler, M., Driver, D., Roe, K. M., & Bedeian, K. (1993). Community interventions to support grandparent caregivers. *The Gerontologist, 33*, 807–811.

Minkler, M., Fuller-Thomson, E., Miller, D., & Diver, D. (1997). Depression in grandparents raising grandchildren. *Archives of Family Medicine, 6*, 445–452.

Minkler, M., Roe, K. M., & Price, M. (1992). The physical and emotional health of the grandmothers raising grandchildren in the crack cocaine epidemic. *The Gerontologist, 32*, 752–761.

Minkler, M. & Roe, K. M. (1993). *Grandmothers as caregivers: Raising children of the crack cocaine epidemic.* Newbury Park, CA: Sage.

Minkler, M. & Roe, K. M. (1996, spring). Grandparents as surrogate parents. *Generations*, 34–38.

Pearlin, L. I., Lieberman, M. A., Menaghan, E. G., & Mullan, J. T. (1981). The stress process. *Journal of Health and Social Behavior, 22*, 337–356.

Pearlin, L. I., & Schooler, C. (1978). The structure of coping. *Journal of Health and Social Behavior, 19*, 2–21.

Pearson, J. L., Hunter, A. G., Cook, J. M., Ialongo, N. S., & Kellam, S. G. (1997). Grandmother involvement in child caregiving in an urban community. *The Gerontologist, 37*, 650–657.

Roe, K. M., Minkler, M., & Barwell, R. S. (1994). The assupmtion of caregiving:

Grandmothers raising the children of the crack cocaine epidemic. *Qualitative Health Research, 4,* 281–303.

Roe, K. M., Minkler, M., & Saunders, F. F. (1995). Combining research, advocacy and education: The methods of the grandparent caregiver study. *Health Education Quarterly, 22,* 458–474.

Roe, K. M., Minkler, M., Saunders, F., & Thomson, G. E. (1996). Health of grandmothers raising children of the crack cocaine epidemic. *Medical Care, 34,* 1072–1084.

Shore, R. J., & Hayslip, B. (1994). Custodial grandparenting implications for the children's development. In A. E. Gottfried & A. W. Gottfried's (Eds.), *Redefining families: Implications for children's development* (pp. 171–218). New York: Plenum.

Strawbridge, W. J., Wallhagen, M. I., Shema, S. J., & Kaplan, G. A. (1997). New burdens or more of the same? Comparing grandparent, spouse, and adult-child caregivers. *The Gerontologist, 37,* 505–510.

Stryker, S. (1987). Identity theory: Developments and extensions. In K. Yardley & T. Honess (Eds.), *Self and identity: Psychological perspectives* (pp. 83–103). New York: Wiley.

Stryker, S., & Serpe, R. T. (1982). Commitment. Identity salience, and role behavior. In W. Ickes & E. S. Knowles (Eds.), *Personality, roles, and social behavior* (pp. 199–218). New York: Springer-Verlag.

Szinovacz, M. E. (1998). Grandparents today: A demographic profile. *The Gerontologist, 38,* 37–52.

U. S. Bureau of the Census. (1993). Marital status and living arrangements: March 1993. *Current Population Reports* (Series P-20, No. 478). Washington, DC: Government Printing Office.

Chapter 6

Risks of Caregiving: Abuse Within the Relationship

Patricia Brownell and Jacquelin Berman

Mrs. M., age 65, began caring for her three grandchildren, ages 5, 7, and 15, 1 year ago when their mother, Mrs. M.'s daughter, died of AIDS, and their father—an IV drug user—abused and neglected them. The two youngest grandchildren are fearful and developmentally delayed—a consequence of the abuse, neglect, and trauma of their mother's illness and death, according to their foster care agency's social worker. Jonathan, the oldest, is aggressive and angry. He takes money from his grandmother's purse without her permission, verbally threatens her when she attempts to discipline him, pushed her on several occasions, and once hit her on her shoulder, causing bruising. Mrs. M. is having difficulty sleeping at night and is experiencing heart palpitations and high blood pressure.

A recent retiree, Mrs. M. has a strong formal support network. She visits a clinic regularly and keeps appointments with the foster care and public child welfare agency caseworkers, the youngest children's therapist, and the high school guidance counselor. Her physician expressed concern about her blood pressure, especially in view of a family history of high blood pressure and congestive heart failure. He cautions her about her diet, and recently prescribed a new medication for high blood pressure and a mild sedative to help her sleep at night. He said her symptoms were common in people of her age, implying they were a normal part of the aging process.

The grandchildren's foster care agency case worker explained to her that the behavior of all the children reflected the impact of a developmental crisis that was affecting them differentially because of their ages. She suggested that Mrs. M. be understanding and supportive of the children's behavior as they worked through the trauma they were experiencing. The public child welfare agency caseworker assigned to the grandchildren expressed concern about the behavior of the oldest grandchild, Jonathan. She said that if this continued, she would have no choice but to remove all the children and put them in the custody of a traditional foster family with skills to manage the children more appropriately. The high school guidance counselor stated that Jonathan's behavior was not unusual, given his early family history, and recommended psychotherapy. Jonathan, however, rejected this option, saying there was nothing wrong with him.

Mrs. M. was left feeling guilty, confused, and helpless. She also felt that she would have to try harder to put her concerns out of her mind so that she could keep the grandchildren she loved with her and not abandon them to strangers. In the back of her mind, she felt that perhaps she was responsible for their problems as she had somehow been responsible for her daughter's problems, which represented a source of shame and embarrassment for her. She could not allow herself to grieve for or harbor anger toward her daughter or her son-in-law. If this meant concealing the pain her oldest grandchild inflicted on her, it was a small price to pay for keeping her daughter's family together.

What Mrs. M. is experiencing is typical of an older caregiver who— through circumstances not of her making or choosing—has entered the child-centered world of foster care. Grandparents raising grandchildren face heightened health and mental health risks and professionals may not recognize these risks as related to the burden of caring for abandoned children. The concerns grandparents in these circumstances are valid.

The term elder abuse often conjures up images of a frail, dependent, defenseless elderly victim of family abuse. Ironically, it is often linked to the popular intergenerational transmission of abuse theory (Wallace, 1998), suggesting—inadvertently, perhaps—that the now frail victim was once abusive to family members. In fact, research has found that elder abuse victims are often caregivers of adult children or grandchildren who are dependent on them for support (Pillemer & Finkelhor, 1988). The theory of intergenerational cycle of violence has been found to explain child abuse more effectively than elder abuse (Korbin, Anetzberger, & Austin, 1997).

The difficulties of raising a grandchild for both the grandparent and the grandchild have been discussed throughout this book. At the same time, the literature mentions abuse and mistreatment of grandparents by grandchildren only anecdotally (Shapiro, 1997) or as reported in analyses of crime report data on violence between people who have intimate relations (Greenfield, 1998). Grandparent abuse has also surfaced incidentally in surveys of elder abuse in the community (Brownell, 1994; Podneiks, 1992a, 1992b). However, to date there has been no effort to frame this as a social problem of concern to researchers, practitioners or policy makers, or any attempt to systematically collect data on incidence, prevalence, and risk factors related to this issue.

For most grandparents and grandchildren, the new relationship presents an opportunity to build a new family on the secure foundation of love, trust and familiarity. However, it can also mask physical and psychological scars, deep disappointment and anger at the perceived failures of missing parents and children, and frustrated hope that the missing parents/ children in the family will reappear, intact, to heal and make whole the ruptured family constellation (Jackson, 1998). The circumstances surrounding the placement of children with grandparents are often considered socially unacceptable and may be a source of shame and secrecy for family members. This shame can inhibit the use of needed services and supports.

Family conflict in circumstances described earlier can escalate into what gerontologists define as elder abuse, particularly if the child is an adolescent. The results may be actions that are understandable in the context of the child's life history but may be a source of pain, fear, and even danger to the grandparent caregiver. Although a child welfare worker may define a child's aggressive or oppositional behavior as representing the acting out of unresolved emotional conflicts or signs of mental illness, a gerontologist may define the same behavior, if directed toward a grandparent, as elder mistreatment or abuse.

Scope of the Problem

Estimates of the percentage of older Americans mistreated by family members range from 4% (Pillemer & Finkelhor, 1988) to 12% (U.S. House of Representatives, 1990). Although these estimates do not address the issue of grandparent abuse in these households, they raise questions about the safety and quality of life of older adults providing care to grandchildren.

Large urban areas such as New York City illustrate the magnitude of the kinship foster care program in some localities. Approximately 15,000 children are in kinship foster homes in New York City (Child Welfare Watch, 1997). Approximately 41.6% of these are headed by a maternal grandmother, and another 11.4% are headed by a paternal grandmother (Bacon, 1997). However, service systems to address the needs of abused and neglected children are not integrated with those intended to support and protect older people suffering from familial mistreatment and stress.

Although some studies of the incidence and prevalence of elder abuse have cited adolescents, including grandchildren, among identified abusers (Podnieks, 1992a, 1992b; Prichard, 1992), none to date have focused on abuse of grandparents by grandchildren. In one study of 319 family crimes against the elderly reported to the New York Police Department, four complaints of grandparent abuse were identified. Of the four, two involved abuse by an adult child of a grandparent caring for the adult child's offspring, one involved a grandchild of undetermined age, and only one involved an adolescent grandchild who had injured a grandparent Although seeking money for drugs (Brownell, 1994).

Most recently, the New York City Department for the Aging's Crime Victim's Unit conducted a telephone survey of older adults reporting family abuse or crimes to the unit in 1998. A questionnaire used to compile information on the crime reports included a question on the presence of a minor in the household and the role of that minor in the reported abuse (Berman, 1998). Approximately 9% of the cases included minors living in the household: 4% included abusive minors. Although the total number of reported cases was small, the abusive minors differed from the nonabusive minors in several ways. The abusive minors were older (average age was 16) and more likely to be black. More of the abusive minors lived exclusively with the grandparents than the nonabusive who lived with both parents and grandparents, Reported forms of grandparent abuse included financial abuse, physical abuse, and psychological abuse. Reported truancy of the abusive minors was also high.

Representative scenarios of the reported abusive minor cases include the following

• Ms. W., a 60-year-old grandmother, called to report that her 17-year-old grandson is threatening to burn down the building where she lives and constantly intimidates her. Mrs. W. has custody of her grandson because her daughter has AIDS and cannot care for him.

- Ms. T., a 76-year-old grandmother, reported that her 16-year-old grandson breaks dishes, has thrown a chair at her, and is taking possessions from her without her permission. She reported feeling threatened by him.
- Ms. J., a 75-year-old grandmother, reported having bruises all over her arms from her 16-year-old granddaughter. The grandmother stated that she believed her granddaughter's behavior was "moodiness," not abuse.

Although no study has examined elder abuse in kinship foster care settings, studies have suggested that children—particularly adolescents—enter both traditional and kinship foster care at increased risk of behavior problems compared with the general population (Dubowitz, Zuravin, Starr, Feigelman, & Harrington, 1993). A study using multiple informants found that both caregivers and adolescents concurred that adolescents in care, particularly boys, exhibit more overall externalizing of problems (Starr, Dubowitz, Harrington, & Feigelman, 1999).

Very little is known about abuse of grandparents by grandchildren living in the same household. Apart from the small convenience sample examined by Berman (1998), no systematic studies have been done on the incidence and prevalence of this issue. Available information is case specific and anecdotal. The reporting process is itself complicated by the fact that grandparents may identify grandchildren's verbal expressions as abusive when in fact they may be normative for that child and not intended to intimidate or humiliate. Conversely, grandparents may also deny the existence of abuse even in the face of strong evidence to the contrary.

Theories That May Explain Abuse

In the 1970s, when abuse of the elderly by family members was first identified as a significant social problem, it was framed as "granny bashing" to suggest the ill treatment of frail, dependent older adults by caregiving family members (McCreadie, 1993). This profile of the abused elder and the vicious or overwhelmed caregiver persisted into the 1980's but gradually gave way to a new profile of the self-supporting and often vigorous older adult who is the caregiver of an impaired adult relative, usually an adult child (Pillemer & Finkelhor, 1988; Podnieks, 1992a).

Grandparents who care for grandchildren in the kinship foster care program, or even informally, are usually strong, vital, and healthy older adults. However, as more recent studies of elder abuse have demonstrated

(Brownell, 1994; Pillemer & Finkelhor, 1988), the empowered older parent and grandparent can be at risk of abuse by dependent relatives who seek to intimidate, exploit, and make unreasonable demands on them.

The categories of behavior as directed toward an older family member (age 60 years or older is often used because it defines "older adult" according to the Older Americans Act) that are defined as elder abuse or mistreatment include *psychological*: threatening, yelling, name calling, menacing, harming animals belonging to the older person; *financial or material abuse*: stealing money, taking possessions without the permission of the older adult; damaging or destroying property or possessions; and *physical*: pushing, shoving, hitting, and assaulting with a weapon (Wolf & Pillemer, 1984).

Symptoms of children and adolescents who have experienced abuse, neglect, or abandonment may include behaviors that can be classified as conduct disorder or oppositional defiant disorder according to the *Diagnostic and Statistical Manual of Mental Disorders* (ed. 4) (Morrison, 1995). Diagnostic criteria for conduct disorder include: has stolen without confrontation of a victim on more than one occasion; has deliberately engaged in fire setting; has deliberately destroyed others' property; has been physically cruel to animals; often initiates physical fights; has stolen with confrontation of a victim; and has been physically cruel to people. The definition of conduct disorder in adolescents is almost a mirror of the definition of elder abuse.

Children and adolescents who are in transition from an abusive or neglectful household situation to a foster care situation with a grandparent may exhibit symptoms of adjustment disorders. Diagnostic criteria can include "within three months of a stressor, and in response to it, . . . materially impaired job, academic, or social functioning" (Morrison, 1995, p. 455). Grandparents anxious to instill discipline and order into their grandchildren's lives may misunderstand these symptoms. As a result, they may precipitate dissention within the household if the grandparents misinterpret the behaviors as disobedient and willful rather than reactive to prior trauma (Holman, 1998).

Neutralization theory (Quinn & Tomita, 1997); abuser pathology (Pillemer & Finkelhor, 1988); and intergenerational transmission of violence (Breckman & Abelman) have been proposed to explain abuse of older adults by family members. Luepnitz (1998), uses a psychoanalytic framework to explain interfamilial abuse, including that of grandchild against grandparent. Peer group influence has also been used to explain elder abuse (Prichard, 1993).

Quinn and Tomita (1997) state that neutralization theory can explain elder abuse by adult children and grandchildren. This theory "attempts to explain acts of denial and rationalization" (p. 201) and was developed in the 1950s by Sykes and Matza (1978) to explain juvenile delinquency. It suggests that adolescents who commit delinquent acts understand that these acts are wrong and feel shame and guilt over them. However, they rationalize or neutralize these feelings using five techniques: denying responsibility, denying serious injury as a result of their actions, denying value of the victim to the larger society, blaming the victim, and appealing to a higher loyalty (the peer group over the family).

The abuser pathology theory is based on the assumption that abusers suffer impairments that may predispose them to violence or mistreatment of older family members (Pillemer & Finkelhor, 1988). Mental illness, substance abuse, and other emotional and neurological impairments may precipitate irrational or abusive behavior that is unrelated to any provocation on the part of the victim. Depression has been recognized as a more serious problem among young people that previously realized. Although adolescence is usually a time of rapid cognitive development, some clinicians suggest that the ability to detach from and observe one's own thinking may be poorly developed in depressed adolescents (Temple, 1997).

Luepnitz (1998) proposes the hypothesis that violence is a form of mourning: children—especially adolescents—may lash out at family members who are present out of overwhelming and unresolved feelings of loss and rejection by a missing family member. The issue of loss is significant as both grandparent and grandchild have suffered enormous loss and each generation may be left with self-doubts. Grandparents have lost children with whom they have felt great pride and hopes. They have lost both their ideal and their real child, especially if that adult child has died. For the adolescent, they have lost both their ideal and real parent (Luepnitz, 1998).

Implications for the future are significant as both grandparents and grandchildren fear that the grandchild will turn out like the parent. The question on the minds of both generations is: Will history repeat itself? The result may be that the grandparent is hypervigilent and controlling, watching every move of the grandchild. However, it is normal that when adolescents feel they are being clamped down on, they rebel. The adolescent may also share the grandparent's fears, as parents are children's first role models (Holman, 1998).

Services and Interventions for Abuse in Kinship Families

The rapid expansion of kinship foster care as a formal caregiving arrangement within public child welfare in the United States has forced changes in both public and voluntary sector child welfare service sectors (Jackson, 1999; Wilson, 1999). In response, this has stimulated the need for training and procedural changes in public child welfare agencies (Gleeson, 1999; Scannapieco, 1999).

The value of kinship care has been recognized as achieving important objectives: children in kinship care are reunited with their parents more often than children in traditional care; children in kinship care move less than those in nonkinship care; and children who leave the system from kinship placement are less likely to return to foster care than those in traditional care (Courtney, White, & Kleiman, 1997).

At the same time, studies have shown that kinship foster families are less likely to be offered services than traditional foster families (Scannapieco, 1999). This is despite the fact that forming a reconstituted family is often perceived as traumatic for both grandchild and grandparent. Aging, law enforcement, child welfare, mental health and substance abuse, and adult protective services (APS) systems provide services that may assist kinship family members when grandparent abuse occurs.

Programs and Services Available Through the Aging Service Provider Network

Although self-help groups for older adults have expanded over the past few years, few address the issue of elder abuse, much less grandparent abuse. An exception is the Neighborhood Self-Help by Older Persons Project in the Bronx, New York (Laureano, 1998). The only bilingual self-help support group on elder abuse, it is supported by funding that requires competitive bidding on an annual basis.

Another elder abuse self-help model, the Elderly Abuse Support Project in Rhode Island, recruits, trains, and places volunteers with victims of elder abuse (Filinson, 1993). Although this program is designed for the impaired elderly, and not older caregivers, findings of an evaluation suggest that volunteer advocate programs, in contrast to professionally managed programs, can lead to greater achievement of goals.

Title VII of the Older American Act mandates state and area aging agencies to address senior crime victims' issues and coordinate services with local law enforcement agencies. In New York City, the senior crime victims unit at the local area aging agency (Department for the Aging) counsels older crime and abuse victims and also trains police officers on elder abuse and crimes against the elderly. Opportunities to discuss and address sensitive issues like abuse of grandparents by grandchildren should be provided by professional service providers. Programs should also be offered in common languages, such as Spanish, spoken within the community.

Services and Interventions Available
Through Law Enforcement

Although often used as a last resort, the police are another resource for domestic violence including elder abuse (Brownell, 1998; Heisler, 1991). They are available 24 hours a day and respond to calls after most social service agencies have closed. The community policing initiative provides a neighborhood presence for law enforcement intended to mediate and support community problem solving (Mastrofski, Parks, & Worden, 1998). However, police may not have knowledge of services and other resources that may be needed by a family where grandparent abuse is a factor. One of the most frequent complaints police receive from grandparents caring for grandchildren is "my grandchild does not respect me." These calls often come on Friday nights, when the grandchild wants to go out with friends against the wishes of the grandparent. Grandparents see police as enforcers of their authority. Instead, the police responding to the call can use their authority to diffuse the situation.

Services Available Through the
Child Welfare System

Programs and interventions obtained through the child welfare system that can provide support and services for abused grandparents and abusive adolescent grandchildren who wish to remain together in the community are virtually nonexistent. Remedies remain primarily those geared to the removal of the adolescent from the home, generally to foster boarding homes and other congregate facilities, or some form of detention (Lucas, 1998).

All adolescents search for a sense of identity and acceptance by their peers, so peer pressure can result in defiant behavior such as staying out all night, skipping school and refusing to obey a grandparent's household rules. This can also result in stealing from, talking back to, and hitting grandparents. When grandparents are also the foster parents of the grandchildren in question, they may be reluctant to disclose this behavior and reach out for services in fear of having the children removed from their custody.

Preventive services, although not specifically designed for grandparents, include parent training and family mediation services. Public child welfare agencies often have staff who serve as ombudsman or advocates for both biological and foster care parents. Homemaking services may be available to assist grandparents in caring for grandchildren when the care demands of the children exceed the physical resources of the grandparent.

Some of the more extreme remedies for a grandparent when defiant behavior of a grandchild continues or escalates include persons in need of supervision, petitions through the family court, placement in diagnostic treatment centers for psychiatric evaluation, and voluntary placements through the local child welfare agency. However, once a voluntary placement is made and the grandchild removed from the grandparent's home, this can only be reversed if the child welfare agency decides it is in the best interest of the child. As a result, this step is best not taken without careful planning and thought to the possible consequences.

Across the country, particularly in urban areas, there is an effort to restructure services funded by government and other sources to children and their families, so that community-based coordination among different service providers and sectors can be more effective (Shorr, 1997). If services are neighborhood based, it may be easier to achieve the level of coordination needed for families that include grandparents and grandchildren to remain safely together in the community.

Services Available Through the Mental Health and Substance Abuse Service Systems

Children and adolescents who act out in an impulsive or destructive manner need to be evaluated for serious neurological or biochemical disorders. According to Wexler (1998), approximately half of all children who are undiagnosed and untreated for attention deficit and hyperactivity disorder are diagnosed with conduct disorder in adolescence. About a quarter are eventually diagnosed with antisocial personality disorder in adulthood. Although it may be understandable that children removed from their homes under traumatic circumstances experience emotional disturbances, these could also be symptomatic of more serious underlying disorders (Wexler, 1998). Mental health services for adolescents with signs of serious mental illness include in-patient, residential treatment, partial hospitalization, and clinic programs.

Substance abuse has been highly correlated with domestic violence. Abuse of grandparents by adolescents may be symptomatic of alcohol or drug use and abuse. The substance abuse may be reflective of peer pressure or attempts on the part of the adolescent to self-medicate feelings of anger or depression (Fleisch, 1996).

Treatment for adolescents with both substance abuse and emotional problems include school-based intervention programs, clinic treatment, adolescent female treatment programs, day treatment and partial day treatment, therapeutic foster care and therapeutic communities. Studies of long-term treatment effectiveness stress the importance of a holistic approach that involves the entire family (Fleisch, 1996).

Services Available Through Adult Protective Services

Adult Protective Services (APS) are a potential resource for grandparents who are abused by grandchildren. However, to be eligible for services through APS, the grandparent must have a physical or mental impairment that limits their ability to protect themselves from harm and must be in imminent danger or risk. All 50 states have adult protective service agencies operating locally under state law and regulation.

APS units may not accept referrals if a child is abusing a caregiving grandparent, unless the grandparent being abused is cognitively or physically impaired and, as a consequence, is incapable of self-protection or exercising informed judgement. Exceptions may include APS programs in states with mandatory reporting of elder abuse, where APS workers are charged with the responsibility of investigating reports of elder abuse. In the authors' view, better collaboration and communication between APS and child welfare programs could assist in ensuring that referrals are routed to the appropriate service provider.

Interventions: A Case Example

All interventions into situations involving family violence must be multi-faceted and always consider the level of danger and risk for the victim. However, the needs and concerns of dependent children under the elder victim's care are also critical to consider. Developing a service plan that is acceptable to the older victim and meets the needs of family members is essential to ensure safety and quality of life for all family members. Often a grandparent is extremely protective of even abusive grandchildren, and interventions are most likely to succeed if the needs of the abuser are taken into account as well. As with any crisis, there can be conflict, pain, and loss but also opportunity for growth and mutual understanding. Abusive adolescents must realize that life is not always fair, but they can emerge stronger and better prepared to face their future if they can learn that it is possible to play a bad hand well (Holman, 1998).

Case of Helen P.

Helen P., age 72, is the maternal grandparent of five adolescent and young adult grandchildren, all of whom had experienced sexual and physical abuse and witnessed domestic violence. She felt they did not help her enough with household chores and took advantage of her, but she was also dependent on them for assistance because of a chronic physical ailment. On several occasions, she discovered money was missing from her purse, and there were frequent verbal altercations between her and her two oldest grandsons. On one occasion, one grandson pushed her, causing her to lose her balance and fall—resulting in a bruised hip.

Discussion

With Helen, it was necessary to assess her safety needs, help her develop a safety plan and assess the need for home care to assist her with household chores and personal care, In-home services could help her to stop relying on her grandchildren. In Helen's case, identifying service providers was not easy. APS did not accept a referral as Helen was not cognitively impaired and not in imminent danger at the time of the referral. Although she qualified for Medicaid based on income and resources, initially the plan for home care was not approved as she had family resources in the household.

Eventually, the two older grandsons moved out of the household, which eased the safety crisis. However, she missed them and wanted them to return. For families like this, it is important to consider emotional as well as physical needs, and work toward linking the grandparent to therapeutic as well as concrete services. Assisting the grandparent plan for the entry of grandchildren, especially adolescents, into their household can be helpful in anticipating and planning for conflict before it starts. Questions to be considered include: What kind of child is the adolescent or preadolescent coming into the grandparent's home? What has the child been through? Often grandparents have no idea what kind of lives their grandchildren have lived up to that point. They may not have gotten enough to eat, or enough structure or boundaries set. This can present overwhelming challenges to grandparents unprepared to address these issues.

First, the grandparent must be helped to know what is inside the mind of the grandchild. This includes the family secrets they are coming with and what they have experienced. Often they are survivors of unimaginable circumstances for the grandparent. The grandparents must learn to advocate for their own needs and those of their grandchildren and even their children. If they make demands, they can get services for both themselves and their grandchildren. For grandchildren who have been exposed to abuse, neglect, violence, or extreme deprivation, counseling is critical. Grandparents must become self-empowered: If the services are unavailable or do not exist, grandparents must learn to advocate for them.

For professionals working with grandparents in these situations, it is important to be prepared to accept nontraditional solutions—psychospiritual, meditation, affirmation, and prayer—as well as to be knowledgeable about resources for both grandparents and grandchildren. For grandparents, becoming involved in grandchildren's school grandchildren's schools and service advisory groups is critical to ensuring that policies and decisions about services reflect the actual needs of reconstituted families of grandparents and grandchildren.

Implications for Practice and Policy

Kinship foster care has rapidly risen in recent years (the American Public Welfare Association—now the American Public Human Services Association—states that the caseload doubled from 1986 to 1990) (U. S. House of Representatives, 1998). However, the observed growth has been in communities of color (White-Hispanic and non-White children). Two thirds of kinship caregivers are grandparents, and more than 85% are female (U.S. Department of Health and Human Services, 1997). According to Jackson (1999), this requires a paradigm shift in the child welfare service delivery system. She suggests that it must become more family centered and holistic in its approach to kinship families, and more conscious of cultural relevance. Developing a kinship training program for workers should be a priority as well as the development of specialized competencies. This includes emphasis on the importance of kinship care that emanates from the philosophical base of family preservation (Jackson, 1999).

Although kinship care of dependent children is not new, the child welfare system that has evolved to date is structured to place children in traditional foster care settings and to move children who cannot return home to their biological parents as quickly as possible to permanency (usually meaning adoption). The system is traditionally child centered. Foster parents are considered professional caregivers and are expected to maintain and meet predetermined standards as a condition of placement. Children who act out in care are removed to another foster placement; adolescents are usually moved to congregate care facilities like group homes or into "independent living" situations. Recognizing and respecting the family preservation goal of kinship care is important in developing new program models and treatment modalities that address the problem of grandparent abuse, before it becomes too serious for the adolescent to remain in the family or even the community.

It is essential to begin to integrate the child welfare and aging networks to ensure that older people caring for grandchildren receive the services and support they need to ensure not only the preservation of the family in the community but to ensure their continued safety and well-being. Services that link grandparents to interventions for grandchildren who are suffering as a result of their separation from parents are also critical. Often, grandparents are not able to obtain needed services for grandchildren—particularly adolescents—until they behave in ways to bring them to the attention of the juvenile justice system. By then it may be too late to intervene in a way to ensure the child is able to remain in the community.

All but six states have mandatory reporting laws for elder abuse, modeled after child abuse mandatory reporting laws. Under elder abuse mandatory reporting laws, grandchildren may be identified among possible abusers. For abusive adolescent grandchildren, this could mean entry into the juvenile justice system or even—depending on the state, the age of the grandchild, and the type of offense the abuse represents—prosecution as an adult.

The current trend toward trying juveniles in adult courts for more serious offenses may serve to deter grandparents from reporting abuse by a grandchild. Special consideration of these types of situations by district attorneys that emphasize rehabilitation and not incarceration may encourage more grandparents to use the criminal justice system for serious offenses.

Although the criminal justice system is often the intervention of choice for abusers of older family members if they are abused by adult children or spouses—particularly if frail and dependent, it must be looked on as the intervention of last resort for abusive juveniles. The "get tough on juveniles" laws most states have passed or are considering enacting could be especially harmful and insensitive to the needs and concerns of adolescents in care because their parents abused or abandoned them. At the same time, older caregivers—often grandparents—are entitled to live lives free of intimidation and abuse. The formulation of programs and policies that can assist all family members live free of abuse should be the primary goal of both child welfare and aging service systems and the practitioners within them.

Finally, services offered kinship families where abuse of grandparents is a factor must be culturally sensitive. Studies have suggested that older persons' perceptions of elder abuse—including financial and verbal abuse—are mediated through a cultural lens (Brown, 1989; Nandlal & Wood, 1997). Understanding the ways in which grandparents interpret particular behaviors, such as a lack of respect, is fundamental to the design of interventions.

Conclusion

The problem of grandparent abuse within the kinship and informal care systems is a hidden but real one. The challenge for aging and child welfare advocates alike is to frame the issue in a sensitive way that can suggest effective solutions culminating in keeping families together in the community. The greatest dangers include ignoring the problem and exacerbating the suffering of grandparents caring for troubled grandchildren, or vilifying the grandchildren, further victimizing both grandchild and grandparent.

Data on the incidence and prevalence of grandparent abuse are needed. Using existing definitions of abuse developed by Wolf and Pillemer (1984) could help to compare these data with findings from other surveys of the general older population (Pillemer & Finkelhor, 1988; Podneiks, 1995). Measures of incidence and prevalence of abuse should incorporate information on the category (financial, psychological or verbal, and physical) and the intensity of the abuse. This is important for two reasons: to obtain a richer picture of the identified abuse and to examine the extent to which it reflects criminal behavior as defined in state law. For example, felony level domestic crimes are dealt with more severely than in the past. Juveniles who are abusive to their caregivers are at risk of incurring serious penalties such as incarceration and even prosecution in adult courts.

Data on profiles of abusers and victims are also important. All domestic violence involves dyads and characteristics of family situations where abuse is a factor can have predictive value for risk assessment and for development of preventive measures and interventions. As this chapter suggests, a clearer understanding of the scope and nature of this problem—beyond that of the anecdotal is needed to develop humane and sensitive interventions and services that address the needs and concerns of both grandparent and grandchild.

References

Bacon, W. (1997). *Kinship care study.* New York City: Administration for Children's Services. (Unpublished).

Berman, J. (1998). *Preliminary report on senior crime victims and grandparent abuse.* New York: Department for the Aging.

Breckman, R., & Adelman, R. (1988). Strategies for intervention into elder abuse. Newbury Park, CA: Sage.

Brown, A. (1989). A survey of elder abuse at one Native American tribe. *Journal of Elder Abuse and Neglect, 1,* 17–37.

Brownell, P. (1998). Elder abuse: Protective and empowerment strategies for crisis intervention. In A. R. Roberts (Ed.), *Battered women and their families: Intervention and treatment strategies.* New York: Springer.

Brownell, P. (1998). *Family crimes against the elderly: A study of elder abuse and the criminal justice system.* New York: Garland.

Brownell, P. (1994). *Family crimes against the elderly: A study of elder abuse and the New York Police Department.* Dissertation, Fordham University Graduate School of Social Service.

Courtney, J., White, A., & Keliman, V. S. (Eds.), (1997, Spring). *Child welfare watch.* New York City: Center for an Urban Future and the New York Forum.

Deater-Deck, K., & Dodge, K. A. (1997). Externalizing behavior problems and disruptions revisited: Non-linear effects and variations by culture and gender. *Psychological Inquiry, 8,* 161–175.

Dubowitz, H., Zuravin, S., Starr, Jr., R., Feigelman, S. & Harrington, D. (1993). Behavior problems of children in kinship care. *Journal of Developmental and Behavioral Pediatrics, 14,* 386–393.

Erikson, E. H. (1997). *The life cycle completed.* New York: Norton.

Everett, J. E., Chipungu, S. S., & Leashore, B. (1991). *Child welfare: An afrocentric perspective.* New Brunswick: Rutgers University Press.

Filinson, R. (1993). An evaluation of a program of volunteer advocates for elder abuse victims. *Journal of Elder Abuse and Neglect, 5,* 77–93.

Fleisch, B. (1996). *Approaches in the treatment of adolescents with emotional and substance abuse problems.* U. S. Department of Health and Human Services,

Substance Abuse and Mental Health Services Administration. Rockville, MD: Government Printing Office.

Gleeson, J. A. (1995). Kinship care and public child welfare: Challenges and opportunities for social work education. *Journal of Social Work Education, 31*, 182–193.

Gleeson, J. A. (1999). Kinship care as a child welfare system: Emerging policy issues and trends. In R. L. Hegal, & M. Scannapieco (Eds.), *Kinship foster care: Policy, practice and research* (pp. 29–53). New York: Oxford University Press.

Greenfield, L. (1998). *Violence by intimates*. Washington, DC: U.S. Department of Justice.

Hegar, R. L. (1999). The cultural roots of kinship care. In R. L. Hegar, & M. Scannapieco (Eds.), Kinship foster care: Policy, practice, and research (pp. 17–27). New York: Oxford University Press.

Heisler, C. J. (1991). The role of the criminal justice system in elder abuse cases. *Journal of Elder Abuse and Neglect, 3*, 5–33.

Holman, D. (1998, June 19). Paper presented at the New York City Elder Abuse Coalition. "Addressing the missing Generation".

Jackson, S. M. (1999). *Paradigm shift: Training staff to provide services to the kinship dyad.* In R. L. Hegar, and M. Scannapieco, (Eds.), *Kinship foster care: Policy, practice and research* (pp. 93–111). New York: Oxford University Press.

Korbin, J. E., Anetzberger, G., & Austin, C. (1995). The intergenerational cycle of violence in child and elder abuse. *Journal of Elder Abuse and Neglect, 7*, 1–15.

Korbin, J. E., Anetzberger, G. J., & Eckert, J. K. (1989). Elder abuse and child abuse: A consideration of similarities and differences in intergenerational family violence. *Journal of Elder Abuse and Neglect, 1*, 1–14.

Laureano, E. R. (1998, April 23). *Unrecognized and unreported: The dilemma of elder abuse.* Testimony at the Public Hearing on Elder Abuse in New York State.

Lucas, H. (1998, June 19). Paper presented at the New York City Coalition on Elder Abuse.

Luepnitz, D. A. (1998, September 8). When violence is a substitute for mourning: The curative use of family therapy. Paper presented at the World Conference on Family Violence, Singapore,

Mastrofski, S., Parks, R. B., & Worden, R. E. (1998, June). Community policing in action: Lessons from an observational study. In *Research review.* Washington, DC: National Institute of Justice.

McCreadie, C. (1993). From granny battering to elder abuse: A critique of U.K. writing, 1975–1992. *Journal of Elder Abuse and Neglect, 5*, 7–25.

Morrison, J. (1995). *DSM-IV made easy.* New York: Guilford.

Nandlal, J. M., & Wood, L. A. (1997). Older people's understandings of verbal abuse. *Journal of Elder Abuse and Neglect, 9*, 17–31.

Pillemer, K., & Finkelhor, D. (1988). The prevalence of elder abuse: A random sample survey. *The Gerontologist, 28,* 51–57.

Podneiks, E. (1992). Emerging themes from a follow-up study of Canadian victims of elder abuse. *Journal of Elder Abuse and Neglect, 4*(1/2), 59–111.

Podneiks, E. (1992). National survey on abuse of the elderly in Canada. *Journal of Elder Abuse and Neglect, 4,* 5–58.

Prichard, J. (1993). Dispelling some myths. *Journal of Elder Abuse and Neglect, 5,* 27–37.

Quinn, M. J., & Tomita, S. K. (1997). *Elder abuse and neglect: Causes, diagnosis, and intervention strategies* (2nd ed.). New York: Springer.

Rhode, D. (1998, November 9). Youth, 16, goes on trial in part slaying. *New York Times,* B4.

Rodriguez, O. (1996, May). The new immigrant hispanic population: An integrated approach to preventing delinquency and crime. In *Risk factors in hispanic delinquency.* Washington, DC: U.S. Department of Justice, Office of Justice Programs, National Institute of Justice.

Scannapieco, M. (1999). Kinship care in the public child welfare system: A systemic review of the research. In R.L. Hegar, & M. Scannapieco (Eds.), *Kinship foster care: Policy, practice, and research* (pp. 141–154). New York: Oxford University Press.

Scannapieco, M. & Hegar, R. L. (1999). Kinship foster care in context. In R. L. Hegar, & M. Scannapieco, (Eds.), *Kinship foster care: Policy, practice, and research* (pp. 1–13). New York: Oxford University Press.

Schorr, L. B. (1997). *Common purpose: Strengthening families and neighborhoods to rebuild America.* New York: Anchor Books.

Shapiro, C. (1997). New project seeks to help and get help from the hidden victims of drug abuse. *Community Corrections Report, 4,* 1–29.

Starr, R. H., Dubowitz, H., Harrington, D., & Feigelman, S. (1999). Behavior problems of teens in kinship care: Cross-informant reports. In R. L. Hegar, & M. Scannapieco (Eds.), *Kinship foster care: Policy, practice, and research* (pp. 193–207). New York: Oxford University Press.

Steinmetz, S. K. (1988). *Duty bound: Elder abuse and family care.* Newbury Park, CA: Sage.

Sykes, G. M. & Matza, D. (1978). Techniques of neutralization: A theory of delinquency. *American Sociological Review, 11,* 664–670.

Temple, S. (1997). *Brief therapy for adolescent depression.* Sarasota, FL: Professional Resource Press.

U.S. House Select Committee on Aging (1990). *Elder abuse: A decade of shame and inaction* (Publication No. 101–752). Washington, DC: U.S. Government Printing Office.

Wallace, H. (1999). *Family violence: Legal, medical, and social perspectives* (2nd ed.). Boston: Allyn & Bacon.

Wallace, H. (1998). *Victimology: Legal, psychological and social perspectives.* Boston: Allyn & Bacon.

Wilson, D. B. (1999). Kinship care in family serving agencies. In M. Scannapieco, & R. L Hegar (Eds.), *Kinship foster care: Policy, practice and research* (pp. 84–92). New York: Oxford University Press.

Wolf, R. S., & Pillemer, K. (1984). *Working with abused elders: Assessment, advocacy and interventions intervention.* University Center on Aging, University of Massachusetts Medical Center, Worchester.

Policy Issues

Chapter 7

Grandparents and Welfare Reform

Faith Mullen

Many grandparents find themselves unprepared to face the financial burden of supporting grandchildren. More than half (56%) of grandparent-headed households, where no parent is present and where the grandparent is at least 45 years old, have annual incomes below $20,000 (Chalfie, 1994). Nearly half of these households, in turn, live at or below the poverty level, which was $10,030 for a family of two in 1998 (Federal Register, 1998). Even grandparents with higher incomes may find themselves financially unable to meet all of their grandchildren's needs. Public benefits, including cash, medical care, and food assistance, can help grandparents who assume responsibility for the care of their grandchildren.

The presence or absence of a parent from a grandparent-headed household is one of the most important factors in determining a grandchild's eligibility for public benefits. If a parent is present and older than age 18 (age 22 for food stamp purposes), the grandparent's presence in the household is irrelevant in determining a grandchild's eligibility for benefits. In other words, eligibility for benefits is based solely on the parent's eligibility. This is true even if the parent has totally abdicated the care of the grandchild to the grandparent. If no parent is physically present, eligibility for benefits (except food stamps, which have household eligibility standards) is based either on the grandparent's eligibility or on the child's own eligibility.

Enactment of the Personal Responsibility and Work Opportunities Act of 1996 (PRA), also known as welfare reform, however, may make it more difficult for grandparents to obtain public benefits on behalf of their grandchildren. The purpose of the PRA was to increase the flexibility of the states in administering their public benefit programs, to reduce the incidence of out-of-wedlock pregnancies, and to end dependency on welfare (42 U.S.C. § 601[a]. With its emphasis on children being raised in poverty by single mothers, the PRA has resulted in policies that were never intended to address the needs of the growing number of children who are being raised by grandparents with no parent present in the household.

This chapter addresses some of the provisions of the PRA that are likely to have significant consequences for grandparent-headed households where no parent is present. The material in this chapter is organized around programs and policies affected by the PRA—Temporary Assistance for Needy Families, Medicaid, Supplemental Security Income, child support enforcement, food stamps, and public benefits for aliens. This chapter examines how welfare reform has served, or failed to serve, children who are in a grandparent's custody. The chapter concludes with recommendations for advocacy.

Temporary Assistance to Needy Families (TANF)

For decades, the single largest source of cash assistance to needy families has been the AFDC program, Aid to Families with Dependent Children. AFDC was established by the Social Security Act of 1935 to provide support for needy children and for others living with them. In August 1996, Congress repealed the AFDC program and replaced it with the TANF program, Temporary Assistance for Needy Families. Like AFDC, TANF is a needs-based program in which only families with limited income and resources can qualify for benefits.

Description of the Benefits

To obtain TANF on behalf of a grandchild, a grandparent must establish several things. First, the grandparent must prove that the child has been deprived of parental support or care by the death, continued absence, unemployment, or incapacity of a parent.

Second, the grandparent must prove that he or she is a "caretaker relative." Caretaker relatives include a grandchild's parents, grandparents, siblings, stepparents, aunts, uncles, and first cousins, and persons of preceding generations as denoted by prefixes of grand-, great-, or great-great-, and the spouse of any of these relatives. It may be difficult for a paternal grandparent to establish caretaker relative status if the father's name does not appear on the grandchild's birth certificate.

Third, the grandparent must prove that the grandchild is living with the grandparent in the grandparent's home. There is no federal requirement that a grandparent obtain legal custody to qualify for benefits.

Finally, the grandparent must prove that the grandchild's income and resources do not exceed the state's eligibility standards. All income received on behalf of a grandchild or by household members who are part of the assistance unit (those in the household who receive TANF benefits) must be included in calculating TANF eligibility. A few states impose a family cap or provide one benefit amount regardless of household size. Most states, however, base the amount of cash assistance on the number of people in the assistance unit—more people in the assistance unit results in more cash assistance. For example, Colorado, like most states, increases the amount of cash assistance as the size of the assistance unit increases. In 1997, a two-person family in Colorado that was eligible for the maximum TANF benefit would have received $280 per month; a three-person family would have received $356 (U.S. Congress, House Committee on Ways and Means, 1998).

Even in states where the amount of cash assistance increases if there are more people in the assistance unit, there are two reasons a grandparent might choose not to participate. First, the grandparent may have income or assets that exceed the state eligibility standard, and may simply not be eligible for benefits. A grandparent with as little as $900 monthly income or $1500 in savings would not qualify for TANF assistance in most states. If the grandparent is not part of the assistance unit, and the grandchild meets the eligibility requirements, the grandchild can still qualify for benefits. Second, a grandparent who is not part of the assistance unit is not subject to the other conditions of program participation, such as time limits and work requirements.

Effect of Welfare Reform

The federal government turned over much of the responsibility for design and administration of the TANF program to the states. But states do not have complete discretion in how they operate their TANF programs. The federal government continues to impose strict requirements with regard to maintenance of effort, time limits, work requirements, and child support enforcement. If a state fails to meet the requirements, the federal government can impose some harsh financial penalties. All of these changes—ending entitlements, block granting, time limits, work requirements, and the associated caseload reduction—may have serious consequences for grandparent-headed households.

Ending Entitlement

The PRA ends all entitlement to assistance. This means that even if a grandchild meets every eligibility requirement of the TANF program, the state has no obligation to provide assistance. The federal statute specifies that the PRA "shall not be interpreted to entitle any individual or family to assistance" from any state program funded under the act (42 U.S.C. § 601[b]). Almost half the states have adopted a similar provision in their own law (Mannix & Cohan, 1998).

Ending entitlements does not mean that states can totally eliminate their assistance to needy families. States are required to maintain 80% of their AFDC spending level. This maintenance of effort drops to 75% if the state meets federal work participation targets. States can satisfy the maintenance of effort requirement in a variety of ways including spending on education and job training. State funds used to assist persons who are ineligible for TANF because they have exhausted their lifetime benefit limit, or because they are not citizens, also count toward the maintenance of effort requirement.

Block Granting

The PRA repealed three programs—Aid to Families with Dependent Children (AFDC), Emergency Assistance for Needy Families (EA), and the Job Opportunities and Basics Skills Training (JOBS) program—and replaced them with TANF, a block grant to states. This block grant structure is a fundamental difference between AFDC and TANF. Under AFDC, states were entitled to unlimited federal funds for a percentage of their expenditures for AFDC, EA, and JOBS programs. The more of its own dollars a state spent on these programs, the more federal dollars it received. Under TANF, the federal obligation to reimburse states for a percentage of their spending has become a fixed block grant, and the federal contribution is based not on current state spending, but on a calculation of recent federal spending in that state. The amount of federal funding states will receive to assist needy families is fixed until the year 2002.

States have always had the authority to establish benefit levels and income eligibility for AFDC within federal guidelines. As a result, there was a great variation among states in AFDC expenditures. For example, in 1996 the maximum AFDC grant for a family of three living in Vermont equaled 58% of the federal poverty level, or $639. If that same family had moved to Missouri, the maximum AFDC grant would have been only 26% of the federal poverty level or $292 (U.S. Congress House Committee on Ways and Means, 1996). Nationally in 1996, the median monthly AFDC benefit for a family of three was $379 but ranged from a low of $120 in Mississippi to a high of $923 in Alaska. Because TANF block grants depend on a state's prior AFDC spending level, the higher the historic spending level the more generous the TANF benefit will be and the greater flexibility the state will have. Conversely, states with historically low benefit levels are unlikely to become more generous. As a consequence, the disparity in state spending is likely to become permanent under block granting.

Although TANF gives states great discretion in how they administer their cash assistance programs, that discretion is not absolute. There are federal conditions attached to the TANF block grant. These include maintenance of effort rules described earlier, time limits, work requirements, child support enforcement, and restrictions on assistance to legal aliens.

Time Limits

TANF cannot be used to provide assistance to a family that includes an adult who has received TANF assistance for 60 months. This is a lifetime limit. It does not matter if the benefits were received continuously or a month at a time over the course of decades. The limit does not apply to individuals who received benefits when they were children, unless they received benefits in their capacity as a minor household head or a minor married to a household head.

The 60-month time limit does not apply to grandparent-headed households where no parent is present, if the grandparent applies for "child-only" benefits. Grandparents of any age who are eligible for TANF can choose to exclude themselves from participation in the TANF assistance unit. Parents do not have that choice. The time limits do not apply to grandparents who obtain a child-only grant because the assistance unit does not include an adult who has received TANF assistance for 60-months. Grandparents must weigh their family's need for the additional cash assistance they would receive as part of the assistance unit against their grandchild's need for benefits beyond the time limits. In many states, the additional cash assistance is less than $100 per month.

Second, grandparents who are older than age 65 should never be part of the assistance unit. A grandparent who is poor enough to qualify as part of the assistance unit will be poor enough to qualify for Supplemental Security Income (SSI) benefits, and at age 65 will be eligible for SSI based on age (42 U.S.C. § 1381). There are several reasons why it is more desirable for a grandparent to participate in SSI than in TANF. Participation in the SSI program is not time limited or subject to work requirements. SSI automatically entitles a grandparent to Medicaid benefits. SSI benefits are likely to be more generous than a grandparent's share of a TANF grant.

States may offer an exemption from the 60-month limit based on hardship to not more than 20% of families that receive assistance. States may or may not elect to use their limited hardship exemptions on children who are in a grandparent's care. The 20% limit on exemptions bears no relationship to the growing number of grandparents who care for grandchildren, or to the number of custodial parents who would otherwise qualify for a hardship exemption.

Work Requirements

One of the main goals of the PRA is to move beneficiaries from welfare to work. Grandparents who are part of the assistance unit, like other caretaker relatives, are required to engage in work activities no later than 24 months after receiving assistance. States can exempt grandparents with children under age one, or up to age 6 when there is no available child care. As a condition of receiving federal TANF dollars, states must meet annual work participation rates for their TANF caseloads. In 1999, states must guarantee that 35% of families receiving aid participate in work activities for at least 25 hours per week. By 2002, that rate increases to 50% of the caseload engaged in work activities for at least 30 hours per week.

The PRA specifies the following activities as counting toward a state's participation rate: unsubsidized employment, subsidized private or public sector work, on-the-job training, job search and job readiness assistance, community service programs, education directly related to employment of recipients who do not have high school diplomas, satisfactory attendance at secondary school, and provision of child care services to a TANF recipient who is participating in a community service program.

The PRA links these work requirements to the state's receipt of federal funds and the penalties for failing to meet the requirements are stiff. If a state falls short of the required work participation rate for a fiscal year, its TANF block grant for the next year must be reduced by 5%. If the failure to reach work participation rates continues, there is an additional 2% penalty each year. So, in the second year, the penalty would be 7%; in the third year, it would rise to 9%; and so on, up to a maximum penalty of 21% in any 1 year.

This puts states under enormous pressure to meet the federal work participation rate. In turn, states must pressure beneficiaries to participate. States must sanction beneficiaries who refuse to engage in work. Sanctions take the form of reducing or eliminating benefits for the family. Formerly, if an adult refused to participate in work activities, the family grant was reduced by that adult's portion. Under TANF rules, the entire household could lose eligibility.

Reduction in Welfare Caseloads

When the PRA was enacted, there was concern that states would have more eligible families than TANF funds could support and that states would need a mechanism for rationing benefits (Mullen, 1996). States have not yet confronted the issue because the dramatic decline in caseloads has made rationing benefits unnecessary. Between August 1996 and June 1998, there was a 32% national decline in welfare caseloads (Administration on Children and Families, 1998).

Two practices in the administration of TANF that may account for some of the decline in caseloads are diversion payments and "work-first" rules. These practices have serious implications for grandparent-headed households.

One practice, diversion payments, may help some grandparents meet the needs of their grandchildren. Diversion payments are one-time lump-sum payments. They are made to prevent otherwise eligible families from needing regular monthly cash assistance by solving the problem that caused the family to apply. Diversion payments are commonly used to address barriers to self-sufficiency, such as the cost of repairing the car that a household member uses to get to work.

Approximately 20 states have authorized diversion payment programs (Center on Budget and Policy Priorities, 1998). A family that receives a diversion payment will be ineligible for cash assistance for some number of months after they receive a diversion payment. In some states, diversion payments are treated as an advance against the family's future eligibility for public assistance. Although these payments can be helpful to grandparents faced with a financial crisis associated with adding a grandchild to the household, it is important that grandparents weigh the value of these one-time payments against the value of ongoing cash assistance.

The other practice, "work first," may divert eligible grandparents from receiving assistance. Many states are phasing in work first programs, in which applicants are directed to participate in a job search prior to the approval for benefits. Applicants are required to make a specific number of job contacts each week and provide written documentation of their job search. It is important that grandparents, particularly those who are applying for child-only assistance, not be deflected from the application process by work first policies. There is a risk that a grandparent who tries to apply for TANF will be told to look for work but not be advised that work requirements do not apply to the child-only grants.

Medicaid

Although the PRA did not block grant or otherwise change fundamental aspects of the Medicaid program, it may have a major effect on how states enroll Medicaid beneficiaries and on who receives benefits. In the past, eligibility for cash assistance and Medicaid have been linked, and grandchildren who received AFDC were automatically entitled to Medicaid. The PRA severs that link (42 U.S.C. § 1396u-1). Although most grandchildren who live in grandparent-headed households with no parent present will still be eligible for Medicaid, they will no longer be automatically enrolled. This could result in a number of grandchildren who are eligible for Medicaid but not receiving benefits.

Description of the Benefit

A major concern for grandparents raising grandchildren is obtaining medical coverage for the children in their care. Medicaid pays for some essential medical services. Of particular importance to grandparents and their grandchildren are inpatient and outpatient hospital services, laboratory and x-ray services, and physician and nursing services.

As with TANF, to obtain Medicaid for a grandchild, a grandparent must establish that he or she is a caretaker relative and that the child is in fact in the grandparent's care. There is no requirement that a grandparent obtain legal custody for the grandchild to qualify for benefits. The grandparent need only show that the grandchild is deprived of parental care and support as defined by the AFDC regulations that were in effect on July 16, 1996, and that the grandchild meets the Medicaid eligibility standards that were in effect on that date.

Effect of Welfare Reform

Before enactment of the PRA, there were essentially two ways to obtain Medicaid for a grandchild. The first was eligibility based on family income. The second was automatic eligibility for children who qualified for AFDC cash assistance or for SSI benefits.

The first route to Medicaid eligibility continues today. A grandchild younger than 6 is eligible for Medicaid if the family income is below 133% of the federal poverty level (42 U.S.C. § 1396(a)(1). In 1998, that was approximately $1,500 per month for a family of three (Federal Register, 1998). Medicaid coverage is being gradually phased in for children older than age 6 in families with incomes below 100% of the poverty level, $1,137 per month for a family of three. The phase-in is achieved by limiting this eligibility to children born after September 30, 1983. Thus, by October 1998, Medicaid benefits were available to all children between age 6 to 14 whose family income was below 100% of the poverty level. By October 2002, all children age 6 through 18 with family incomes under 100% of the poverty line will be Medicaid eligible.

The second route to Medicaid eligibility, and the most important route for grandchildren who are in a grandparent's care, has been altered by the PRA. Formerly, states were required to provide Medicaid to grandchildren who received AFDC. The PRA eliminated the automatic link between cash assistance and Medicaid but retained the AFDC eligibility standards for determining Medicaid eligibility (42 U.S.C. § 1396u-1). Under the PRA, states must provide Medicaid benefits to grandchildren who would be eligible for AFDC cash aid if the program still existed, under the standards of the AFDC program as it existed on July 16, 1996. States must continue to use AFDC standards to determine Medicaid eligibility, even though AFDC no longer exists.

The continued use of AFDC standards was designed to prevent low-income families from losing Medicaid coverage as a result of changes in the cash assistance program. Consequently, grandchildren will not lose their eligibility merely because their state adopts more rigorous TANF eligibility standards or because their family loses TANF benefits owing to work requirements or time limits.

The main concern with this approach is that even if grandchildren are eligible for Medicaid, they may not actually receive the benefit. Studies have shown that children in families who do not receive cash aid are much less likely to enroll in the Medicaid program. In 1994, only 38% of children under age 11 who did not receive cash assistance but were eligible for Medicaid were enrolled in the Medicaid program (Summer, Parrott, & Mann, 1997).

The Department of Health and Human Services has urged states to conduct aggressive outreach to ensure that Medicaid-eligible children are enrolled in the program (DeParle, 1998). States can take several steps to ensure that grandchildren who receive cash aid and who are eligible for Medicaid actually receive Medicaid. For example, states can provide automatic Medicaid eligibility to TANF recipients or develop mechanisms to ensure that families receiving diversion payments are encouraged to apply for Medicaid. In some communities, child care agencies, schools, and health care providers help enroll eligible families. The extent to which states ensure that eligible grandchildren are enrolled in Medicaid will have serious consequences for grandparent-headed households.

Child Support Enforcement

Parents have a legal obligation to support their children. When a grandparent assumes custody of a grandchild, the grandparent has the right to receive child support from the noncustodial parents. If the grandparent receives TANF, Medicaid, or (at state option) food stamps on behalf of a grandchild, the grandparent must assign the right to child support to the state. This means that grandparents must transfer to the state their right to bring legal action against the noncustodial parent, or parents, for child support. States in turn use the dollars recovered from noncustodial parents to reimburse their assistance program budgets.

Formerly under AFDC, and now under the PRA, grandparents are required to cooperate with state child support enforcement efforts. Cooperation means providing specific information about the identity and location of the absent parent or parents, making the grandchild available for blood tests to establish paternity, and appearing at interviews and court hearings.

The policy rationale for requiring cooperation is sound; public dollars should not be used to support children when their parents are able but simply decline to do so. Application of the cooperation rules, however, poses a unique problem for grandparents. Any effort to establish paternity or obtain child support has the potential to destabilize informal custody arrangements and trigger a custody battle. Parents who allow a grandparent to have informal custody may balk at that arrangement if ordered to pay child support. A grandparent who considers applying for public assistance on behalf of a grandchild must evaluate the risk that an angry parent may come and take the child away. State custody laws offer grandparents very little protection. Absent a showing of unfitness, a grandparent may lose a custody contest even if the parent has been indifferent to the child's welfare for years.

Effect of Welfare Reform

Passage of the PRA infused paternity and support enforcement efforts with a new urgency. States must try to recover every possible dollar of assistance paid on behalf of any child whose parents have failed to provide support. In the past, states have had limited success with support enforcement. Even the most successful states, Arkansas and Idaho, had a support enforcement rate of less than $40 for every $100 spent on AFDC (U.S. Department of Health and Human Services, 1998).

If states fail to demonstrate that families are cooperating with the child support enforcement agency, they can lose up to 5% of the federal dollars payable to the state (42 U.S.C. § 409 [a][5] and 341[a]). Conversely, if states show an increase in the number of paternity adjudications, they can gain additional matching payments for child support activities. The pressure on states to establish paternity and collect support is great, and it is likely to make states less sympathetic to the problems that support enforcement can create for grandparents.

The PRA allows states to grant a limited number of "good cause" exemptions. AFDC allowed an exemption when there was the potential for emotional or physical harm to the child or the grandparent. States are no longer required to grant an exemption based on fear of harassment or the threat of psychological or emotional harm. Even under the broader good cause standards of AFDC, good cause was rarely alleged. In 1995, 7,830 claims for good cause were reported by states. Good cause was found in only 4,819 cases (U.S. Department of Health and Human Services, 1998).

Supplemental Security Income (SSI)

The PRA changed the SSI program eligibility rules for children. Under the PRA, close to 100,000 children will lose SSI benefits because of new definitions of disability (SSA's Implementation, 1998).

Description of the Benefit

The SSI program provides a cash benefit for grandchildren who are severely disabled. In 1998, the monthly federal benefit rate was $484 (Social Security Administration [SSA], SSA Handbook, 1998). This is significantly higher than the TANF benefits offered in many states. SSI benefits also include automatic enrollment in Medicaid. A grandchild cannot receive both SSI and TANF benefits.

Effect of Welfare Reform

The PRA established a strict definition of disability for children that is no longer based on comparability with the adult standard (42 U.S.C. § 1382c). The new definition of disability requires a grandchild to have a physical or mental condition that can be medically proved and that results in marked and severe functional limitations. The condition must last or be expected to last at least 12 months or be expected to result in death.

The PRA eliminated the Individual Functional Assessment (IFA). The IFA evaluated how a disability affected the grandchild's ability to perform daily activities, such as playing, studying, eating, and dressing. The IFA was controversial. Critics claimed it allowed children to "fake" disabilities, especially emotional and behavioral problems, to qualify for benefits. However, none of the studies of the IFA found evidence to support allegations of widespread abuse (SSA's Implementation, 1998). Elimination of the IFA will make it more difficult for grandchildren with mental and emotional disorders to obtain benefits.

Initially, the SSA estimated that among the one million children receiving benefits, 288,000 would need to have their eligibility redetermined under the new law, and that 135,000 would eventually be determined ineligible for SSI benefits. The SSA now estimates that 100,000 children will be found ineligible after all appeals are completed (SSA's Implementation, 1998).

Food Stamps

The Food Stamps program was developed to enable low-income households to buy a nutritionally adequate low-cost diet (7 U.S.C. § 2011). Participating households are expected to spend 30% of their countable monthly income on food. Food stamp benefits then make up the difference between the household's expected contribution to its food costs and an amount judged to be sufficient to buy a nutritionally adequate low-cost diet.

Description of the Benefit

The Food Stamps program is a federal, needs-based program. Grandparents must have low incomes and limited resources to qualify. The federal government bears the full cost of the benefits and 50% of the states' administrative costs. The state food stamp agencies determine eligibility, calculate the amount of assistance, and issue food stamps.

Food stamps are distributed in the form of coupons or electronic benefit cards. In the past, food stamps were issued only in coupon booklets. Some states now use a debit card system to deliver food stamps, and by October 2002, all states are required to implement an electronic benefit transfer system. Food stamps can be used to purchase food for home preparation and consumption.

Eligible households receive food stamps in amounts ranging from $10 up to the maximum monthly food stamp allotment for their household size. The monthly amount of food stamps a household receives is determined by household size and income. The maximum benefit increases several dollars each year. For October 1998 to September 1999, the maximum monthly food stamp allotment for a grandparent with two grandchildren is $329. For a grandparent with one grandchild, the maximum monthly allotment is $230 (United States Department of Agriculture, 1998).

There are no child-only food stamp benefits. Generally, individuals who live under one roof are members of the same food stamp household if they regularly purchase food and prepare meals together. Grandchildren who live in households maintained by their grandparents, with no parents present, are automatically treated as if they buy and prepare food with their grandparents.

Effect of Welfare Reform

The PRA cut the Food Stamps program more than $27 billion over six years. Most of those savings will be realized by limiting the eligibility of childless adults between the ages of 18 and 50. Childless adults in this age range are now eligible for only 3 months of food stamp benefits every 36 months unless they are working half-time or participating in a job program. The 3 month time limits do not apply to grandparent-headed households or other households where children are present.

For grandparent-headed households, the most important changes to the Food Stamps program are those changes affecting benefit amounts and how income and resources are counted in determining eligibility (7 U.S.C. § 2014). As noted earlier, families are expected to devote 30% of their countable income to the purchase of food, and food stamps are intended to make up the difference between this amount and the cost of a nutritionally adequate diet. The PRA eliminated a previously scheduled 3% increase in what was considered the cost of a minimally adequate diet. It also fixed the standard income deduction at $134, capped the shelter deductions at $275, and froze the vehicle allowance at $4,650. The earnings of a grandchild who is in high school count as income once the grandchild reaches age 18. Prior law excluded the income until the student's 22nd birthday. All of these changes affect the amount of food stamps a grandparent-headed household will receive.

Grandparent-headed households that include a legal immigrant may experience a sharp drop in eligibility for food stamps. With few exceptions, legal immigrants are not eligible for food stamps. However, the PRA allows states to count all or part of the income of ineligible legal immigrants in calculating a household's food stamp allotment (7 U.S.C. § 2015[f]). Including the income of the ineligible immigrant can significantly decrease or even eliminate a household's food stamp allotment.

The PRA eliminated requirements concerning application forms, verification requirements, in-person and home interviews, and special application processes for elderly, disabled, rural, homeless, and non- English–speaking populations. These requirements were helpful to grandparents who had difficulty traveling to the food stamp office or otherwise navigating the food stamp system. Instead, states are required to establish procedures for fair and accurate services and for meeting the needs of special populations.

Welfare and Public Benefits for Legal Aliens

Under the PRA most legal aliens are ineligible for cash welfare, including TANF, Medicaid, food stamps, SSI, and other programs that benefit grandparents and grandchildren (8 U.S.C. § 1611). With the exception of emergency medical care and limited public health assistance, states can make both legal and illegal aliens ineligible for public benefits.

The PRA has a variety of exceptions to the prohibition on granting benefits to legal aliens including time-limited exemptions for refugees and asylees, exemptions for certain permanent resident aliens who have accumulated 50 quarters of coverage as defined by the Social Security Act, and exemptions for some veterans. It may be difficult or impossible for grandparents who do not read well or speak fluent English to know whether they are eligible.

The prohibition on giving benefits to legal aliens presents three additional problems for grandparents whose grandchildren are United States citizens. First, grandparents whose immigration status precludes their own eligibility might not realize they can obtain child-only benefits on behalf of their grandchildren, except for food stamps where program rules require the household to be eligible. These grandparents may be discouraged from applying for benefits on behalf of a qualified grandchild because of misinformation about the availability of benefits.

Second, the PRA eliminates any prohibition on communication between states and the Immigration and Naturalization service regarding an individual's immigration status. Grandparents who are illegal aliens may be reluctant to apply for benefits on behalf of grandchildren who are citizens, if they believe they risk deportation by doing so.

Finally, some grandparents lack birth certificates and may have difficulty proving their own citizenship. This may present an additional barrier to obtaining assistance for their grandchildren. At a minimum, they may experience delay in receiving benefits while they attempt to prove that they are, in fact, U.S. citizens.

Conclusions

The PRA fundamentally changed the nature of the American welfare system. It swept away three decades of welfare policies and practices. Though far from perfect, the former welfare system had evolved over the last past 30 years and, to some degree, accommodated grandparents. Issues that had been clearly resolved, like how to calculate the eligibility for cash assistance for unrelated children in a grandparent's household, have now become unsettled.

These changes raise several issues that are of particular importance to grandparents. First, the fundamental nature of public benefits changed. The administration of the program devolved to the states. Although states have great discretion in how their programs are structured, they are under pressure to comply with federal requirements—to meet work participation rates, to limit the number of families who receive aid for more than 60 months, and to obtain and enforce child support orders. The pressure states are under to meet federal standards cannot help but translate into pressure on beneficiaries.

Second, it is difficult to predict what effect policies targeted at young single mothers will have on older grandparents. Requirements that prompt a 22-year-old parent to enter the work force may present an impossible challenge to a 63-year-old grandmother who has just taken on responsibility for three grandchildren. Furthermore, if a policy has a significant effect on one group of beneficiaries, it is likely to have unexpected and possibly harmful consequences for other groups. The 5-year time limits on TANF may prompt some parents to turn over custody of their children to grandparents. It remains to be seen whether there will be a surge in the number of grandparent-headed households once parents exhaust their eligibility for benefits.

Third, instead of uniform federal standards, each state has the authority to create its own system for administering benefits and its own rules for determining eligibility. These new rules are accompanied by a level of uncertainty. A grandparent who is thinking about obtaining aid on behalf of a grandchild not only needs to ascertain which benefits might be useful to that grandchild—food, medical care, and cash assistance—but must also figure out the often contradictory eligibility standards for each program.

Because these programs are need based and need is defined differently for each program, it can be daunting for grandparents to collect the information required to make an application. Some benefits, like food stamps, which are based on countable income, require disclosure of a large amount of personal information—the value of the grandparent's car, the amount of any uncompensated medical bills, the names of other family members in the household who are neither eligible nor applying for the benefits, and so on. Others, like Medicaid, require only that a grandparent prove the grandchild is deprived of parental care and does not have income or assets that exceed the eligibility standard.

Given the complexity of the programs and the number of choices available to a state, it is often difficult for grandparents to know what the rules are and whether they are being applied correctly. It is much more difficult to know when a grandparent has grounds to challenge a decision made by a local welfare office. Some practices that were formerly prohibited, like cutting benefits without advance notice, are now allowed. These changes interject a high level of uncertainty into what the rules are and how they should be applied to grandparent-headed households.

Finally, the PRA may have the effect of freezing benefits at inadequate levels. AFDC has always offered only modest cash assistance. In more than half the states, benefits do not bring recipients up to 50% of the federal poverty level. Block granting has bound states to choices they made in the past, because the amount of money they will receive for the TANF program is related to the amount they have historically spent on the AFDC program. It is unlikely that benefit levels will increase, even as the cost of living rises.

To date, most states have turned their attention to addressing basic welfare reform issues like what to count as work activity or how to enhance child support enforcement. States have largely neglected the question of how these policies affect grandparent-headed households. As the numbers of these households increase and as other welfare issues are resolved, states are more likely to focus on the concerns of these households. Now is the time for advocates to urge states to adopt policies that will protect and serve grandparents and children in their care. Some of those policies include the following:

- Establishing a separate application process for grandparents where they will be advised about the availability of the child-only grants, and where they will be insulated from practices that do not apply to their particular situation.
- Using a single application form to determine eligibility under both TANF and Medicaid and a single agency to make the eligibility determination.
- Keeping the basic financial eligibility rules for TANF and for Medicaid consistent.
- Not requiring grandparents to complete an application for more than one kind of benefit. A grandparent who wishes to obtain Medicaid on a grandchild's behalf should not be forced to disclose the income an immigrant relative who lives in the household, merely because that question is appropriately asked in connection with a food stamp application.

- Supporting outreach for Medicaid, particularly for children who do not receive either TANF or SSI cash assistance. These efforts should include allowing health care providers and schools to enroll children in Medicaid.
- Ensuring that children and grandparents who did not qualify for TANF-funded assistance are separately evaluated for Medicaid eligibility.
- Developing simple, clear written materials explaining what the child support enforcement system is about and how it works. The materials should explain the cooperation obligation, the consequences for failing to cooperate, and the good cause exemptions.
- Training all TANF workers in identifying domestic violence issues that may affect grandparents.
- Training all TANF workers on child custody and visitation issues so that they can better assist grandparents when a parent threatens to take a grandchild in response to support enforcement activities.
- Conducting outreach to grandparents on TANF, Medicaid, and food stamps.

Most important, states must establish clear, fair, and consistent policies for implementing the programs that are under their control. Grandparents are not well served when they do not know what the rules are or how they will be applied. Caseworkers should not be faced with trying to fit grandparents' circumstances into rules that were never designed to accommodate them. States should give serious consideration to the policies and procedures that affect grandparent-headed households, and they should try to anticipate which policies would best meet the needs of those households.

References

Administration for Children and Families, DHHS. *Change in Welfare caseloads since enactment of the New Welfare Law*, 1998: www.acf.dhhs.gov/news/aug-jun.htm).

Center on Budget and Policy Priorities (1998, July 17). *USDA permits TANF diversion payments to be excluded from Food Stamp income calculations*.

Chalfie, D. (1994). *Going it alone, a closer look at grandparents parenting grandchildren*. Washington, DC: American Association of Retired Persons.

DeParle, N. A. M. (1998, June 5). Administrator Health Care Financing Administration, Letter to state Medicaid Directors and TANF sdministrators.

1998 HHS Poverty Guidelines." In *Federal Register* (Vol. 63, No. 36, February 24, 1998. pp. 9235–9238).

Mannix, M., & Cohan, M. (1998). Welfare litigation developments since the PRA. *Clearinghouse Review*, *31*, 435–453.

Mullen, F. (1996). Welcome to Procrustes' house: Welfare reform and grandparents raising grandchildren. *Clearinghouse Review*, *30*, 511–520.

Personal Responsibility and Work Opportunity Reconciliation Act of 1996 (PRA) (Pub. L. No. 104–193, codified in part at 42 U.S.C. § 601 et seq.)

Summer, L., Parrott, S., & C. Mann. (1997). Millions of uninsured and underinsured children are eligible for medicaid. Center on Budget and Policy Priorities: www.cbpp.org/mcaidprt.htm.).

Social Security Administration. *SSA handbook*. (2171 Federal SSI payments): www.ssa.gov/OP_Home/handbook/handbook.21/hbk-2171.htm.

Social Security Administration. *SSA's implementation of the new SSI childhood disability law*:www.ssa.gov/policy/childoo4.htm.

U.S. Congress, House Committee on Ways and Means. (1996, July 15). *Overview of Entitlement Program: 1996 green book* (p. 416). Washington, DC: 103rd Cong., 2d sess.

U.S. Congress, House Committee on Ways and Means. (1998, May 19). *Overview of Entitlement Program: 1998 green book* (p. 419). Washington, DC: 105th Cong., 2d sess.

U. S. Department of Agriculture. Food Stamp program monthly allotments and deductions, October 1998–September 1999: www.usda.gov/fcs/stamps/99allot.htm.

U.S. Department of Health and Human Service. (1998, August). *Twenty-first annual report to Congress for the period ending September 30, 1996. (p. 99).*

7 U.S.C. § 2011.

7 U.S.C. § 2014.

7 U.S.C. § 2015(f).

8 U.S.C. § 1611.

42 U.S.C. § 409(a)(5) and 341(a).

42 U.S.C. § 601(a).

42 U.S.C. § 601(b).

42 U.S.C. § 1381.

42 U.S.C. § 1382c.

42 U.S.C. § 1396(a)(l).

42 U.S.C. § 1396u-1.

Chapter 8

Grandparent Caregiving: Legal Status Issues and State Policy

Melinda Perez-Porter
and Margaret M. Flint

The right of parents, both mothers and fathers, to raise their children is a right traced by the United States Supreme Court to the United States Constitution. Generally, parents have the right to raise their children without state interference unless it can be shown that the parent is unfit or other extraordinary circumstances exist which compel a consideration of the child's best interests.

If a child's parents were married, the rights and responsibilities of the mother and father are equal and shared, unless modified through divorce or a separation agreement. If the parents were not married, steps must be taken to give the father legal status. This can happen either through a legal proceeding brought by the father, mother, or welfare official or by the conduct of the father who openly acknowledges paternity and acts accordingly. Children born during a marriage are presumed to be fathered by the husband, unless proved otherwise in a legal proceeding.

The law gives parents broad discretion to make decisions inherent in raising children. Generally, parents are presumed to be acting in the best interests of their children when they make decisions concerning the medical care, education, religious upbringing, and social contacts of their children. Laws that impact on a parent's choices are generally narrowly construed and may be waived if they conflict with parents' religious beliefs. For example, mandatory education laws allow parents to choose religious schools or state-supervised home schooling. Consent of parents to medical treatment for their children is generally required and, if withheld, can be challenged only if the failure to treat is clearly life threatening. Generally, parents may decide with whom their children may socialize; under common law, even close family members have no right to access to children if the children's parents object. Grandparent visitation laws give some grandparents access to grandchildren over the parent's objection, but only after the grandparent proves that the contact is in the child's best interest and in many cases only if the grandparent's child has died or is not the custodial parent.

The law recognizes that some parents are not able to raise their children. Each state has enacted its own laws that provide for the care of children who cannot be cared for by their parents because of the death of the parents, abandonment, abuse or persistent neglect. Legal mechanisms exist that enable parents to delegate their parental responsibilities to others. We will discuss these mechanisms first because we believe that parents should be encouraged and assisted to make plans for the care of their children in advance of their disability or death. We also believe that even parents who have not planned in advance should, to the extent possible, be given the opportunity to participate in the decisions concerning the care of their children when they are not able to assume full responsibility for their care.

Planning for the Care of Children by Others

Guardianship

Parents can ensure that their children are taken care of when they are unable to care for them with guardianships. Guardianships are formal legal relationships awarded by a court and can be immensely helpful to parents who want to convey to grandparents the authority to make decisions for the child in the parent's absence because of incapacity, incarceration, or death. Guardianship options include legal guardianships, standby guardianships, and testamentary guardianships. The availability of these options varies from state to state. Advocates should find out which of these options are available in their states to assist parents who wish to plan for the care of their children.[1]

Legal Guardianship

A judge may appoint a legal guardian for a child when the parents consent or are otherwise unable to care for their children because of incapacity, absence, unfitness, or death, if the court finds that it is in the child's best interests to have a guardian appointed.

When a third party, such as a grandparent, is awarded guardianship of a child, the parent's rights are not terminated, they are suspended. Parents remain legally responsible for the support of their children and may be ordered to provide health insurance. Parents cannot remove their children from the home of the guardian without the guardian's permission, unless the parents first go to court and prove a change in the circumstances that prompted the court to appoint the guardian.

Grandparents who have legal guardianship are able to make all day to day decisions regarding the care of their grandchildren and may enroll them in school, consent to their participation in school activities, and consent to their medical care. Grandparents who are legal guardians are also able to apply for public benefits, such as Social Security benefits, SSI, or TANF, Food Stamps for the family, and Medicaid for the children in their care. Legal guardians can also pursue child support payments from the children's parents if such award was not made when guardianship was granted.

Legal guardianship is not a permanent relationship. It can end when a child marries, turns age 18, or the court finds that circumstances have changed and that the best interests of the child are served by removing the guardian and returning the child to the parent.

Standby Guardianship

Where available,[2] standby guardianship laws authorize parents who are not ready to give up their decision-making authority, to designate an adult to act as the children's guardian when the parents are no longer able to care for their children because of illness or death.

Standby Guardianship legislation was enacted in New York State in response to the AIDS/HIV epidemic. Parents wanted to plan for the care of their children when they were incapable of caring for them but did not want to immediately give up their right to make decisions and to care for their children. New York State's Standby Guardianship law allows the creation of a standby guardian in two ways: The parent can file a petition in court for the appointment of a Standby Guardian or can designate the standby guardian in a written document without going to court. If the Standby Guardian is appointed by a court, the guardianship becomes effective when the parent consents, becomes mentally incapacitated or dies. If the parent makes a written designation, the standby guardian must go to court to be formally appointed within 60 days when the parent dies or is no longer able to care for her children.

Written designations of standby guardians are very useful when the parents are unable or unwilling to go to court. However, parents should know that when making a designation, they are making a recommendation to the court as to who should be the child's guardian. The court is not required to approve the designated standby guardian but will appoint that person only if it finds that the appointment would be in the child's best interests. The risk with designations is that the parent will not be around to defend his or her choice of guardian if the designation is later contested by someone else or rejected by the court. The best way to ensure that the chosen standby guardian becomes the child's guardian is to have that person appointed the standby guardian by the court before the parent's death or incapacity.

Parents can decide when the standby guardianship becomes effective and can consent to the commencement of the guardianship at any time. Their rights are not terminated when a standby guardian becomes the child's guardian. Rather, the parent and the guardian have concurrent authority to act. Alternative guardians can also be named in case the chosen guardian in unable or unwilling to serve.

Testamentary Guardianships

Parents who want to plan for the care of their children upon their death can also designate a guardian in their last will and testament, called a testamentary guardianship. When parents name a guardian in their will, they are recommending to the court that a particular person be named the guardian of their children when they die. The nomination has no effect until the will is admitted to probate after the parent dies. If a will is not probated, the person named as the guardian will not have authority to make decisions on behalf of the child. There is also no guarantee that the court will appoint the person nominated in the will as the child's guardian. The court must decide whether the child's best interests will be promoted by appointing the chosen guardian. Parents are not around to defend their choice of guardian if the will or the nomination of the guardian is contested. In addition, because it takes time for a will to be probated—proven valid or invalid—the person nominated as guardian in the will may not exercise that power immediately. A temporary guardian may have to be appointed or the children may be forced into the foster care system until a guardian is appointed if other informal arrangements are not made for the children's care.

For all of these reasons, a testamentary guardianship is less useful than a standby guardianship for parents who anticipate the need to choose a guardian for their children. However, if standby guardianship is not an option in the state, appointing a guardian in a will is one way for parents to make plans for the future care of their children after the parent's death.

Temporary and Limited Delegation of Parental Authority

A parent whose children are being cared for by a grandparent may be unwilling to agree to the grandparent becoming the child's legal guardian. However, the parent may be willing to give the grandparent limited authority to make certain decisions or carry out certain parental obligations.

Some states have enacted laws that authorize parents to convey the authority to make medical and educational decisions to an adult on behalf of their children, without going to court or consenting to the appointment of a guardian. In some states, this delegation can be made through a general or special power of attorney. In others, the law provides for special forms to be completed by parents. In a few states, grandparent caregivers are given some limited powers to consent to medical treatment if the parents are absent or do not object.

Powers of Attorney

Powers of attorney are written documents that authorize another person (the "agent" or "attorney in fact") to perform some duty for the person giving the power of attorney (the "principal"). By signing a power of attorney, parents can authorize other adults to make decisions on behalf of their minor children when they are absent or otherwise unable to handle such matters themselves.

Some states have enacted laws that explicitly give parents the right to delegate decision-making concerning their children to others for a limited period, by executing a power of attorney. In these states, a parent or guardian of a minor may delegate to another person, for a period ranging from between 60 days to 1 year, any powers regarding the care, custody or property of a child, except for the power to consent to the child's marriage or adoption.[3]

In other states, parents may be able to use general powers of attorney to give grandparents decision-making powers during their absence. In these states, powers of attorney are most often used to provide authority over financial decisions and may not be uniformly accepted in places where grandparents would use them—in schools to enroll children or in hospitals to consent to the children's medical care. New York State's power of attorney law, for example, provides for a statutory short form power of attorney lists a series of transactions that the principal can convey to the agent. Among the list of transactions is a provision that allows the principal to grant the agent authority over "personal relationships and affairs." The form itself does not define this term. However, the law defines "personal relationships and affairs" as the authority "to provide usual educational facilities" and "to provide, whenever necessary, medical, dental and surgical care, hospitalization and custodial care for the spouse, children and other dependents of the principal."

Powers of attorney can be *durable*—to last during the principal's incapacity—and *springing*—to become effective upon a certain date or event. The rights of the parents are not terminated with powers of attorney, parents still have legal custody of their children and the powers can be revoked by the parent at any time.

Consent Legislation

Some states have enacted legislation that specifically allows parents to authorize an adult to consent to school enrollment or medical care for their children without first going to court. Consent legislation usually involves authorization to act on behalf of a child, which can be effective for a certain period, or until terminated by the parent. Hospitals, doctors, or other health care practitioners are not held liable for reasonably relying on properly executed affidavits granting such authority.

Washington, DC, has responded to the need to give grandparents and other relative caregivers the authority to consent to medical care, without court involvement, by enabling parents, legal guardians or legal custodians of minor children to give the authority to consent to the immunization, medical, surgical, dental, developmental screening, or mental health examination or treatment of a child, to an adult, through a written statement or by use of a sample form.[4] Once the document is signed, it must be honored by providers who will not be held liable for relying on the document to treat minors if the reliance was reasonable.

California's **Caregiver's Authorization Affidavit**[5] authorizes a nonparent to enroll a child in school and consent to school-related, dental, and other medical care. California's statute is unique in that it has two parts. Part one allows a parent, a legal guardian, or a person with legal custody to authorize another adult to enroll a child in school and to consent to school related and other medical care. The law also provides for situations where parents are not available to convey the needed authority. Part two of California's law authorizes grandparents and other relative caregivers to consent to school enrollment and medical care for the children in their care in the absence of the parent. Caregivers may consent after signing an affidavit that states either that they have advised one or both parents of their intent to obtain the authority to consent and have received no objection, or that they are unable to contact the parent or parents.

This two-part legislation is important because it provides for two scenarios: one where the parents are available and planning for their children's care and also for when the parents are not available or not acting on behalf of their children. The California affidavit is signed under penalty of perjury, is valid for one year after the date it is signed and persons who rely on the affidavit in good faith and in the absence of actual knowledge to the contrary, face no liability. The law is attractive because it provides for a temporary delegation of parental authority and a way for grandparents and other relatives to get the needed authority without having to go to court. The parents' rights are not terminated or suspended and children receive the educational and medical care they need.

Legislation that removes the barriers to medical and educational care for children being cared by grandparents and other relative caregivers is imperative where relatives are the primary caregivers of children, do not have a legal relationship to them and are having difficulty enrolling children in school and consenting to their medical care. Consent legislation is an attractive option to parents because their rights are not terminated or suspended, the authority they convey is revocable at will, after a brief or extended period, and they do not have to go to court. The legislation is also attractive to grandparents and other relative caregivers because they obtain the ability to adequately provide for the child's educational and medical care without first having to go through an adversarial proceeding with the child's parents to get the legal authority to make decisions on behalf of the children in their care.

Consent legislation similar to California law has opponents who believe that such laws interfere with a parent's right to custody of their children because it allows caregivers to obtain the right to make legal decisions on behalf of children—something that only parents can do—without a court order. Where the parents are dead, grandparents should be advised to seek guardianship—the legal right to make decisions on behalf of their grandchildren in their parent's absence. However, where grandparents who are the primary caregivers of their grandchildren do not wish to go to court because they wish to avoid an adversarial proceeding with their children and where parents are unwilling to convey the proper authority to the grandparent, it is helpful to have a mechanism that will temporarily allow grandparents and other relatives the ability to respond properly to the needs of the children in their care. Consent legislation ensures that children receive the educational and medical care they need when in their grandparents' care. The legislation allows grandparents to avoid adversarial proceedings to obtain the legal right to make decisions and properly care for their grandchildren while at the same time safeguards the right of the parents.

Notarized Documents

Some parents give grandparents notarized documents conveying the authority to consent to medical care or school enrollment for their children. Although these documents may not give grandparents the legal right to make decisions on behalf of their grandchildren, they may in fact help grandparents enroll their grandchildren in school, apply for benefits, and get some medical care for them. Notarized letters do not affect the rights of parents to make decisions on behalf of their children and allow parents to return and regain custody of their children at any time, without first going to court.

Voluntary Foster Care Placement

When parents are unable to care for their children because of illness, homelessness, or other reasons, voluntary placement in foster care may be an option. A child can enter the foster care system involuntarily—through an abuse or neglect proceeding—or voluntarily—as when parents voluntarily place their children with a child welfare agency.

Voluntary placement agreements are documents signed by the parent, legal guardian, or other person responsible for the child which transfer legal custody of the child to a child welfare agency. The agreement can provide for the return of the child upon a specific date or event and can state who will be allowed to visit the child or even who should take care of the child. The agreement can also provide for visits between the child and the parent. In some states, like New York, the child welfare agency must try to locate relatives, like grandparents, to care for the child if the parent has not specified who should care for the child. The parent's rights are not terminated under a Voluntary Placement Agreement. Parents should consult with a lawyer before voluntarily placing a child in foster care to ensure that they understand and agree to the terms and conditions under which they are making the placement. It is important that parents understand that the agency, may, on being asked by the parent to return the child, institute proceedings to show abuse or neglect and thereby delay or prevent the return of the child to the parent.

Grandparents in whose care a child is placed under a voluntary placement agreement may be eligible for a foster care subsidy to help them with the child's needs, as the child is legally in the custody of the state. Voluntary placements allow parents to plan for the care of their children when they are unable to care for them and may provide relatives with financial assistance pending the parent's resumption of care. Placement in foster care is meant to be a temporary arrangement. If the parent is not able to resume care for the child within a specified period, the parent's rights may be terminated in a court proceeding. If the grandparent foster parent is not willing to adopt the child, the child may be placed with another adoptive family.

Open Adoptions

Adoptions are formal legal arrangements that sever the rights and responsibilities of biological parents and that allow other persons to acquire the rights and incur the responsibilities of a parent in relation to a child. The consent of parents to the adoption is required, otherwise the biological parent's rights must be terminated in a legal proceeding by proving, for example, abandonment, surrender, mental illness, or retardation.

In an open adoption, the adoptive parent becomes the child's legal parent and is responsible for the support and care of the child. The biological parent agrees to give the child up for adoption and have his or her parental rights terminated contingent on an agreement with the adoptive parent that the biological parent may have some contact with the child after the adoption. Reserving the ability to communicate with the child does not give the biological parents an automatic right to the communication but gives them the right to go to court to request the communication if it is denied by the adoptive parent. Even in open adoptions, the court will only order visitation if it finds that it is in the child's best interest. This option often appeals to parents, who will still have some communication with their children, and to grandparents who want to give their grandchildren stability but also wish to maintain a relationship with the child's biological parents.[6]

Where Parents Have Not Planned for the Care of Their Children by Others

When a child's parents have died, have abandoned the child, or are absent from the home and planning for the future care of the child has not occurred, a legal vacuum, if not an actual vacuum, exists that must be filled. If grandparents or other relatives are willing to assume responsibility for the child, the actual vacuum may be filled quickly, as when grandparents move into the home of the deceased or absent parent or take the child to the grandparents' home and begin to care for the child. (If no adult assumes informal responsibility for the child, child welfare authorities are required to take custody of the child.) However, the legal vacuum still exists, and if legal steps are not taken to fill that legal vacuum, grandparents may experience difficulties carrying out some of their caretaking responsibilities. For example, grandparents may have difficulty enrolling their grandchildren in school, obtaining medical treatment, or obtaining government benefits for their grandchild. Even if planning has occurred, legal steps may be necessary to effectuate the planning. For example, a designated standby guardian will have to go to court to be appointed the child's guardian; a guardian nominated in a will must be appointed guardian by the probate court.

If a child's parents are deceased or have abandoned the child, a guardian may be appointed to assume caretaking responsibilities. Depending on the circumstances, a guardian may be appointed over the child's person, property, or both. Most state statutes require that the child's parents either be deceased or consent to the guardianship. If the parent has abandoned the child and his or her whereabouts are unknown, a court may appoint a guardian without that parent's consent. In other states, a guardian may be appointed if the parent is found to be unfit and the appointment of a guardian is in the child's best interests.

A guardian of the person may generally make any decisions concerning the upbringing of the child. A guardian of the property may manage the income and assets belonging to the child, usually with court supervision. A guardian is a fiduciary, owing a duty of care to the child and accountable to the court. A guardian may be removed if he or she fails to competently perform his or her duties. In some states, after he or she is appointed, a guardian may designate a standby guardian to assume the duties of guardianship in the event that he or she dies or becomes incapacitated while the ward is still a minor.[7]

A guardian does not assume financial responsibility for the child. Therefore, the child will be eligible for public benefits without regard to the guardian's income or resources.

In some states, the caretaker of a child whose parents are deceased or absent may file for custody. Custody is generally regarded as a mechanism that provides for physical care of the child without compromising other rights the parent might have to make major decisions. Grandparents with legal custody generally have no power to manage the finances of a child, but for a child with no property that needs to be managed, there may not be any practical difference between custody and guardianship.

Grandparents who have legal custody also do not assume financial responsibility for the child and the child will be eligible for public benefits without regard to their grandparent's income or assets.

Involuntary Procedures

There are also times when the child's parent is still alive and may not be able to appropriately care for the child but is also unwilling to delegate decision-making responsibility to another person who is in fact taking care of the child on a day-to-day basis. The parent may be physically or mentally ill, addicted to drugs or alcohol, or simply too young to be able to be a parent. Grandparents in this situation faces difficult dilemmas. Their caretaking is made difficult by the fact that they have no legal authority to make the everyday decisions that need to be made. However, to the extent that their child allows them to make decisions and care for their grandchild, they are able to accomplish much that needs to be done for their grandchild. If they attempt to obtain legal authority to act over the objection of their child, they may lose the ability to do anything and their grandchildren may be placed in a more vulnerable position with an abusive parent or removed to foster care with strangers. Many grandparents are reluctant to cause their children to lose legal custody of their children or to lose their parental rights.

Because of the risks inherent in involuntary solutions, we advise that every attempt be made to enlist the cooperation of the parent, using the mechanisms described in the previous sections. When involuntary solutions are considered, grandparents should be thoroughly counseled about the risks and benefits to themselves, their child, and their grandchild.

Informal Arrangements

Many grandparents choose to continue to act as informal caretakers without legal authority. If the parent is available, the parent can consent to medical treatment, when necessary, and enroll the child in school. The parent can be involved to the extent possible in the day to day decisions and grandparents can step in when necessary. Depending on the community, grandparents may be informally recognized as the real decision makers and caretakers.

A few states have laws that specifically authorize grandparents to consent to medical care in the absence of the parent.[8] Parents do not have to delegate the authority to consent, the consent is available in the parent's absence and there is no liability to the provider for treating the child. The laws are not uniform and contribute to the confusion over when grandparents can consent to medical care if they have not been appointed the guardian or do not have legal custody of their grandchildren.

Kinship Foster Care

In some states, grandparents become formal caretakers for their grandchildren through the foster care system. All states have a mechanism for protecting children who are neglected or abused by their parents. In most states, when children are removed from their parents because of abuse or neglect, the preferred solution is placement on a short or longer-term basis with a relative who is approved as a foster parent.[9]

In most cases, the state child welfare agency has custody and control of the child, and the grandparent foster parents report to the child welfare agency or a private foster care agency. The grandparent foster parents do not have the right to make medical decisions for the child, must get permission to travel out of the state with the child, and may be prohibited from using corporal punishment. The child may be removed from the grandparent foster parents if the child welfare agency believes that the foster parents are not providing appropriate care. In most states with large kinship foster care programs, grandparent foster parents receive a foster care payment that is much larger than they would receive if they were the guardians and the child were on public assistance.

Generally, grandparents who have voluntarily assumed responsibility for a child are not able to become a foster parent. It is only after children have been removed from their parents by the state child welfare agency that foster care placement with grandparents is possible. If the child is already living with grandparents in a safe environment, removal from the parents is not required.

Foster care is supposed to be a short-term solution for children who cannot be cared for by their parents. For many children in foster care, reunification with their parents is the goal. When the child welfare agency believes that the child's parent is able to care for the child and the child will be safe, the child will be returned to the parent. If a court determines that the parent will not be able to care for the child, the parent's rights may be terminated and the child's permanency goal changed to adoption. In that case, if the grandparent does not wish to adopt the child, the child may be placed with other adoptive parents and, once adopted, ties to the grandparent may be severed.

Subsidized Guardianship

Grandparent who have been foster parents may be able to become the child's guardian.[10] In that case, foster care payments would end as, in some cases, would the supervision of the child welfare agency. A few states are experimenting with the idea of subsidized guardianship. When a state has a subsidized guardianship program, if children who have been in foster care are not able to return to their parents, and their grandparents are not willing to adopt the children, the grandparents can be appointed the children's guardian. These guardians receive payments that may be less that the foster care payment but more that the public assistance payment.[11] Because of the cost to the states, very few states are implementing subsidized guardianship programs.

Ex-Parte Temporary Custody Orders

Ex-parte temporary custody orders are granted by a court upon the application of one party, like a grandparent, in the absence of notice to the party who is adversely affected, like the parent or legal guardian of a child. These orders allow grandparents to obtain legal custody on a temporary basis, without first going through a custody proceeding, when parents come back into the picture and try to resume custody of the child. Ex-parte temporary custody orders are important in situations where grandparents need immediate relief to protect their grandchildren, like in situations where drug-addicted or abusive parents return home and want to regain custody of their children. In states where these orders are available, grandparents can go to court to get temporary custody of their grandchildren by showing that it would be in the child's best interests to award temporary custody to them.

Minnesota's Relative ex-parte custody order[12] presumes that it is in the child's best interest to grant temporary custody to a relative in whose home the child has resided for a period of 12 months or more under certain circumstances, including where the parent has not had contact with the child on a regular basis, has not participated in the child's well-being for 6 months, or has not provided the child with food, clothing, shelter, health care, education, and other care for the child's physical, emotional health, or development. Parents must be served and a court hearing is then held to determine legal custody. At this hearing, if the judge finds that the parent has had contact with the child on a regular basis for 6 months, the child is returned to the parent; if temporary physical custody is ordered because of the parent's failure to provide for the child, the court will then determine custody.

Connecticut allows an application for immediate temporary custody to be granted ex-parte only where the caretaker of the child signs an affidavit, under penalty of perjury, which states how custody was obtained, the length of time they have had custody and specific facts that would justify granting immediate temporary custody without the required hearing.[13] The court grants the application if it finds that the child was not taken from or kept from the parent or guardian, that there is substantial risk that the child would be taken away from the jurisdiction of the court before the hearing or that the child would have serious physical illness or injury before a court hearing could be held. If the ex-parte temporary custody is granted, notice of the hearing is sent to both parents at least 5 days before the hearing.

Oregon's ex-parte temporary order of custody[14] is available only if the individual requesting the order is present in court and presents an affidavit that alleges the child is in immediate danger. If the court finds, based on the testimony and affidavit, that the child is in immediate danger, the temporary order of custody will be granted. The individual requesting custody must provide the court with their telephone number and an address where they can be reached and a copy of the order, and the affidavit must be served on the parent or other party, who may then request a hearing with the court while the order is in effect. The hearing is held within 14 to 21 days after it is requested.

Where available, ex-parte custody orders ensure the safety of the children until the court can determine whether a change in custody is warranted.

Custody

In some states, grandparents who have voluntarily assumed responsibility for a grandchild can ask a court to award them custody of the grandchild. If the parent of the child objects, the grandparents must prove that the parent is unfit or has abandoned the child and that custody with the grandparent is in the grandchild's best interests. In a custody proceeding, parents may have the right to a court-appointed lawyer if they cannot afford a lawyer. Depending on the circumstances, a lawyer or guardian ad litem may be appointed for the child. It may be difficult for grandparents to get a lawyer to represent them if they cannot afford to hire a one.

Adoption

Adoption is the way to permanently give parental rights to a nonparent. Generally, the biological parents must either be deceased, consent to the adoption, or their parental rights must be terminated by a court before a child may be adopted. When children are in foster care and cannot be reunited with their biological parents, the foster care agency may go to court to terminate the parents' parental rights, thus freeing the child for adoption. In many states, foster parents who have been caring for a child for a certain period have priority to be adoptive parents, once the biological parents' rights have been terminated. Many children who have been in foster care are eligible for subsidies if they are adopted.

Adoption usually ends all contact between the child and the child's biological family, but in some states, contact between the child and biological relatives may be maintained, if such contacts are found to be in the child's best interest. Grandparents who adopt their grandchildren assume all the rights and responsibilities of the biological parents including the duty to provide financial support to the children. Thus, children who have been adopted by a grandparent will receive only public assistance if their grandparents qualify for public assistance. Adoption ensures that there will no longer be challenges to a grandparent's custody and that children have a permanent home.

Conclusion

The legal system often imperfectly responds to the needs of grandparents who are taking care of their grandchildren. Grandparents who are the primary caretakers of their grandchildren need to be informed about the legal options available to them which may assist them in their caretaking responsibilities. In this chapter, we have discussed the legal options that may be available to grandparent caregivers and when they might be appropriate. It is important to remember that many of these options will be possible only if the parents agree, are found to be unfit, or have already died. Whenever possible, grandparents should be encouraged to work with their children to obtain the legal authority necessary to appropriately take care of their grandchildren. When adversary proceedings are necessary, grandparents should be clear about the risks and benefits before proceeding. Finally, if the child's parents will never be able to care for them, grandparents should be encouraged to take steps to provide long-term stability for their grandchild and make plans for the care of the child should the grandparent be unable to do so.

Notes

1. One way to access particular state law relevant to grandparent caregivers is to access the web site *Grandparent caregivers: A national guide*: www.igc.org/justice/cjc/lspc.manual/cover.html.

2. Standby Guardianship laws exist in the following states: California (Cal. Prob. Code ß 2105(f) (West 1991); Connecticut (Conn. Gen. Stat. Ann. ß 45(a)-624 et seq. (West 1998)); Florida (Fla. Stat. Ann. § 744.304 (West 1996)); Illinois (755 Ill. Ann. Stat. § 5/11-5.3 (Smith-Hurd 1996)); Iowa (Iowa Code Ann. § 633.560 et seq. (West 1992)); Maryland (Md. Code Ann. Est. & Trust § 13-901 et seq. (Supp. 1995)); Massachusetts (Mass. Gen. Laws Ann. ch. 201, § 2A (West Supp. 1996)); New Jersey (N.J. Stat. Ann. § 3B:12-68 et seq (West Supp. 1996)); and New York (N.Y. Surr. Ct. Proc. Act §1726 (McKinney 1996)).

3. The states are Arizona: Ariz. Rev. Stat. Ann. § 14-51-4 (West 1991)(6 months); Alaska: Alaska Stat. § 13.26.020 (1991) (1 year); Colorado: Colo. Rev. Stat. Ann § 15-14-104 (West 1991) (9 months); Idaho: Idaho Code § 15-5-104 (1992) (6 months; 12 months if parent is in the military serving outside the U.S.); Maine: Me. Rev. Stat. Ann. tit. 18-A § 5-104 (West 1991) (6 months); Michigan: Mich. Comp. Laws Ann. § 700.405 (West 1992) (6 months); Minnesota: Minn. Stat. Ann. § 524.5-505 (West 1992) (6 months); Missouri: Mo. Ann. Stat. § 475.024 (Vernon 1992) (1 year); Montana: Mont. Code Ann. § 72-5-103 (1991) (6 months); Nebraska: Neb. Rev. Stat. § 30-2604 (1991) (6 months); New Jersey: N.J. Stat. Ann. § 3B:12-39 (West 1992) (6 months); North Dakota: N.D. Cent. Code § 30.1-26-04 (1992); Oregon: Or. Rev. Stat.

§ 126.030 (1991) (6 months; or 12 months if to a school administrator); Utah: Utah Code Ann. § 75-5-103 (1992) (6 months); Indiana: Ind. Code Ann. § 29-3-9-1 (West 1992) (60 days during which the parent is physically incapacitated or absent from the parent's resident); Alabama (Ala Code § 26-2A-7 (1991) (1 year).

4. D.C. Code Ann. § 16-4701 (1981). The parent, legal guardian, or legal custodian can convey the authority in a written statement. The written statement does not have to have any specific language to convey the authority. The legislation includes a suggested form that can be distributed to interested parties to ensure education and availability.

5. Cal. Family Code § 6550 (West 1998), Cal. Educ. Code § 48204 (West 1998).

6. For a discussion of open adoptions and the adoptive parent's perspective see Siegal, D. L. (1993, January). Open adoptions of infants: Adoptive parents perceptions of advantages and disadvantages, *Journal of the National Association of Social Workers, 38*, 15

7. See e.g., N.Y. Surr. Ct Proc. Act. §§ 1726.3(a), 1726.3(b) (McKinney 1996); Conn. Gen. Stat. § 45a-624 (West 1998).

8. The states are Texas (see Tex. Fam. Code §32.001 (1996)), Florida (see Fla. Stat. Ann. §743.0645 [West 1998]), and Mississippi (see Miss. Code Ann. §41-41-3 [1993, 1998 Supp.]).

9. Relatives may not be prohibited from becoming foster parents, Miller v. Youakim, 440 U.S. 125 (1974); however, some states, notably, New York, Illinois, and California, have created special programs for relatives who are foster parents.

10. See Adoption and Safe Families Act of 1977, which allows states to seek the appointment of a guardian of a child in foster care who cannot be reunited with her parents rather than terminate parental rights and place the child up for adoption. 42 U.S.C. § 675 as amended by PL 105-89.

11. The states are Alaska, California, Colorado, Hawaii, Illinois, Massachusetts, Nebraska, New Mexico, South Dakota, and Washington States. California pays subsidies only to nonrelative guardians.

12. See Minn. Stat. § 518.158 (1997). See also Cal. Fam. Code § 3062 (West 1994); Ark. Stat. Ann. § 28-65-207 (1991); Conn. Gen. Stat. § 45a-607 (1993, 1998 Supp.); Oregon Revised Statutes § 107.097 (1995).

13. Conn. Gen. Stat. §45a-607 (1997).

14. Oregon Revised Statutes § 107.097 (1995).

Chapter 9

Planning for Permanence

Martha Johns

Permanency planning, the guiding principle of the child welfare system, is intended to limit the number of children who enter foster care and reduce the amount of time children spend in out-of-home care (Sudia, 1986; Seaberg, 1988). It encompasses a mix of family-centered casework and legal strategies designed to assure that children have safe, caring, stable and lifetime families in which to grow up. It recognizes the importance of family and family life to the healthy development of a child. Permanency planning aims to reduce the trauma that separation and loss have on children when they enter foster care as well as the detrimental effects on children of remaining in foster care for extended periods.

Although the permanency planning process was first legislated with the passage of the federal Adoption Assistance and Child Welfare Act of 1980, Public Law 96-272, the movement to find safety and stability for children can be traced back to the early development of the child welfare system. Permanency planning as a strategy to preserve families cannot be examined without including the role of kin, specifically grandparents, as a part of the extended family caregiving system.

This chapter examines the evolution of permanency planning within the child welfare system, reviews the laws that govern its application, explores the dilemmas that confront grandparents and other kinship care providers and finally discusses practice and policy implications.

What Is Meant by Permanency Planning

Effective permanency planning requires that family members, caretakers, and professionals work together in partnership to pursue the common goals of protection, permanence and well-being for children. This mutual effort recognizes the strengths within the family system and the importance of family relationships, culture, and community.

Multiple definitions of permanency planning have emerged in the literature. It has been described as a philosophy:

- Permanency planning as a philosophy seeks first to preserve and support the child's biological family as the most natural environment and when this is not possible, to secure an adoptive family (Cole, 1985).
- [A]s a process . . . it is the systemic process of carrying out, within a brief time-limited period a set of goal-directed activities designed to help children live in families that offer continuity of relationships with nurturing parents or caretakers and an opportunity to establish lifetime relationships (Maluccio & Fein, 1983). It is a process of helping a child live in a home which offers the hope of establishing lifetime relationships . . . all children have a right to a permanent family. [A]s a collection of programs: . . . delivered in behalf of children, in the effort to secure for each child a caring, legally recognized, continuous family in which to grow up (Cole, 1985).
- Permanency planning acknowledges the value of rearing children in a family setting, recognizes the primacy of parent-child attachment and the significance of the biological family in human connectedness, it also incorporates the view that stability and continuity promote a child's development (Anderson, 1995).

The struggle to define permanency planning reflects the fact that the child welfare system's permanency goal and the permanency goal of families in the system are often in conflict. For families who enter the system either voluntarily or as the result of an involuntary removal, the precipitating problem is often one that requires long-term intervention. The time frames established by the child welfare system assume that families who enter the system require short-term interventions to resolve their problems

Foster care was designed as such a temporary measure—an opportunity for short-term crisis driven intervention that would allow parents to either reestablish their care giving/provider role or free their children for alternative care or adoption. The foster care system has not lived up to this promise; children continue to languish in care far too long without either reunification with their birth parents or adoption by caregivers who can provide them with lifetime families.

Permanency planning is guided by a set of beliefs about the importance of family life, consistent relationships, and community connections for children's healthy growth and development. It recognizes that families are society's primary source of strength, support, education, and socialization for children and that children's well-being is intimately linked to families well-being. Although families have the primary responsibility for their children's development, all families need community resources and supports to enable them to fulfill their responsibilities effectively.

Historical Development

An early study, "Children in Need of Parents" (Maas & Engler, 1959), of the public and voluntary child welfare system indicated that children removed from their birth parents and placed with foster families for what was presumed to be temporary care often lingered for long periods of time; an average of three years, in these "temporary" placements.

Results of the study also founded neglect and abandonment the most common reasons for placement, followed by death, illness, economic hardship and marital conflict. Even though many of the children in care had at least one parent alive, parents did not visit and generally had no plans for resuming care of their children. Two thirds were unlikely to return home and most of the children experienced numerous placements while in care. Foster care, developed as a temporary arrangement for children while providing help to their parents in order to hasten reunification of the family, was not meeting its goals.

These studies and subsequent research documented children's lengthy stays in care, lack of contact between social worker and family, a paucity of visiting between child and family, and the neediness of families with children in care (Fanshel & Shinn, 1978; Shyne & Schroeder, 1978; Wiltse & Gambrill, 1974). Foster care, designed as temporary care, was not only being used as long-term care, it was failing to fulfill its mandate to reunite children with their families.

It was not until the 1973 Oregon project, "Freeing Children for Permanent Placement," that the concept of permanency planning became a widely accepted practice strategy. The Oregon project found that, through aggressive casework and planning techniques, children placed in foster care could be returned to their biological families or could be placed through adoption (Pike, 1976).

Foster care drift, identified as large numbers of children removed from their families, remaining in foster care and drifting from one placement to another, continued throughout the 1970s (Fanshel & Shinn 1978). The trauma of separation and loss experienced by many of these children, might have been avoided if focused, in-home prevention efforts had been made with their families prior to placement. Child welfare advocates and professionals recognized that these children were spending too many years "lost in the system, growing up without attachment to family and belonging to no one—despite the fact that both research and practical experience underscored the need for secure attachment for the healthy, long-term development of children" (Bowlby, 1963).

During the 1970s, the permanency planning movement continued to gain momentum. Advocates for children pushed for legislation that would address the developmental needs of the close to 500,000 children who were currently in the child welfare system.

Passage of the Adoption Assistance and Child Welfare Act of 1980, Public Law (P. L.) 96-272, represented the first major federal legislation to address the complex issues of permanency planning in child welfare. It set forth placement goals as (a) reunification, (b) adoption, (c) guardianship, and (d) long term out-of-home care. Its broad goal was to reform the framework of the child welfare system by developing and encouraging practices that would strengthen families to avoid placements or reunite children with their birth parents (NRCPP legislative summary). This legislation addressed the issue of permanency and foster care drift, long a concern of child welfare advocates.

Federal Laws

During 1980 to1997, several major legislative initiatives have attempted to address concerns in the child welfare system around the numbers of children in care and the length of time they spend in care without either returning to their birth families or finding new families. Before this period, Congress, in 1974, passed the Child Abuse Prevention and Treatment Act (CAPTA), which provided funds to states to develop programs and services for abused and neglected children and tied these federal funds to state laws establishing a system for identifying and responding to child abuse and neglect. The passage of CAPTA was in response to growing awareness of child abuse and the link between child abuse and placement in foster care.

In addition to these developments in child protection, the civil rights and deinstitutionalization movements led to a greater emphasis on "least restrictive placements" and the rights of children, biological families, foster and adoptive parents. Definitions of "adoptable" children were expanded to include older and disabled children. Concurrently many human service professionals began to embrace an "ecological perspective," rather than focusing on a child in isolation, these practitioners were concerned with understanding the child within the context of the family and the family within the context of their community, culture, and social setting.

The Indian Child Welfare Act (ICWA) P. L. 95-608 passed in 1978 recognized tribal courts as having jurisdiction in child welfare issues involving Native Americans and was the first legislation to acknowledge a child's right to ethnic and cultural identity. ICWA makes no specific reference to kinship care, although the provision of the act that recommended placement in the "least restrictive" and "most family-like" setting has been interpreted by many state policy makers as justifying or mandating a relative preference (U.S. DHSS 1997). Together, these related social trends promoted a focus on permanence in child welfare practice and eventually resulted in state and federal child welfare legislation.

The Adoption Assistance and Child Welfare Act of 1980, P. L. 96-272, guided by the philosophy of permanency planning, provided federal funding to the states to support efforts to restore children to their birth families or free them for adoption. The major provisions of 96-272 required states to:

Prevent Out-of-Home Placement

- Making reasonable efforts in each case prior to the placement of a child in foster care to prevent or eliminate the need for removal of the child from his or her home.
- Preventing the unnecessary separation of children from their families by identifying family problems, assisting families in resolving their problems, and preventing break-up of the family where the prevention of child removal is desirable or possible.

Promote Family Restoration

- Making reasonable efforts in each case to make it possible for the child to return home and directing social services toward the accomplishment of restoring to their families children who have been removed, by the provision of services to the child and the families.

Implementing Placement Guidelines

- Assuring that the child's placement is (a) in the least restrictive (most family-like) setting available; (b) in close proximity to the parents' home; and (c) is consistent with the best interests and special needs of the child.

Other Placement Outcomes

- Placing children in suitable adoptive homes, in cases where restoration to the biological family is not possible or appropriate.
- Assuring the adequate care of children away from their homes, in cases where the child cannot be returned home or cannot be placed for adoption.

Other Provisions

- Establishing planning and review mechanisms (case plan, administrative review) and financial aid (adoption assistance, foster care maintenance).
- P. L. 96-272 required state departments of social services to demonstrate to the appropriate court that they had made reasonable efforts to prevent out-of-home placement and to reunify the family to be eligible for federal funding.

There are at least two compelling reasons why permanency planning is the primary view point of American child welfare; (a) child development knowledge of the importance of attachment signified that it was *in the best interests* of children to be raised within a family that offers hope of life-long relationships and continuity; (b) three decades of studies of children's experiences in out-of-home care documented the troubling effects of drifting aimlessly in foster care. Entry into out-of-home care appeared at times to be precipitous or at least preventable if appropriate services or supports were available to families in crisis. Achieving permanence for children in a continuous relationship with a caring adult *reduced the harm to children* and families that resulted from unnecessary separations or unnecessary prolongation of out-of-home care (Anderson 1997).

Unfortunately the passage of P. L. 96-272 did not bring about significant change in the child welfare system, as the mandated services that were required to promote family reunification frequently were not provided. A study of children who were returned to their biological families found that a majority of the families needed housing, medical and dental services, income, counseling, special education, legal services, recreation services and employment training or counseling (Fein et al,. 1983).

The broad reductions in federal spending for social programs during the Reagan administration, ended support for major demonstration programs that were designed to respond to the needs of reunified families. As a consequence, the funds to provide these services were never provided.

Despite a lack of funding for social programs in the early 1980s, permanency planning began to have an impact—reducing the numbers of children in foster care through increased efforts to reunify children with their families and by more aggressive recruitment of adoptive homes for children who could not return to their birth families.

By 1985, the national foster care population had been reduced to 265,000 children from a high in 1980 of more than 500,000 children. In addition many public and private agencies began to pilot innovative family support and family preservation services aimed at preventing unnecessary out-of-home placement while strengthening the ability of families to safely care for their children.

However, as the 1980s progressed, the number of children in foster care began to climb dramatically because of the combined effects of persistent poverty, the increased accessibility of inexpensive and highly addictive drugs, the emergence of HIV and AIDS, unplanned teen pregnancies, lack of decent and affordable housing in distressed communities, and increases in domestic and community violence. Nationally close to 500,000 children were once again in foster care.

During the same period and into the early 1990s, there was a growing national dissatisfaction with child welfare efforts. Several factors contributed to this including a number of high profile child deaths, foster care caseloads that had risen again to 1980s heights, less access to needed services for an increased number of high-risk families, a financial system that at times seemed to promote long stays in foster care, and rules and practices that made it difficult for some parents to adopt foster children awaiting families.

P. L. 96-272, required states to make reasonable efforts to prevent the need for removal of children from their homes or to reunify them with their families. However, over a number of years, multiple interpretations, practices and judicial rulings resulted in confusion about how to balance efforts to preserve children's families with their need for safety.

Given these concerns, on November 19, 1997, President Clinton signed the Adoption and Safe Families Act, P. L. 105-89, (ASFA) into law. ASFA represents a bipartisan effort to effect change in the foster care system. It is the most significant child welfare reform since the Adoption Assistance and Child Welfare Act of 1980. The legislation attempts to refocus attention on child safety, to reduce overly long stays in foster care by moving children promptly into permanent homes, and to facilitate adoption of waiting children (NRCPP Legislative Summary). The legislation modifies the reasonable efforts requirements of 96-272, enacts adoption incentives and reauthorizes funding for family support and preservation programs.

The major provisions of ASFA are the following:

Enhancing the Safety of Children in
Home and in Out-of Home Care

- ASFA clarifies that a child's health and safety are paramount concerns in making decision about removing a child from or returning a child home.
- ASFA requires specific attention to safety in case planning, services, and case reviews for children in care or receiving services through the Title IV-B child welfare services program.
- Criminal record checks are required for perspective foster and adoptive parents before final placement of a child (unless a state opts out of the provision).

Reducing Foster Care Delays and Moving
Children into Permanent Homes

- Agencies may engage in concurrent planning, working simultaneously toward family reunification and adoption, without violating federal reasonable efforts requirements.
- The date by which a permanency planning hearing must be held is moved up from 18 to 12 months after a child's placement in foster care. It must be held within 30 days if a court decides that reasonable efforts to reunite child and family are not required. Foster parents, pre-adoptive parents and relatives caring for the child must be given notice of foster reviews and permanency planning hearing and allowed to participate. (They need not be made full parties, however).

Reasonable efforts must be made to implement the child's permanency plan. The steps taken must be documented in the child's case plan. States must use child specific recruitment efforts such as use of state, regional and national adoption exchanges (including electronic exchange systems) in finding adoptive homes.

Improving Permanency Options for Children

• ASFA seeks to reduce the use of long-term foster care by limiting permanency options at the 12 month hearing to return home (by a specified date), placement for adoption (with termination petition filed by a specified date), or establishment of legal guardianship. A child may be placed in another planned, permanent living arrangement only when compelling reasons for doing so are documented to the court, none of the prior options is appropriate, and no suitable relative is available to take custody.

• "Legal guardianship" is defined as a judicially created relationship between child and caretaker which is intended to be permanent and self-sustaining. The guardian given responsibility for the protection, custody, education, care and decision making for the child. (No change is made from prior law regarding funding for guardianships).

Efforts to Speed Permanency for Children

Mandatory filing of Termination of Parental Rights Petitions

States must initiate or join proceedings to terminate parental rights in three groups of cases, unless an exception applies. Concurrently, the state must identify, recruit, process and approve a qualified family to adopt each child. This is required when

• The child has been in state foster care for 15 of the most recent 22 months.

• A court has determined that a child is an abandoned infant under state law.

• One of the reasons for not pursuing reasonable efforts (other than aggravated circumstances) has been established (e.g., murder or manslaughter of another child, felony assault on child, or parental rights of a sibling terminated).

Exceptions: The exceptions follow:

- The child is being cared for by a relative (if the state has identified this as a reason for not terminating parental rights).
- There is a compelling reason why terminating parental rights would not be in the child's best interests (and the reason is documented in the case plan, available for court review).
- Reunification services were not provided to the child's family within the timeframe required by the child's case plan. (Dodson, 1998).

Provisions in the ASFA legislation recognize for the first time the role of relatives in out-of-home care, and as permanency resources. The shortened time frames for the termination of parental rights are modified when children are placed with relatives.

Legal guardianship is also recognized as a permanency option. A large percentage of children who live with grandparents or other relatives are in the legal custody of these caregivers. This arrangement is sanctioned by ASFA. Finally, relatives must be given notice of foster care reviews and permanency planning hearings (they need not be made full parties to, i.e. do not require legal representation). This change in the law is an important gain for grandparents who previously did not receive notice of hearings even though the outcome of these hearings effected the children in their care.

The Adoption and Safe Families Act holds out the promise for speeding adoption and reducing foster care stays for many children who are unable to return home and who might otherwise wait for years in foster care. States are faced with the challenge of implementing ASFA in ways that will ensure the safety of children while increasing families' access to services. As necessary changes are made in child welfare practice and systems, they must be governed by a philosophy that is family centered, culturally sensitive, and community based.

Permanency and Grandparent Caregivers

Planning for permanency with grandparents and other kinship caregivers poses a particular challenge. Placement within the kinship network is often perceived by the caregiver as a permanent arrangement. The concept of "permanency" as defined by the formal child welfare system is frequently at odds with the families' view of caregiving.

Despite the fact that close to 1 million children are being raised by their grandparents, the efforts of these grandparents were largely ignored by the child welfare system and in the laws that govern placements. Additionally, children who have been removed from their parents as a result of abuse or neglect are disproportionately minority and more often than not are placed with kin, primarily grandparents.

Approximately 85% of kinship caregivers in the formal kinship system are African-American grandmothers many of whom come from a long tradition of kin caregiving. It is widely recognized that parenting by kin has historically been employed as a survival strategy by a large number of African-American families (Hays & Mindel, 1973; Hill, 1977; Martin & Martin, 1978; Stack, 1974; Sudarkasa, 1988; Thornton, 1987).

The placement of children with relatives is not new, but before the 1980s this was not a typical arrangement in the formal child welfare system (Kusserow, 1992). Kinship care placements, as a permanency option, maintain children in their birth families, are more stable than traditional foster care placements and address the need for continuity of relationships, which is critical to the healthy growth and development of children.

The use of kinship care as a formal child welfare service dramatically increased in recent years as a result of many parents who are unable to care for their children due to substance abuse, HIV/AIDS, persistent poverty, homelessness, teenage pregnancy, family violence and disruption, divorce, mental illness, and incarceration of parents. The more complex the reason for children entering care, the more difficult the task of developing a plan for permanency that is consistent with the intent of the law and that recognizes the rights of families.

U.S. Census figures estimate that 4.3 million children live with grandparents or other relatives. Whereas most of these children live with their mothers in the homes of relatives, 878,000 live apart from both parents in their grandparents' homes. Of the approximately 400,000 children in the formal foster care system, nationally 150,000 live with relatives, primarily grandparents (CWLA, 1997).

This increase in the number of children coming into care and the increase in kinship placements posed new challenges to an already overburdened system. Kinship placements were disproportionately composed of minority children being cared for by relatives who were generally older than non–kin caregivers, with limited financial resources and two thirds of whom were also single grandmothers.

Using systems theory, Joe Crumbley (1997), examines some of the issues of separation and loss that impinge on the relationships between and among caregivers, birth parents and children in kinship care. Each member of the triad experiences a series of losses that include interruptions in the lifecycle; the future plans of the caregiver are put on hold, the caregiver suffers a loss of privacy, moves from supportive to primary caregiver, from friend to authority and feels a need to atone for birth parent's inadequate parenting.

The birth parent suffers a loss of relationships, roles, and purpose; moves from parent to relative; and is angry and resentful at the relative caregiver and agency as well as birth child for becoming attached. The child suffers similar feelings of loss and separation from the parent, emotional detachment and withdrawal, feels unwanted by birth parent, internalizes fault for causing the birth parent to give him or her away, and is angry at the birth parent for abandonment. The child is also embarrassed at being raised by a relative and the often visible differences indicating the relative caregiver is not the parent (i.e., age).

The following case example exemplifies these issues:

Ann E. is a 57-year-old single grandmother raising three grandchildren who are 3, 6, and 11 years old. The children have been in her care for the past 2 years. The children's mother, Pat, is currently in drug rehabilitation, her third such program in the past 4 years (this time she says it will work). Ann has another daughter and a son who have their own families and even though they try to help, they find it difficult to do so on a regular basis. Ann planned to return to school to pursue a degree in early childhood education when her kids were "grown and gone," but that now seems unlikely. Unfortunately, they are grown and gone, but she is left with three youngsters to raise.

The kinship allowance provides some assistance, the children are pretty well behaved, but miss their mother and want to know when she will come to see them. When she comes, it is like a visiting empress has arrived. Ann struggles with her feelings of anger at her daughter. She knows that if she does not make it this time that it is highly unlikely that she will ever be free of drugs. For the sake of her grandchildren, she would like to see their mother off drugs.

This is not the life that Ann had anticipated, "I did all that I could do for my children. . . . I did not expect to spend this time of my life as a caregiver." "I miss the life I used to have, I would give anything to have it back." Ann knows that she will have to a make a decision about what kind of long-term commitment she is willing to make for the children. The thought of terminating her daughter's parental rights does not "sit right with her." Her worker has begun to talk to her about making a decision, she is not sure that she has a choice. Her youngest grandson has asthma and a hearing loss, her grand-daughter is beginning to notice boys, the thought of going through adolescence again is a pretty frightening thought.

Ann says that at night she is so tired that when the kids go to bed, she follows. She feels caught in a maze and does not see a way out in the forseeable future.

Ann's plight represents the plight of the vast majority of grandparents in the child welfare system. In New York City, of the approximately 22,000 children in foster care, 11,000 are in kinship foster care. Of this number, 90% are Black, 4% are Latino, and 6.9% are White. The social, legal, financial, and emotional need of these families are of concern to the formal and to the informal system of care.

The quest for permanence in the placement of children initially focused on securing adoptive homes for children needing out-of-home care. More recently, this quest has come to focus on the need to preserve families of origin. These two strategies, although an essential part of an effective permanency effort, will not, by themselves, provide security for those children at risk of out-of-home placement. An analysis of each is needed to develop a holistic approach for meeting the permanency needs of African American as well as other children (Williams, 1991).

For African-American families who have historically cared for kin, the transition from informal care to formal care holds many challenges. LeProhn (1994) suggests that kin foster parents behaved more like biological parents by assuming more of the affective parenting responsibilities than nonrelative foster parents. A major benefit of kinship care is that it involves less disruption to the child because the child remains connected to their existing personal support network, community, and cultural background.

Conversely, several concerns have also been raised about kinship care. Fein and Maluccio (1992) suggest that there is the potential risk associated with contact with parents who may still be engaged in lifestyles that may pose a danger to the child and caregiver. An additional concern is that foster care payments may serve as a disincentive to reunification (Meyer & Link, 1990).

The attendant monitoring of relative caregivers necessitated by the receipt of foster care payments can be intimidating. Although families need the financial assistance, the designation of the home as a "kinship foster home" and the authority and control issues that emerge from this can create an atmosphere fraught with tension. For grandparent caregivers, the reality that the children in their care are actually in the custody of the state is difficult to accept. The restrictions and the need for approval of decisions regarding the child that were previously made independently brings the caregiver face to face with her loss of authority and control. The embarrassment of needing permission to take the grandchild out of the city or have an "approved" baby-sitter is one more opportunity to feel at fault—surely if she had been a better parent, her child would be capable of parenting her own child. The shame often attached to having to raise the grandchild and needing assistance to do so compounds feelings of helplessness.

Conclusion

Moving children through the child welfare system quicker is a laudable goal, the concern is that this fast track will not allow enough time for families to make appropriate decisions about the youngsters in their care. Is 12 months to permanency an unrealistic or an achievable goal? And if it is the former, what services need to be in place to achieve this goal? Approximately, 75% of the children who come into care do so because of substance abuse, either directly or as a result of having been neglected by substance abusing parents. What are the realities that confront parents who want to get off drugs? Is the formal system able to provide the necessary supports and services to birth parents to enable them to resume their roles as parents.

Planning for permanency with relative caregivers is a complex task, complicated by familial relationships that are incongruent with the demands of the child welfare system. These inconsistencies are a result of trying to fit what has been an informal system of care into a system that was designed to work with voluntary care providers who sought the responsibility of caregiving and understood the role that the child welfare system would play in their lives. This is but one of the problems of trying to fit a response to a social anomaly into a system of care that was developed without thought or consideration of birth familes.

Should a separate system of care be designed for relative caregivers? What have we learned about these families, and how they fit within the current system during the past seven years? Do we believe that the recent changes brought about by the ASFA will encourage families to make permanency decisions that coincide with the child welfare system's view of permanency? Or will we find that families who opt out of the system will become more impoverished and children in these families will suffer unnecessarily? Are we then creating a large permanent underclass composed of largely minority youngsters and their caregivers who have no hope of ever realizing the American dream?

If permanency is a viable option for children in the formal child welfare system, then we must take on the responsibility of assuring all children an equal opportunity for a lifetime, nurturing family, preferably within their family of birth. Absent appropriate caregivers within their family system, then every effort should be made to recruit an adoptive family that will meet their needs for nurturance and a safe secure future.

References

Anderson, G. A., Ryan, A. S., & Leashore, B. R. (Eds.). (1997). *The challenge of permanency planning in a Mulicultural society.* New York: Haworth.

Child Welfare League of America. Washington Social Legislation Bulletin. (1997, July). *Report on formal and informal kinship care* (Vol. 35). Washington, DC.

Crumbley, J., & Little, R. L. (1997). *Relatives raising children: An overview of Kinship care.* Washington, DC: Child Welfare League of America.

Fanshel, D., & Shinn, E. (1978). *Children in foster care: A longitudinal Investigation.* New York: Columbia University Press.

Kusserow,R. P. (1992). *Using relatives for foster care.* Washington DC; U.S. Department of Health and Human Services, Office of the Inspector General (OEI-06-90-02390).

Le Prohn, N. S. (1994). The role of the kinship foster parent: A comparison of Relative and non-relative foster parents. *Children and Youth Services Review 16,* 65–84.

Maas, H., & Engler, R. (1959). *Children in need of parents.* New York: Columbia University Press.

Maluccio, A. N., Fein, E., & Olmstead, K. A. (1986). *Permanency planning for children: Concepts and methods.* New York: Tavistock.

U.S. House of Representatives, Select Committee on Children, Youth and Families. (1989). *No place to call home: Discarded children in America.*Washington, DC: U.S. Government Printing Office.

Grandparenting Among Diverse Populations

Chapter 10

Grandparents Raising Children Orphaned and Affected By HIV/AIDS

Daphne Joslin

Nearing the end of its second decade, HIV/AIDS is a family disease with multigenerational and intergenerational impact and implications. Yet despite interest in older adults who have become surrogate parents to young relatives, grandparents raising children orphaned and affected by HIV/AIDS are all but invisible in recent gerontological literature. The purpose of this chapter is to bring this neglected population of custodial and caregiving grandparents into view so that research, program and policy initiatives can address their special needs. Why do grandparents parenting in the wake of HIV/AIDS warrant singular attention? In its course in the United States and around the globe, the HIV pandemic continues to impose parental surrogacy upon large numbers of grandparents, typically grandmothers. If program and policy efforts targeting late life surrogate parents are to be effective, the needs of those affected by the HIV epidemic must be addressed. This chapter examines the unique circumstances of HIV-related surrogate parenting by grandparents, presents recent research that identifies risks to their health and well-being, and makes program and policy recommendations.

Demographic and Epidemiological Patterns

Catastrophic illness and death have always been a prime reason for grandparents raising their son or daughter's children. Yet as Michaels and Levine observed, "AIDS has come to rival or surpass other important causes of death in taking the lives of mothers of young children" (Michaels & Levine, 1992). Demographic and epidemiological projections of AIDS orphans and children affected by parental HIV infection are alarming indicators of the persistent need for grandparents and other third- and fourth-generation relatives to assume parental surrogacy. Between 82,000 and 125,000 children and adolescents in the United States are likely to be orphaned by HIV disease as we enter the 21st century (Michaels & Levine, 1992). Grandmothers are typical surrogate parents to children losing a primary parent to HIV disease (Draimin, 1995) and were serving as parental surrogates as many as one third of families in an urban, comprehensive AIDS center (Mevi-Triano, 1997). Using this proportion as a rough parameter, it can be estimated that as many as 27,060 to 41,250 orphaned AIDS children will be raised by grandmothers by the year 2000. Recent research has found that AIDS-affected grandmothers raise, on average, two children (Joslin, Mevi-Triano, & Berman, 1997). Conservatively, then, an estimated 13,530 to 20,625 grandmothers in the United States will be primary parents to AIDS orphaned children in the United States by the year 2001.

Because AIDS is the third leading cause of death among women of child bearing age (i.e., between 25 and 44 years) in the United States, the number of children orphaned by the epidemic is not likely to decrease, despite the hope generated by the new combination antiretroviral therapies. The recent decline in AIDS mortality rates has been much less dramatic among women, especially Blacks and Latinas (Altman,1997), where rates of infection are much higher than for White women (CDC, 1994). Infected women's reduced survival time after diagnosis and more rapid progression of HIV disease is associated with poor access to care and delayed presentation for clinical care rather than gender differences per se (Brettle & Leen, 1991; Landesman & Holman, 1995).. Infected women are more likely to be low income (Chu, Buehler, & Berkleman, 1990), to have a lifetime of poorer health and inadequate health care and poorer self-care behaviors (i.e., stress management, not smoking, and minimal alcohol use), that promote immune function. Poverty and family responsibilities undercut their capacity to adhere to the complicated regiments of the new combination antiretroviral therapies. Frequently, their own health needs are often secondary to those of an infected male partner or child for whom they are the caregiver (O'Hara, 1995).

There are no estimates of the number of grandmothers raising HIV affected and infected whose infected mother is still alive yet too debilitated from HIV disease to fully parent. Given female infection incidence, especially among women of color, the number of children affected by maternal HIV disease will not diminish over the coming decades. HIV infection among women has been rising more rapidly than among other populations (Ickovics & Rodin, 1992), and the proportion of American women who have HIV disease, or AIDS, continues to grow (CDC, 1995), especially among African American and Latina women (CDC, 1994). Hundreds of thousands of children and adolescents will be living with an infected mother who is coping with disease symptoms, complicated drug therapies, numerous remissions, and debilitating medication side effects. Because of the effectiveness of ziduvodine (AZT) in decreasing maternal transmission of the HIV virus (Connor et al., 1994) the number of infected children has decreased. With maternal transmission via pregnancy, labor and delivery and breast feeding estimated to be 20% to 30%, there are approximately 1,500 to 2,000 infected children born each year (Simonds & Oxtoby, 1995), with at least one half being raised by grandmothers.

The intergenerational responsibilities imposed by HIV disease on grandparents and other third- and fourth-generation relatives, such as great grandmothers and great aunts, will continue to be especially harsh in African-American and Latino communities, given the infection rate among African-American and Latina women. Because older adults living in these communities are more likely to be poor and to be in poorer health, the assumption of surrogate parenting in the wake of HIV/AIDS imposes new burdens in the absence of adequate resources.

Invisible Caregivers

Conceptually, caregiving grandparents in the HIV epidemic are located at the intersection of two groups: HIV/AIDS caregivers and "grandparents as parents." Yet assumption of parental responsibility for HIV affected and orphaned children has not earned them research, program or policy attention. Nearly invisible within both gerontological and HIV/AIDS literature, they have barely been acknowledged as part of the group of HIV caregivers (Poindexter & Linsk, 1997a, 1998b) and "grandparents as parents" (Burnette, 1997; Jendrick, 1994). To date, only one published study has focused specifically on parental surrogacy for HIV affected and orphaned children (Joslin & Harrison, 1998). Given the burgeoning of research on custodial and caregiving grandparents, it is difficult to identify why they have been neglected. The intensity of HIV caregiving, coupled with child rearing, may make them less accessible to primary research studies. Recent bereavement and the internalized stigma of HIV/AIDS (Poindexter & Linsk, 1998) may dampen willingness to participate in research.

Notable in neglect by HIV caregiving research are the multiple, often simultaneous, caregiving roles many assume for infected adult children and grandchildren. Others have a protracted HIV caregiving "career," burying a daughter, and then caring for infected infants, children, and adolescents. Absent from the literature on HIV caregiving stress (Clipp, Adinolfi, Forrest, & Bennett, 1995; LeBlanc, London, & Aneshenel, 1997; Pearlin, Semple, & Turner, 1988; Theis, Cohen, Forrest & Zelewsky, 1997;) is research on physical and psychological symptoms among those caregivng for multiple family members, infected women, and children. This neglect may be partially explained by the predominant number of HIV caregiving studies conducted on caregivers to infected gay men. Yet even in research focused on infected women and children where the caregiving role of the grandparent is noted (Goicoechea-Balbona, 1998; Hackl, Somlai, Kelly, & Kalichman, 1997), the older generation is overlooked even in their capacity to continue caregiving.

HIV/AIDS: More Than the Reason for Parental Surrogacy

Like other custodial grandparents, those raising HIV affected and orphaned children face financial problems, lack available and affordable child care, have inadequate housing, and cope with discipline issues and the loss of personal time and privacy. However, as a progressive, debilitating and ultimately fatal disease, HIV imposes a convergence of its own powerful challenges: diagnosis and disclosure, social stigma and isolation, disease progression, treatment management, anticipated death, dying, and bereavement. HIV disease is more than just the reason for parental surrogacy.

With new antiretroviral therapies extending the time between HIV diagnosis and terminal illness, grandparents often assume the dual roles of surrogate parent and HIV caregiver simultaneously. Some grandmothers may be caring for two generations of infected family members: adult child(ren) and grandchild(ren). With disease progression and the unpredictable "roller coaster" of HIV disease, with periods of relapse and plateau (Mason, Preisinger, & Donohue, 1995), grandparent(s) assume greater responsibility for the infected person's household and children. Among a sample of poor infected mothers of young children, more than four fifths identi-fied their own mother as part of their support network (Williams, Shahryarinejad, Andrews, & Alcabes, 1997) helping them cope with symp-toms, treatment regimens and side effects, and often providing intensive care in the final stages of the disease. In a convenience sample of HIV affected grandparents (Joslin, Mevi-Trianco, & Berman, 1997) only three out of twenty surrogate parents had not directly cared for the children's infected and dying mother.

This section examines three of the central challenges faced by HIV affected grandparents: the stigma of HIV infection, disease caregiving, and death and bereavement. In describing how each impacts on parental sur-rogacy, qualitative data will be presented from an exploratory study con-ducted in northern New Jersey of 20 older adults who were raising children affected and orphaned by AIDS. The caregivers ranged in age from 47 to 72 years, with a mean of 59. Eighty percent were grandmothers; one care-giver was a great aunt, another a grandfather with primary parental respon-sibility. The purpose of the study, reported elsewhere (Joslin & Harrison, 1998) was to gather descriptive information about physical and emotional health, physical and psychological stress, and self-care behaviors.

AIDS Stigma

Ms. N. is a 54-year-old African-American woman who is raising her 4-year-old infected grand-daughter, Michelle, whose mother is dying of AIDS. Although a college graduate, Ms. N. is not immune to the toxic effects of AIDS stigma. Rather than place her grand-daughter in day care, her sister is Michelle's baby-sitter. "It gives me peace of mind if I'm run-ning late. But if I start to look for regular day care, it means that I have to tell them she's infected and I don't want to. I will have to tell them [her HIV status] when she starts school."

Family members of HIV infected individuals confront a range of emo-tions including fear, anger, denial, despair, confusion, anguish, and uncer-tainty (Macklin, 1989). Because HIV disease symbolizes deviance—homosexuality, drug use, promiscuity (Tibler, Walker & Rolland, 1989)—shame and stigma add to the emotional "timebomb" (Roth, Siegal, & Black, 1994) felt by both infected and affected. Unlike grandparents rais-ing children who have lost parents to cancer or other causes, HIV stigma casts a shadow over the uninfected, including caregivers and affected chil-dren, threatening self-esteem and social support.

Ms. B is raising an infected 3-year-old grand-daughter and four other grandchildren. Her daughter and infant grandson died of AIDS the prior year. Mrs. B's only social outlet is going to church, yet she never talks with church friends about her daughter's and grandson's deaths. Shame and feared ostracism isolate Mrs. B. from potential supports, who may be judgmental and rejecting, given the view by some that AIDS is "God's punishment" for a deviant lifestyle (Tiblier, Walker, & Rolland, 1989). The wariness with which grandparents approach HIV disclosure is not unfounded as the stigma extends beyond the infected person to caregivers and uninfected family members (Christ & Wiender, 1994; Fair, Spencer, & Winer, 1995; Herek & Capitanio, 1993; Land & Haragody, 1990; Lesar, Gerber & Semmel, 1995–96; Macks, 1990; Maj, 1991; McGinn, 1996; Poindexter & Linsk, 1998a; Roth, Siegal, & Black, 1994). Shame and feared rejection further isolate grandparents from potential informal and formal supports (Poindexter & Linsk, 1998a) which can buffer stressful circumstances.

Typical of the shame and secrecy that develops within families, a 72-year-old grandmother describes having to comply with her infected daughter's wishes to tell no one about her disease including her infected 11-year-old granddaughter. Maintaining secrecy prohibited the grandmother from seeking formal support until after her daughter's death. Social isolation, in response to AIDS stigma, was a powerful and consistent theme in the study. A 63-year-old grandmother, caring for an infected 37-year-old daughter and 2-year-old infected granddaughter doesn't go out socially because "I don't have many people I can trust." Another describes helping her grandsons cope with the taunts of other children. " 'Your mother has AIDS.' It was thrown up in their faces. They wanted to move."

Caring for the HIV Infected

Some surrogate parents to HIV affected and orphaned children may be raising uninfected children whose infected mothers died elsewhere and received no assistance from the grandparent or if still living with HIV disease, receives care from another relative. However, among the 20 surrogate parents in the exploratory study, all were, or had been, directly involved in the some aspect of HIV infection or disease. This ranged from one 74-year-old grandmother's anxiety over whether to have her 8-year-old granddaughter tested for HIV, after the AIDS death of the child's mother to two grandmothers caring for HIV infected daughters and their infected children. Others were managing medications and coordinating medical care for infected but healthy grandchildren or caring for dying adult daughters. Several who were raising uninfected children had been the primary caregiver to an infected daughter as HIV disease weakened, debilitated, and ultimately took her life.

The new antiretroviral therapies have not reduced the complexity of HIV disease, nor eliminated its catastrophic impact on the infected person and her or his caregiver(s). With greater chronicity of HIV disease, its course is still uncertain and unpredictable. Caregivers may provide assistance over a longer period, as caregiving requirements shift in length and intensity (Theis, Cohen, Forrest, & Zelewsky, 1997).

Studies of HIV caregiving amply document the physical and psychological toll on caregivers, despite satisfaction they receive in caring for a loved one or family member (LeBlanc, London, & Anenshensel, 1997; Pearlin, Anenshensel, & LeBlanc, 1997; Walker, Pomeroy, & Franklin, 1996). Chronic fatigue and physical exhaustion (Turner & Pearlin, 1989), emotional exhaustion (Turner, Catania, & Gagnon, 1994), depression (LeBlanc, Anashensel, & Wright, 1995) and somatic physical and psychological stress symptoms (LeBlanc, London, & Aneshensel, 1997; Trice, 1988) are common, as parents, partners, spouses, siblings, children, friends, and other informal supports assist with bathing, toileting, dressing, and feeding, coordinate medical and social service appointments, help the infected person to cope with intermittent, unpredictable, and sudden illnesses (Holzemer, Rothenberg, & Fish, 1995), and with disease symptoms and treatment side effects, such as loss of appetite, fatigue, pain, nausea, vomiting, diarrhea, and headaches that intefere with normal, daily activities.

In addition to direct patient care and instrumental assistance (shopping, laundry, transportation, cooking, and bill paying), caregivers also provide emotional support and help to manage irritability, confusion, and depression (Clipp, Adinolfi, Forrest, & Bennett, 1995). They learn how to address the special nutritional and feeding needs of infected children and adults (Marder & Linsk, 1995; Miller, Turner, & Moses, 1990; Shevlov, 1994), and assist with medication adherence, especially with combination antiretroviral therapies. Meticulous attention must given to reducing the risk of viral transmission in the handing of the infected person's blood and bodily wastes and in preventing and managing even minor illnesses such as colds and the flu because of the virus' suppression of the immune system. One grandmother raising an infected 13-year-old granddaughter described a constant vigilance to the normal aches, pains, and sickness of childhood.

Death and Dying

AIDS is now the leading cause of death for African-American and Latino women ages 25 to 44 in the United States and the third leading cause of death for all women in that age group (CDC, 1997). It ranked seventh in causes of death to children ages 1 to 4 in the United States. Among African American children in New York and New Jersey, only accidents surpassed AIDS as the leading cause of death for children in this age group (Chu, Buehler, Oxtoby, & Kilbourne, 1991). Loss, grief, and bereavement are paramount issues in the lives of HIV affected grandparents. Although deaths may occur over a period of several years, it is not uncommon for deaths to occur in a cascade affect, with a mother and infant or toddler dying within a few months of one another, especially in poor communities (Honey, 1988). Two grandmothers each buried a daughter and a grandchild within the same year and one was also caring for an ill 3-year-old granddaughter.

In burying the family's younger generation(s), grandparents are survivors in an epidemic that has disordered the normal phases of the life cycle (Tiblier, Walker & Rolland, 1989). Mothers of adult children who have died of AIDS may feel guilt and inadequacy that they failed to protect the child from life choices that seemed were responsible for her death (Tiblier, Walker, & Rolland, 1989). Intense, prolonged and incomparable grief is associated with the loss of even an adult child (Gorer, 1965; Levine-Perkell, 1996). A daughter's death may have its own unparalleled grief, intensified by the realization that a potential caregiver to the grandparent's own later life has died.

Grandparents raising children whose infected mother is still living, cope with anticipated death of their daughter or daughter-in-law, often caring for her as she dies. They must attend to the children's grief, confusion, rage, and despair as they watch their mother's physical and often mental deterioration. Often grandparents put their own need to grieve "on hold" to attend to the emotional needs of the dying parent and her children. Although many custodial grandparents worry whether they will live long enough to raise the child(ren) to maturity, those raising HIV infected children, may express a sentiment similar to that of one 72-year-old grandmother raising her infected 13-year-old granddaughter: "I sometimes wonder which one of us will die first. Either is more than I can bear to think about."

Unlike other causes of parental death, HIV disease casts its stigmatized shadow even in bereavement. Because shame and rejection are so common, family members mourning an AIDS-related death of a parent, sibling, child or grandchild may experience "disenfranchised grief" (Doka, 1989), where the cause of death cannot be disclosed. Under these circumstances, a grandmother may not be able to tell friends, church and community associates, neighbors, or even other relatives that she has lost her daughter to AIDS, thereby losing potential social support during bereavement. The grieving process for surviving children, whether HIV infected or uninfected, may also be disturbed by secrecy and shame (Doka, 1989). Grandparents and children may be bound tightly in a "conspiracy of silence," fearful that the cause of death will be revealed (Dane, 1993). Orphaned children must be helped through one of the most stressful experiences a child can face. Anger, guilt, behavioral problems, denial, depression, and suicide attempts are common in AIDS-bereaved children and adolescents (Dane, 1993).

Caregiver Well-Being

Recent studies of custodial and primary care giving grandparents point toward heightened risk for compromised physical and psychological health (Burton, 1992; Fuller-Thompson, Minkler, & Driver, 1997; Joslin & Brouard, 1995; Joslin & Harrison, 1998; Kelly, 1993; Minkler, Roe, & Price, 1992; Strawbridge, Wallhagen, Shema, & Kaplan, 1997). Quantitative and qualitative data from the exploratory study conducted with older adults raising HIV affected and orphaned children in New Jersey indicate that caregiver physical and emotional well-being may be diminished for this group of "grandparents as parents." Although quantitative data from a small, convenience sample must be interpreted with caution, findings from the exploratory suggest that HIV caregivers had poorer self-reported health than Oakland, California, grandparents raising children in the crack cocaine epidemic. Forty-five percent of the HIV-affected grandparents reported their health as excellent or good compared with 54% of the crack cocaine affected grandmothers. HIV-affected grandparents were more likely to report their health as having declined over the past year: 55% compared with 28% of non-HIV grandparents (Minkler & Roe, 1993). More than two thirds of those raising an HIV infected child experienced a decline in health over the past year compared with 29% of those raising uninfected children. In both studies, it is noteworthy that these older surrogate parents were less likely to report excellent or "good" health, 45% (New Jersey) and 55% (California), compared with 70% of a national sample of those age sixty and above (National Center for Health Statistics, 1990).

Data from the exploratory study underscore the vulnerability to physical health problems among HIV-affected grandparents who reported an average of three chronic health problems. At least 90% had one chronic health condition, hypertension, arthritis, or diabetes being most prevalent. A greater number of chronic health conditions, a decline in global health over the past year and poorer self-reported health, were more likely among those who were raising children alone, raising more than one child, with low incomes, raising an HIV infected child, or age 59 or younger. These patterns suggest "pockets" of greater vulnerability whose family, caregiving, or socioeconomic circumstances place them at added risk for poorer health (Joslin, Mevi-Triano, & Berman, 1997). Not surprisingly, those who had lost a family member to HIV disease within the past year reported a greater number of physical and psychological stress symptoms. The relatively better self-reported health among grandparents 60 years and older can be misleading when viewed only in comparison with the younger group who tended to have lower incomes. Although older caregivers had fewer chronic health conditions, nearly one half rated their health as fair or "poor," and 56% reported their health to have deteriorated over the past year. Older adults often reframe their perception of health in reference to peers, their own functional capacity, and the aging process. Those raising HIV orphaned and affected children may also compare their own health with that of their own child, dead or dying from HIV disease. Even those in good health report that their physical stamina is sorely taxed by surrogate parenting responsibilities. Only one third reported having enough time to for their own health because of caregiving responsibilities.

Qualitative data reported elsewhere (Joslin & Harrison, 1998) provided a profile of systemic and psychosocial barriers to self care (i.e., "the intentional behavior that a lay person takes on his or her own behalf . . . to promote health or to treat illness") (Levin, Katz, & Holst, 1979). As "hidden patient(s)" (Joslin & Harrison, 1998), HIV affected grandparents are likely to minimize their own health problems, to be reluctant or unable to seek medical attention as well as to make time for promoting their own well-being, whether through relaxation and socialization, or adopting healthier lifestyle behaviors (i.e., quitting smoking or exercise). Factors that reduce their capacity for self-care to prevent or manage chronic health problems include the lack of health insurance, lack of respite, poverty's crushing impact on daily priorities, and fear that attention to one's own health will signal their inability to parent their grandchildren.

The catastrophic and all-consuming nature of HIV disease can overshadow the needs of caregivers who are raising an infected child or also caring for an adult child with HIV disease. Cultural beliefs about the priority of family needs can also be barriers to self-care. As stated by one 60-year-old Puerto Rican grandmother who was raising a 15-year-old infected grandson whose parents had recently died of AIDS, "I must put other's needs ahead of my own. I have other people to think about." Caregiver depression also undermines motivation to take action on behalf of one own well-being. A grandmother caring for a daughter and granddaughter, both ill with HIV disease, described herself as "a little depressed." Her hopeless about the future extended to her sense of futility about her own health. "I've gained 10 pounds from eating ice cream. It's like I don't care."

Program and Policy Implications

As Minkler and Roe observed (1993), grandmothers raising grandchildren of the crack cocaine epidemic may be a self-selected group—heartier and healthier—whose internal and external resources support parental surrogacy. Their resolve to maintain a profile of competence in the face of daunting circumstances, often downplaying their own needs, was visible among those raising HIV orphaned and affected grandchildren. Their reluctance to make their needs known to social service agencies contributes to their invisibility and neglect. Public eagerness to applaud older adults as resources for their families and the fulcrum of community stability can also mute the articulation of custodial grandparents' needs. In this final section, policy and program implications will be presented, addressing three areas: health promotion; creation of a responsive service system; and public policy.

Health Promotion

Neglect of one's health is detrimental to well-being at any age, but for older adults it may ultimately rob them of functional capacity and independence. Poor health may compromise the capacity of parental surrogate to continue in this role. Because grandparents often express anxiety about living long enough to see the grandchildren fully grown, professionals who come into contact with them can use this concern as a basis for counseling and education regarding the importance of self-care (e.g., seeking regular medical care and using respite, day care, afterschool and volunteer services) to attend to their own preventive and chronic health needs. Grandparents can be encouraged to see that practicing self-care is a means of caring for their families rather than a selfish distraction. Referrals for medical care, assistance in accessing health insurance or charity care, respite, child care, and transportation may be necessary. The exploratory study found that one quarter had no health insurance. These caregivers were younger than age

65 and either not covered if working or ineligible for Medicaid although unable to purchase private health insurance. Access to primary health care is a programmatic issue that can be addressed through innovation at the community level by establishing collaborative arrangements with local health care providers and by bringing health care to the caregiver (i.e., home visits by a geriatric nurse practitioner).

Creating a Responsive Service System

Lack of systematic research on HIV affected grandparents has been paralleled by an absence of programs designed to address their unique needs (Joslin & DeGraw, 1997). As this chapter has shown, although they share much in common with other grandparents raising grandchildren, HIV disease imposes its own constellation of burdens which require sensitivity in client outreach, familiarity with HIV testing and diagnosis, disease progression, symptoms, and treatment, experience with dying and bereavement issues in adults and children, and ability to access services from the aging, HIV/AIDS, and child welfare systems (Joslin & DeGraw, 1997; Joslin & DeGraw, 1998).

Programmatic neglect of these custodial and caregiving grandparents must be examined in relationship to the two service systems that would be the most logical service providers: the aging network, that is, programs funded under the Older Americans Act, and the HIV/AIDS care network, funded through the Ryan Whyte Comprehensive Resources Emergency (CARE) Act of 1990. In looking at the aging network, that is, public and private agencies whose mission under federal mandate is to serve persons sixty years of age and older, what is striking is how much they reflect the sociocultural milieu in which they exist. Although public and private aging agencies in the California Bay area; Dade County, Florida; northern New Jersey; and New York City have been active in the creation of HIV/AIDS and Aging task forces and coalitions (Joslin & Nazon, 1996), AIDS phobia remains strong among staff of county offices on aging and other programs serving older adults, such as senior centers. Outreach conducted by one supportive service and case management program for HIV affected surrogate parents was met with the response, "There's no AIDS here" and "This doesn't affect seniors." Nearly a decade after Lloyd (1989) observed that AIDS-phobia had infected the aging network as well, such misinformation and prejudice continues to exist.

Although HIV/AIDS agency staff may be concerned about grandparent well-being, the catastrophic nature of HIV disease and federal guidelines under the Ryan Whyte CARE Act restrict professional attention and time to the medical management of the infected person and her or his psychosocial needs. CARE funded case management and mental health services are available only as they assist the caregiver in meeting the needs of the *infected* child or grandchild. Services must be terminated once the infected person dies. In addition to restrictions under the CARE Act, with the hope generated by the new combination therapies, the decline in overall mortality rates and a profile of HIV as a more chronic than terminal disease, in home supportive services, such as housekeeping and personal care that serve as respite for parental surrogates, are being sharply curtailed by state agencies unless the infected person has acute medical needs (Coalition on AIDS in Passaic County Membership Meeting, October 1997).

Neglect of grandparent needs by HIV/AIDS staff also reflects the lack of gerontological training and experience. Narrow client categories, age-determined eligibility criteria for aging network services and Medicare, and a lack of uniform eligibility criteria confuse grandparents and professionals, with the result being a lack of service and advocacy (Mellor, 1996). Building relationships across the HIV/AIDS and aging networks is essential for client outreach and referral, staff development, effective case management, collaborative program development and service integration. Ad hoc coalitions and task forces on issues such as HIV/AIDS and aging can create a network of professionals committed to education, program and policy initiatives (Joslin & Nazon, 1996; Nazon & Levine-Perkell, 1996).

Such a system is especially important in reducing the isolation of these custodial and caregiving grandparents. HIV stigma, disease caregiving, death and bereavement conspire to make grandparents particularly isolated from informal supports as well as create barriers to helpseeking from formal agencies. Although grandparent support groups are an important resource (Bell & Garner, 1996; Minkler & Roe, 1996). HIV affected grandparents may be unable to attend meetings, given their HIV caregiving responsibilities per se and the isolation and shame fostered by HIV stigma. A generic support group may be viewed cautiously because grandparents may fear rejection and stigma from those whose lives are not affected by HIV. Reducing social isolation among these grandparent caregivers is an important service goal and calls for close attention to reducing both client and system barriers (Poindexter & Linsk, 1998a). The experience of the OASIS Project, a supportive service program developed by the Coalition on AIDS in Passaic County, New Jersey, for older caregivers to HIV affected and orphaned children, found that an intensity of case management service, including in-home assessment and counseling, was required to establish caregiver trust so that a care plan could be developed (Joslin & De Graw, 1998).

Public Policy

Public policy issues identified by the study reported here include those affecting a broad range of custodial and caregiving grandparents, such as the lack of health insurance as well as those related specifically to HIV-affected families. Lack of universal health insurance was a two fold problem among the New Jersey grandparents raising HIV affected and orphaned children. One quarter were too young for Medicare but unable to afford private insurance. Their lack of insurance was paralleled by uninfected grandchildren who were not eligible for Medicaid and who could not be covered under their grandparent's insurance policy. Access barriers to supportive and information and referral services funded by the Older Americans Act were also raised. Chronological definitions of "elder" limit OAA funded services to those age 60 and older. Clearly, with greater numbers of older adults assuming the *elder* generational responsibility of child rearing, regardless of their chronological age, serious consideration must be given by the aging network about public responsibility for these caregivers.

Programs to address the needs of custodial and caregiving grandparents affected by HIV can be supported through the OAA and as well as through Ryan White CARE (Poindexter & Linsk, 1998b). Aggressive training, through Title IV of OAA, is needed to overcome AIDS phobia within the aging network and to sponsor collaborative training with the HIV/AIDS network. Supportive services, such as respite and counseling, could be developed through CARE, under guidelines for women, children, and families (Poindexter & Linsk, 1998a).

The caregiving needs of HIV-affected grandparents make them allies with advocates for long-term care. Care of the chronically and terminally ill infected person has been termed a "hidden cost of HIV" (LeBlanc, London, & Aneshensel, 1997), which these grandparents, like other family caregivers, shoulder in the absence of adequate community based long-term care. (Kane & Kane, 1983). The improved quality of life and survival of some HIV infected, coupled with declining mortality rates, has led to a redefinition of HIV as a chronic, that than terminal, disease. With this redefinition has come the erosion of publicly funded in-home services. Such recent ebb and flow of Medicare funded home care has dramatized the burdens to those living with debilitating chronic conditions and their families. Narrowing eligibility categories in the existing limited pool of community-based long-term care continues to underscore the need for a universal, public long-term care policy. From a societal point of view, AIDS-affected caregivers, including grandparents, absorb the hidden psychological, physical, social, and financial costs of the HIV epidemic.

Social policies to support grandparent caregivers do not always fall neatly within the classification of "aging policies." As gerontological research draws attention to HIV/AIDS, the crack cocaine epidemic, and the incarceration of mothers (Dressel & Barnhill, 1994) as the circumstances which determine late life surrogate parenting for growing numbers of older adults in the United States, the fault lines of American social policies, including aging and welfare policies, may be exposed. Dressel and Barnhill (1994) argue that attention to the service needs of grandmothers raising children of incarcerated women exposes the limits of current gerontological thought. Their conceptual critique suggests that aging policies themselves may need to be evaluated in the context of older caregivers raising grandchildren, particularly those who are economically marginal.

Grandparents as parents places older adults in new arena of social policy, not as care recipients, but as intergenerational resources for their family and community. At the same time, because these grandparents tend to be poor, female, and from communities of color (Fuller-Thompson, Minkler, & Driver, 1997), gerontological thought is challenged to see these older adults within families whose lives and limited life chances are structured by the inequality and injustice of the broader society. Serving as resources for their families, their needs expose the lack of both a comprehensive family policy, including universal health insurance. As the United States enters the next millennium, more inclusive family and aging policies will be needed to respond to the diverse family structures involving older adults. Gerontologists can advocate for the design of polices that address the issues faced by third- and fourth-generation caregivers in the HIV/AIDS epidemic who are representatives largely of the poor, working class, and communities of color.

References

Bell, W., & Garner, J. (1996) Kincare. *Journal of Gerontological Social Work*, *25*, 11–20.

Brettle, R. P. & Leen, C. L. (1991) The natural hisotiry of HIV and AIDS in women. *AIDS*, *5*, 1283–1292.

Centers for Disease Control and Prevention. (1997, July). HIV/AIDS and Women in the United States. *CDC Update*.

Centers for Disease Control and Prevention. (1995). Update: AIDS among women—United States, 1994. *Morbidity and MortalityReport, 44,* 81–84.

Chu, S., Buehler, J., & Berkelman, R. (1990). Impact of the human immunodeficiency virus epidemic on mortality in women of reproductive age, United States. *Journal of the American Medical Association, 264,* 225–229.

Chu, S., Buehler, J., Oxtoby, M. J., & Kilbourne, B. W. (1991). Impact of the human immunodeficiency virus epidemic on mortality in children, United States. *Pediatrics, 87,* 806–810.

Clipp, E. C., Adinolfi, A. J., Forrest, L., & Bennett, C. L. (1995). Informal caregivers of persons with AIDS. *Journal of Palliative Care, 11,* 10–18.

Connor, E., Sperling, R., Kiselev, P., Scott, G., O'Sullivan, M., Van Dyke, R. Bey, R., Shearer, W., Jacobson, R., Jiming, E., O'Neill, E., Bazin, B., Deepaissey, J., Culnane, M., Coombs, R., Elkens, M., Moye, M., Stratton, P., & Balsey. J. (1994). Reduction of maternal-infant transmission of human immunodeficiency virus type 1 with zidovudine treatment. *New England Journal of Medicine, 331,* 1173–1180.

Dane, B. (1993). Mourning in secret: How youngsters experience a family death from AIDS. In C. Levine. (Ed.), *Orphans of the HIV epidemic.* New York: United Hospital Fund.

Goicoechea-Balbona, A. (1998). Children with HIV/AIDS and their families, *Health & Social War, 23,* 61–69.

Holemer, S. P., Rothenberg, R., & Fish, C. A. (1995). Continuity of care. In P. Kelly, S. Holman, R. Rothenberg, & S. P. Holzemer (Eds.) *Primary care of women and children with HIV infection.* Boston: Jones & Bartlett

Honey, E. (1988). AIDS and the inner city. *Social Casework. 69,* 365–370.

Ickovics, J., & Rodin, J. (1992). Women and AIDS in the United States: Epidemiology, natural history and mediating mechanisms. *Health Psychology, 11,* 1–16.

Joslin, D. & DeGraw, C. (1998). *OASIS final report.* Palerson, NJ,: Coalition on AIDS in Passaic County.

Joslin, D., & Harrison, R. (1998). The "hidden patient": Older relatives raising children orphaned by AIDS. *Journal of the American Medical Women's Association. 53,* 65–71.

Kelly, S. J. (1993). Caregiver stress in grandparents raising grandchildren. *IMAGE: Journal of Nursing Scholarship, 25,* 331–337.

Landesman, S. H., & Holman, S. (1995). Epidemiology and natural history of HIV infection in women. In P. Kelly, S. Holman, R. Rothenberg, & S. P. Holzemer (Eds.) *Primary care of women and children with HIV infection.* Boston: Jones & Bartlett.

LeBlanc, A. J., London, A. S., & Aneshensel, C. S. (1997). The physical costs of AIDS caregiving. *Social Science in Medicine, 45,* 915–923

Levin, L. S., Katz, A. H., & Holst, E. (1979). *Self-care: Lay initiatives in health.* New York: Prodist.

Levine, C. (1995). Orphans of the HIV epidemic: Unmet needs in six US cities. *AIDS Care*, 7 (Suppl. 1), 557–562.

Macklin, E. D. (1989). Introduction. In E.D. Macklin (Ed.), *AIDS and families*. New York: Harrington Park.

Martin, J. L. (1988). Psychological consequences of AIDS-related bereavement among gay men. *Journal of Consulting Clinical Psychology*, 56, 856–862.

Mason, J. W., Preisinger, J. E, & Donohue, M. (1995). Women and their families: Psychosocial stages of HIV infection. In P. Kelly, S. Holman, R. Rothenberg, & S. P. Holzemer (Eds.), *Primary care of women and children with HIV infection*. Boston: Jones & Bartlett.

Mellor, J. (1996). Special populations among older persons. *Journal of Gerontological Social Work*, 25, 1–10.

Michaels, D., & Levine, C. (1992). Estimates of the number of motherless youth orphaned by AIDS in the United States. *Journal of the American Medical Association*, 268, 3456–3461.

Minkler, M., & Roe, K. (1993). *Grandmothers as caregivers: raising children of the crack cocaine epidemic*. Thousand Oaks, CA: Sage.

Minkler, M., & Roe, K. (1996). Grandparents as surrogate parents. *Generations*, 20, 34–38.

National Center for Health Statistics. (1990). Current estimates from the National Health Interview Survey: U.S. 1989. *Vital and Health Statistics* (Series 10), 176. Washington: U.S. Government Printing Office.

O'Hara, M. J. (1995). Care of children with HIV infection. In P. Kelly, S. Holman, R. Rothenberg, & S. P. Holzemer (Eds.) *Primary care of women and children with HIV infection*. Boston: Jones & Bartlett.

Pearlin, L. I., Semple, S., Turner, H. (1988). Stress of AIDS caregiving: A preliminary overview of the issues. *Death Studies*, 12, 501–517.

Poindexter, C., & Linsk, N. (1998a). Sources of support in a sample of HIV-affected older minority caregivers. *Families in Society*, V. 79, 491–503

Poindexter, C., & Linsk, N. (1998b). HIV-related stigma in the lives of a sample of HIV-affected minority caregivers. *Social Work*, 44, 46–61.

Roth, J., Siegal, R., & Black, S. (1994). Identifying the mental health needs of children living in families with AIDS or HIV infection. *Community Mental Health Journal*, 30, 581–592.

Simonds, R. J., & Oxtoby, M. J. (1995). Epidemiology and natural history of HIV infection in children. In P. Kelly, S. Holman, R. Rothenberg, & S. P. Holzemer (Eds.), *Primary care of women and children with HIV infection*. Boston: Jones & Bartlett.

Theis, S. L., Cohen, F. L., Forrest, J., & Zelewsky, M. (1997) Needs assessment of caregivers of people with HIV/AIDS. *Journal of the Association of Nurses in AIDS Care*, 8, 76–84.

Tiblier, K. B., Walker, G., & Rolland, J. (1989). Therapeutic issues when working with families of persons with AIDS. In Macklin (Ed.), *AIDS and families*. New York: Harrington.

Chapter 11

Special Situation of Incarcerated Parents

Jeff Porterfield, Paula Dressel, and Sandra Barnhill

Over the past 20 years, an unprecedented and costly expansion in prison construction has been under way in the United States. The cost of construction has averaged $80,000 per bed; another $20,000 is spent annually to imprison an individual (Camp & Camp, 1996). Construction and spending, however, have not been able to keep pace with the corrections system's growing propensity to incarcerate. A 345% increase in the rate of incarceration since 1980 (Beck & Gilliard, 1995) has inundated the American penal system. Initiatives aimed at a focus on confinement and extended time served, such as "three strikes—you're out" legislation, mandatory sentencing guidelines, and truth-in-sentencing mandates, have all been instrumental in increasing prison populations.

Among the host of social issues related to growing rates and duration of incarceration is the toll such policies and practices take on families. In particular, this chapter is concerned with the consequences of the absence of a middle generation of caregivers because of their imprisonment (Dressel & Barnhill, 1994; Minkler & Roe, 1993). Approximately 800,000 men and women among the incarcerated are parents (Johnson & Gabel,

1995). Efforts on the part of grandparents, particularly grandmothers, to assume the caregiver roles of their adult incarcerated children have exposed the intergenerational effects of incarceration (Barnhill, 1994). The problems of parental incarceration extend into families in complex ways (Johnson, 1995a; Reed and Reed, 1997). Yet efforts to address the peripheral effects of parental incarceration are lacking in comparison with the demand for incarceration.

This chapter has four major sections. In the first section we examine the dynamics and effects of parental incarceration to provide context for our focus on grandparent caregiving. In the second section, we discuss the challenges of grandparents as caregivers in these circumstances. The third section gives consideration to policies and practices that would attend more directly and effectively to the issues raised in the preceding sections. Finally, we conclude with attention to the bigger picture within which these issues unfold: the nation's lack of family-focused social policies and its coupling of poverty and punishment.

Parental Incarceration as the Context for Grandparent Caregiving

---

Magnitude of Parental Incarceration

Given that no uniform mechanisms are in place to document parental incarceration, exact figures on the number of incarcerated parents are nonexistent. The basic approach to soliciting such data is to gather information from the incarcerated population. When this information is requested, it is often optional and relies primarily on self-report. Nonetheless, many studies (Beck & Gilliard, 1995; Greenfield & Minor-Harper, 1991; USDJ, 1994) provide workable estimates that fall within a similar range.

Estimates pertaining to the children of incarcerated parents (Bloom and Steinhart, 1993; Johnson, 1991; Johnson & Gabel, 1995) have been drawn from the 90,000 incarcerated women who report having a total of 145,000 minor children and the 1.23 million incarcerated men who report having 1.38 million minor children. In some cases, both parents are incarcerated and thus potentially report the same children. Even allowing for this situation, it is estimated that there are 1.5 million children with incarcerated parents. The data further indicate that an additional 3.5 million minor children have a mother or a father currently under some type of restriction (e.g, probation, parole, and house arrest) imposed by the corrections system. Another 5 million children have parents with past experiences of supervised restrictions. In sum, it is approximated that an astonishing 10 million children have had their lives impacted in some form or another by a parent's encounter with social control agencies.

Although males constitute more than 90% of the incarcerated population, just over one half have children 18 years of age and younger (Hairston, 1995; USDJ, 1994). Many of these fathers were not the primary caregiver prior to incarceration. Conversely, the growth in overall incarceration has included dramatic growth in the imprisonment of women, two thirds of whom are mothers—many the primary caregiver—of minor children (Baunach, 1985; Bloom & Steinhart, 1993). The female prison population has increased threefold since 1980 (Beck and Gilliard, 1995).

Through processes informed by racism (Dressel, 1994) and the marginalization of the poor, prisons disproportionately house men and women of color who are undereducated or unskilled, unemployed or underemployed, and low-income. Women are most likely to have been imprisoned for nonviolent property crimes and drug-related offenses. The lack of widespread alternatives to incarceration for people convicted of nonviolent crimes means that the state willingly removes parents from their children, even when those parents pose no physical danger to others. The net result of such policy decisions has been an increase in child rearing by foster care providers and relatives, especially maternal grandmothers.

Placement and Care of the Children

Parental incarceration produces a host of family issues encompassing the placement and care of children (Bloom & Steinhart, 1993; Johnson, 1991, 1992), questions of custody and parental equity (Barry, 1995; Johnson, 1995a; Smith, 1995), and matters of child development (Adalist-Estrin, 1986; Johnson, 1991, 1992, 1993; McCall et al., 1985).

On the incidence of a parent's incarceration, most children who have been living with both parents remain with the nonincarcerated parent, thereby experiencing little to no change in placement or care (USDJ, 1994). Children of incarcerated fathers typically experience limited change due to the prevalence of the mother being the primary caregiver prior to the father's incarceration. In contrast, one half of the children of incarcerated mothers are placed with grandparents, one fourth with their father, 15% with friends and relatives, and the remaining 10% in foster care.

As noted in the past (Baunach, 1985; McGowan & Blumenthal, 1978; Zalba, 1964) and reported more recently by the U.S. Department of Justice (1994), the placement of children with their fathers because of maternal incarceration is more common among older, either married or divorced,

European-American women, as opposed to young, single or separated, African- American women. African-American women are more likely to have children placed with relatives. Foster care is more common among children of young European-American women with large families and least common among children of African American women with small families who reside in metropolitan areas.

An additional issue relative to placement and care concerns the separation of siblings. Thirty-three percent of children with incarcerated fathers are separated from their siblings. Twice this percentage of children of imprisoned mothers are separated from their siblings (Barry, 1995; Koban, 1983).

Johnson (1991, 1992, 1993) notes that frequent changes in a child's placement or care are likely with the imprisonment of a mother. Most children experience at least one change in either placement or care during maternal incarceration. Two or more changes in caregiver are experienced by 11% of the children with imprisoned mothers. Because they reside with their natural mother before a father's incarceration, 90% of children with imprisoned fathers do not change placement. Eight percent are relocated to the home of a grandparent (USDJ, 1994). Research reveals significant associations between multiple changes in placement and care and problems with school and behavior (Johnson, 1995).

The juvenile court assumes responsibility for children of incarcerated parents in cases where relatives are not available for placement and care. These children are then placed into foster care. The parent has a specified period in which to meet reunification requirements, that is, to regain custody. If these requirements are not met within that time frame, the state revokes parental rights and seeks long-term guardians for the child. To say the least, reunification requirements are difficult to achieve while incarcerated.

A child is subject to multiple placements in foster care (Kampfner, 1995), and some children may even be separated from their siblings. These issues further add to parents' difficulties in that they may not be aware of the child's placement. The efforts of social service providers become significant at the point. Through provision of economic assistance, transportation for visitation, assistance with communication barriers, and overall development of a comprehensive plan, the social service provider is the key to reunification. Without these services, the physical, emotional, and economic demands are usually too great for the incarcerated parent to overcome (Johnson & Gabel, 1995), and regaining custody becomes all but impossible.

Even when a child is placed with a family member, reunification requirements are frequently placed on the parent (Smith, 1995). Problems between family members may then arise, particularly in terms of equity in rights of authority. Social services are also needed for reunification in these circumstances. However, social service agents may think that since the child is with family members, such services are not needed. On the contrary, family members typically accept child placements out of responsibility and obligation, regardless of their level of resources. Therefore, the need for assistance may be greater for children placed with family members than it is with foster families, who volunteer to provide child care and receive certain levels of assistance as a result.

Impact of Parental Incarceration on the Children

Parental incarceration impacts the social, psychological, and cognitive development of the children (Johnson, 1992, 1995b). The emotional and behavioral disposition of children who have experienced the circumstances of parental crime, arrest, and incarceration are affected (Baunach, 1985), with consequences varying by the age of the child.

The separation of children from parents and perhaps even their siblings can have deleterious consequences (Kampfner, 1995). It is not uncommon for children to be unaware of the true whereabouts of the incarcerated parent (Bloom & Steinhart, 1993). It is even more common for children not to know the details of the circumstances that led to their parent's incarceration. To the extent that such lack of information occurs, an atmosphere of secrecy and shame is created and emotional support for the children gets precluded.

The impact of parental crime and incarceration on children is documented as early as the prenatal stages of development (Egley et al., 1992). Stress, substance abuse, and neglect of prenatal care are common experiences of women involved in certain criminalized circumstances. To the extent that pregnant women participate in such milieus, they potentially expose their unborn children to risks. Numerous studies (Fritsch & Burkhead, 1982; Johnson, 1991, 1992, 1993) have revealed the developmental consequences of parental crime, arrest, and incarceration on children from birth to young adulthood. Within the first two years, children of incarcerated parents may suffer in emotional and intellectual development, specifically as it pertains to trust and bonding. From 2 to 6 years of age, children may not fully develop autonomy and initiative due to their inability to process traumatic experiences associated with their parent's circumstances. The ability to get along with others is likely altered between the ages of 7 and 10. Those children who have not overcome the experiences of parental incarceration by early adolescence (ages 11–14) may exhibit behavior that is indicative of rejecting rules and authority. By late adolescence to early adulthood, the cumulative effect of all experiences may lead to negative attitudes toward law enforcement and even involvement in criminal activities that will eventually lead to their child's own incarceration.

Children's emotional and behavioral responses to the trauma of parental crime, arrest, incarceration and subsequent separation are exhibited in numerous forms (Baunach, 1985; Kampfner, 1995): grief as shown through sadness and excessive crying; fear and anxiety as illustrated in low school performance and drug abuse; shame and stigma through withdrawal and depression; and anger expressed through disciplinary problems and criminal activity. These effects are cumulative as the children age (Johnson, 1995b) and put them at disproportionate risk for engaging in illegal activity, getting arrested, and being subjected to social control agencies themselves (Barnhill, 1994). As many as one half of all incarcerated juveniles report having parents who have been incarcerated (American Correctional Association, 1990).

This section has described the growing need for child care alternatives, given the burgeoning rate of incarceration of adults who are parents. It has also documented the particular challenges of child development faced by young people whose mother or father gets arrested and imprisoned. To be sure, those grandparents who step in to assume child care face circumstances that go well beyond routine parenting responsibilities. One agency that works on behalf of all three generations, Aid to Children of Imprisoned Mothers, Inc. (AIM), in Atlanta has found that caregiving grandparents express concern about the growth and development of the children, the legal circumstances surrounding the incarcerated parent, the adequacy of family resources to accommodate caregiving demands, and the complications of eventual reunification (Barnhill, 1994). These are the issues to which we now turn.

Grandparents as Caregivers to Children of Incarcerated Parents

Some three million children currently live with their grandparents or older relatives (U.S. Census Bureau, 1990). This number constitutes 5% of all children in the U.S. (Fuller-Thomson, Minkler, & Driver, 1997). More than 60,000 children of incarcerated mothers alone were among this group in

1990 (Greenfield & Minor-Harper, 1991), and this figure is expected to double by century's end. Approximately 32,000 grandmothers, who are mostly African American, single, and economically marginalized, have assumed the caregiver role absented by their incarcerated adult daughters (Greenfield and Minor-Harper, 1991; Fuller-Thomson, Minkler, & Driver, 1997). These figures, of course, do not begin to account for children living with their grandparents due to the effects of substance abuse, AIDS, teen pregnancy, unemployment, parental death, or the incarceration of men. Grandparental caregiving is expected to continue to rise, primarily due to the middle generation's inability to achieve socioeconomic status equal to that of their parents and the continued increase in parental incarceration, particularly among women. To be sure, these factors are significantly interrelated. Nonetheless, many grandparents are assuming the costs of these social dislocations through their sense of responsibility for providing child care for their grandchildren.

Caregiver Role

On parental incarceration, the assumption of the caregiver role by grandparents is usually the result of necessity and feelings of obligation (Burton & Bengtson, 1985). The assumption of responsibility by grandparents not only prevents the children from being subject to adoption by nonfamily members, but it also allows the grandparents to forego criticism by other family members for not responding to the needs of their grandchildren. The caregiver role may provide an opportunity for the grandparents to deal with feelings of helplessness and sadness about the parent's incarceration. Indeed, grandparents may even feel some responsibility for their incarcerated adult child's outcome (Minkler & Roe, 1993).

Caregiver responsibilities impose financial burdens on grandparent populations (Minkler and Roe, 1993) that typically are already economically vulnerable. Economic strain ranges from the elimination of discretionary spending to not being able to afford such necessities as food. In many states public assistance programs provide nonrelative foster care parents more benefits than caregiving grandparents (Yorker et al., 1998). Furthermore, grandparents express resentment for being subjected to shame and seemingly endless red tape to acquire meager benefits.

Many grandparents must balance their caregiver responsibilities with their own employment (Minkler & Roe, 1993; Scharlach & Boyd, 1989). This adjustment can require changes in hours, shifts, and even jobs. Some are forced to quit their jobs to meet the demands of full-time caregiving.

Even so, grandparent caregivers still experience pressures relative to time, finances, and conflicting roles. Although the combination of work and child care may not be a new experience—many held jobs while raising their own children and gave intermittent care to their grandchildren—the timing of these newly acquired full-time responsibilities can be disruptive. Indeed, the assumption of child care responsibilities may completely alter the expectations grandparents had for this phase of their lives.

Work and health are interrelated for these grandparents (Burton, 1994), with employed care-providing grandparents being more likely than non-employed care-providing grandparents to report health problems. Issues of age, social class, race, gender, and circumstances surrounding parental incarceration increase the vulnerability of caregiving grandparents in terms of physical and emotional health.

Similar to the circumstances of grandparents raising children as a result of parental substance abuse (Minkler & Roe, 1993), grandparents raising children as a result of parental incarceration report experiences that differ from more routine child care situations (Reed & Reed, 1997). The trauma of the parent's arrest, parent-child separation, and the stigma of incarceration add to the complexities of child rearing. Furthermore, it is not uncommon for grandparents to encounter additional frustration in attempts to secure appropriate social services. Nor is it uncommon for service agencies to display suspicion and distrust for grandparents seeking assistance, in part because of the stigma associated with the plight of incarcerated parents and, in part, because of the question of the children's entitlement to social services. This is particularly the case if the grandparents possess resources.

The foregoing complicate the merger of the grandparent's new or increased role as caregiver with existing roles. As a result, caregiving grandparents have been forced to sacrifice employment, economic security, health, privacy, and leisure to address the needs of their extended families. In the face of these challenges, grandparents generally have demonstrated remarkable resourcefulness in keeping their families together and as secure as circumstances allow. At the same time, many grandparents report joy and gratification from the caregiving experience (Chappell, 1990; Dressel & Barnhill, 1994). Satisfaction is derived from observations of the child's positive growth and development, the child's personal accomplishments, and, more simply, the mere presence of the grandchild in their lives.

Need for Assistance to Support Grandparent Caregiving

Parental incarceration prompts the need for a variety of forms of assistance targeting at least three generations (Dressel & Barnhill, 1994; Reed & Reed, 1997: Johnson, 1992, 1993). A comprehensive plan based on specific family needs is likely to include both material and psychosocial supports. Demand for such assistance exists prior to, during, and after the incarceration of the parent.

First and foremost, grandparents have a need for economic support (Dressel & Barnhill, 1994; Reed & Reed, 1997) whether through TANF, employment, or child support payments and with the assistance (where qualified) of Medicaid, housing subsidies, and in-kind aid (e.g., clothing, school supplies, and transportation). A familiar complaint of these caregivers, which echoes the frustration of parental caregivers reliant on public supports, is the complicated array of bureaucracies that must be navigated to access resources to which one is legislatively entitled. Indeed, the provision of information and referral about available resources is a typical component where services are offered specifically to the families of incarcerated parents.

Grandparents also have legal and psychosocial needs (Reed & Reed, 1997; Johnson, 1992, 1993). The legal circumstances of the incarcerated parent, issues surrounding the grandparents' custody, and occasionally the grandchildrens' encounters with the law are implicated in grandparents' needs for legal services. Support services relative to the psychosocial needs of grandparents include respite from the demands of child care, recognition for their caregiving efforts, reconciliation with their incarcerated adult child, and an understanding of how to respond to their grandchildrens' behaviors and emotions.

Frequently, caregivers are reluctant to seek support from agencies or organizations, such as the church, because of the shame and stigma of the adult child's incarceration. (Minkler & Roe, 1993). Interaction and association, both formal and informal, with other caregiving grandparents in similar situations has been found to enhance grandparents' abilities to manage their circumstances (Dressel and Barnhill, 1994). Caregivers report numerous benefits from these associations. Conversations with individuals having similar problems relieve stress and allow for understanding without judgement. Interacting with individuals with similar burdens not only permits the sharing of problems as a therapeutic process, but it also allows one to compare his or her situation to others and thereby potentially to reframe his or her perspective more positively (Kessler, Price, & Wortman, 1985).

The children of incarcerated parents are also in need of assistance throughout the various phases of their parent's arrest and incarceration. To the extent that such assistance undergirds children's material and psychosocial well-being, the child-rearing challenges for grandparents can at least be lessened. Proper training for law enforcement in the areas of family and child trauma, knowledge of family support agencies, and applicable arrest protocol would work toward reducing the trauma a child faces upon witnessing the arrest of a parent and being transitioned to an alternative caregiver. Arrangements that allow for parent-child contact or communication immediately after arrest (i.e., visitation policies, transportation, and cooperation from personnel at the detention facility) are critical in maintaining the parent-child bond under harsh circumstances. Immediate and long-term effects of parental incarceration can be reduced in this phase with the proper interventions that enable the child to construct an understanding of the situation and to anticipate the eventual return of the parent.

As previously discussed, direct material assistance to the grandparent caregivers during parental incarceration is essential to the child's well-being. The objective of such assistance is to increase the economic stability and living conditions of the child and to the extent possible alleviate the need for multiple placements and the separation of siblings.

Similar to the services that allow for parent-child contact in the arrest/detention process, expanded contact services are needed during the extended separation of incarceration. Several agencies around the United States provide transportation for children to the site of incarceration, which may be hours away from their place of residence. Adequate housing, or funds to accommodate extended visitation, are virtually nonexistent. As noted earlier, the effects of past and ongoing trauma on children are most evident during the period of parental separation. Services that identify and treat or prevent such effects are critical supports for grandparents. Many of the children have been exposed to living environments consisting of domestic violence, neglect, and substance abuse. Depending on the extent of trauma, children may require academic tutoring, behavioral assessments, therapeutic services, support group involvement, and even medical treatment.

Parental release and eventual reunification also require appropriate services. All three generations must be involved in this process to address any existing familial tensions and questions of caregiving authority. Such services should also be attentive to the behaviors and activities that produced incarceration and threaten recidivism (e.g., poverty, substance abuse, and domestic violence). The juncture of reunification is not without the possibility of conflict arising between the soon-to-be-released parent and the grandparent. Although the political movement for grandparent rights advocates on behalf of grandparents on issues such as decision-making authority and custody (Barnhill, 1994; Dressel, 1996; Dressel & Kelley, 1998), the rights and responsibilities of parents must be part of this debate.

Finally, incarcerated parents need assistance toward reducing their likelihood of recidivism and increasing the chances of relieving their parent(s) of care for the grandchild(ren). Training and education with respect to marketable skills for employment upon release may be offered in prison, but too often these are either unavailable to all prisoners or clustered in employment areas that are unlikely to move workers out of poverty. Treatment while incarcerated should address problems, such as addiction that may have been a primary factor leading to incarceration, but too often prisons use medication rather than counseling as a means to address prisoners' personal problems. Frequent family contact through visitation allows for parental involvement and participation in the family during the period of incarceration, but most visits occur under closely guarded and inhospitable conditions that are not conducive to comfortable parent-child interaction. Nevertheless, continuation of parental roles through incarceration, albeit in a more limited capacity, diminishes some interpersonal obstacles toward reunification It is important for all three generations throughout the incarceration to come to agreement about the conditions under which parental custody will be resumed and caregiving responsibilities transitioned from the grandparents to the parent at the time of the parent's release.

Need for Policy and System Reform to Support Grandparent Caregiving

The foregoing context sets the stage for a range of possibilities regarding improved policy and practice for the families of incarcerated parents. It is our position that such an agenda must be philosophically grounded in the affirmation of families and focused on the overarching goal of strengthening families across the generations. Although these premises may seem self evident, they are all too often violated by social control agencies and human service systems.

We also take the position that policies and programs to support grandparent caregivers must start from the vantage point of the incarcerated mother. We focus here on mothers because most incarcerated mothers have expressed a desire to perform parental responsibilities, despite their present circumstances. To the extent that such a desire is expressed by incarcerated fathers, their parental roles, too, should become a centerpiece for policy design and program operation. However, the agenda of fathering from prison is even less developed than that of an agenda on behalf of incarcerated mothers; thus, we offer the latter as a baseline from which the former might build. Research repeatedly documents the stake an incarcerated mother has in her children's welfare during her imprisonment; we maintain, therefore, that she should be closely involved in childrearing and actively engaged in decision making about her children during her incarceration. We believe that it is in the interest of all generations for a mother to fulfill her parenting role, even if it is constrained by her present circumstances.

The objective of an incarcerated mother's (or father's) engagement in childrearing and decision-making is difficult to achieve for a host of reasons. First, the stigma surrounding imprisonment spills over into more general assessments, so that many people feel that a mother (or father) has forfeited her (or his) right to parent. Even if public sentiment stops short of this position, it may come to rest on the conclusion that anyone in prison by definition cannot be a good parent. Although we do not know the precise contours of public opinion on these issues, we do know that policies and practice with regard to imprisoned parents tend to isolate them from the range of possibilities they might have to demonstrate good parenting as well as physically isolating them from their family members.

Second, prisons function in ways that breed dependency rather than self-sufficiency. Circumstances outside of prison such as poverty often preclude parents from being able to maintain their child's well-being at the same time that they also engender actions by adults that put them in jeopardy of imprisonment. Once imprisoned, these same adults are generally deprived of opportunities to prepare for self-sufficiency on release and are conditioned to react to the dictates of the institution. As a consequence, they are likely to come out of prison being no more able, and in some ways perhaps even less able, to be effective parents than when they were imprisoned.

Third, as a society we have not always made the explicit connection that children tend to do better when their parents or other caregivers do well. Investing in incarcerated parents and free world caregivers' abilities to address the needs of children and youth is the best strategy that can be provided to prevent juvenile crime, violence, and the waste of young peoples' potential. At the same time, such an investment can reduce parental recidivism. Research shows that those who maintain strong bonds with their families during their incarceration have lower rates of recidivism than those who cannot (Finney Hairston, 1995).

How, then, can families be affirmed and strengthened, even as they cope with the harsh circumstances of a parent's imprisonment? The remainder of this section identifies paths of policy and system reform that should be pursued toward these ends.

A basic step toward improved policies and systems is the identification of the family configurations of imprisoned parents by the corrections and human service systems. In a report prepared for the Child Welfare League of America, Barnhill (1997) found that almost no state family service units collect data that would enable them to determine the specific population among the families they serve. Not only is it important to assess the magnitude of such families in the service population to assess the level of specialized concerns; such a census would also enable systems to ascertain, appreciate, and support the various shapes that such families take, including the configuration of grandparents as caregivers.

Once such families have been identified, a next reasonable step is to assess policies, system operations, and programs in light of the new data. It is often the case that existing programs require only marginal modifications and few new dollars to be responsive to grandparent caregivers. At the same time, if such an assessment reveals serious gaps, the investment required to address these gaps is likely to be much smaller than the dollars required for addressing even larger problems fostered later by the presence now of serious service gaps.

At both the federal and state levels, family success policies should be adopted. Such a policy framework would simultaneously support a caregiver's ability to provide adequately for children while it also provides flexibility for incarcerated parents to stay active in their children's lives. Family success policies call for both reform in individual systems and cross-system collaboration. Although many systems interact with families, the two which do so most frequently and most detrimentally with the families who are the subject of this chapter are the correctional and the human service systems. Thus, we offer some suggestions about how each could promote family success.

Correctional systems must first be willing to give attention to the parental role of women and men inside institutions. Although we have already mentioned that most visitation of parents by their children occurs in highly controlled, high density settings, in the case of jails, no visitation is allowed. Thus, children are deprived of contact with their parents at this critical transition juncture, a period that is increasing because of increased delays their parents are experiencing in being tried and awaiting sentencing. Furthermore, incarcerated parents must call their children collect, with the family burdened by the higher rate of such calls, if they are able to afford the call at all. Family success-oriented policies would include more hospitable visitation settings, the opportunity for full-family visits in the less restricted settings, and less restrictions on phone privileges.

In addition, although some prisons offer parenting courses, the curriculum is not always realistic in terms of the limitations incarcerated parents experience. Parents in prison have far fewer opportunities, resources, and tools for demonstrating effective parenting than their free-world counterparts. Curricula should start from this vantage point and identify ways that parents who are confined can creatively exercise their skills and desires on behalf of their children.

At the prospect of a parent's release and re-entry into the community, family success policies would focus first on seeking to promote a parent's self-sufficiency, whether the need is for housing, work, or related means of stability. Another immediate need in the case of a released mother is the effort to reintegrate her into a position as caregiver. The mother, the grandparent caregiver, and the children all have issues of transition that would benefit from both individual and family counseling. Indeed, these activities should begin within the prison as the mother is preparing to exit.

Human service systems also require change to foster family success policies. They have a role to play in providing grandparent caregivers, foster parents, and agency staff a basic understanding with regard to the particular and unique features of families of incarcerated parents. We maintain that they should promote kinship care as a first option of child care and pay kin families at least equal to what foster parents receive for care provision. Permanency planning needs to be revisited, as well. With women now receiving longer sentences, the federal law of an 18-month mandate for resolution of the child care situation will only separate more and more mothers from their children.

Finally, cross-systems collaboration should begin with the desire to work together to sustain the prisoner's family. Memoranda of understanding should be developed between and among agencies so that families are no longer subjected to the bureaucratic tangles that now characterize their efforts to create a patchwork of support for their families. If families are truly put at the center of systems' concerns, no major policy decisions in one system would be undertaken without input and advice from representatives of the other systems whose work would be impacted by such change. For families to work better, systems must work together on behalf of families.

The foregoing ideas by no means exhaust the array of change that is implied by the notion of family success policies. The schools, the courts, health care systems, and the like also have critical roles to play on behalf of family success. We have only intended to articulate the basic premises and provide some illustrative examples of how policies and systems can be responsive to the very basic concern for family success.

Attention to the Bigger Picture

In the foregoing sections we have described the growing number of circumstances wherein grandparents assume caregiving responsibilities for the children of their incarcerated offspring. Those circumstances, as we noted, are frequently complex arrangements, filled with both challenges and satisfactions and reflective of strong familial commitments, even as they may also be frought with family struggle and conflict.

Well-Being of Multigenerational Families[1]

Given both the magnitude and the complexities of the phenomenon, it is not surprising that grandparent caregiving both under the circumstances of incarceration as well as more generally is receiving increased attention by advocates and practitioners. For example, the 1995 White House Conference on Aging adopted among its 50 resolutions one which explicitly addresses issues related to grandparents raising grandchildren. Various books offer guidance for grandparent caregivers (e.g., Takas, 1995; deToledo, 1995). The Grandparent Information Center of the American Association of Retired Persons publishes a newsletter entitled, "Parenting Grandchildren: A Voice for Grandparents." A study conducted by Minkler et al. (1993) to locate service models and community programs for grandparent caregivers yielded leads on more than 300 such programs. To be sure, critical structures and outlets are in place to ensure that the issue of grandparent caregiving will remain high profile and that the needs of grandparent caregivers will be advocated. And so they should.

In the enthusiasm for highlighting grandparent caregiving; however, a certain caution is in order. As scholars, advocates, and practitioners, we start our work from the assumption that we wish to promote the well-being of the multigenerational families on whose behalf we work. Thus, the respect we have for grandparents who frequently labor under highly stress-

1. This section is derived largely from Dressel (1996).

ful circumstances must be balanced with an appreciation for the rights and needs of other family members. Recognition of the complexities of family situations may preclude automatic advocacy for one generation instead of or over another. For example, support for an incarcerated mother's opportunity to resume her parental function upon release can conflict with support for grandparent custody preferences. Alternatively, it could be argued that advocacy should be child centered, or focused primarily on the best interests of the child. For instance, if the only parental figure the child has known is a grandmother, should this relationship with the child's primary attachment figure be disrupted when a mother wishes to assume a parenting role after a critical absence? The illustrations pose no ready or automatic conclusions.

Because they do not, we advocate an appreciation of the needs of family *systems*, across generations, in their diversity, with reciprocal rights and responsibilities. This position is not meant to supplant advocacy work on behalf of grandparent caregivers. Rather, we are calling for an orientation to the rights and responsibilities of each generation in these complex and often stressful family arrangements. Such an orientation should enable advocates to avoid the romanticization of grandparent caregiving even as they demonstrate an appreciation for grandparents' contributions to family life. It is our basic contention that policy and practice that attend to a single generation's interests cannot ultimately be good family policy because it is likely to be atomistic and not fully contextual. Families are multigenerational, complex, and dynamic. We should expect good family policy and practice to reflect this understanding.

Linkage Between Imprisonment and Poverty[2]

Why are more and more grandparents having to assume child care because of the incarceration of their offspring? The basic answer to this question is that such circumstances confront us because the U.S. imprisons its population at a rate higher than that of any other industrialized nation. But this statement in and of itself masks major social forces implicated in the issue.

Dressel (1994) contends that imprisonment and poverty, as well as racism, are closely linked in the U.S. Her argument proceeds as follows:

1. When social assistance is not provided at a level that allows for a family's basic needs "some members of the population may be unable

---

2. This section is derived largely from Dressel (1994).

to conduct their lives within the usual legitimized opportunity structures" (p. 8). Thus, they may turn to economically motivated crimes such as bad check writing, welfare fraud, drug sales, prostitution, and theft.

2. Within a political climate that seeks scapegoats and individualized explanations for social problems such as poverty, the means for addressing behaviors like those mentioned focuses on social control rather than social assistance.

3. The convergence of welfare devolution and more punitive TANF regulations on the one hand and the dramatic growth of imprisonment on the other hand are related dynamics that reflect the political climate just described.

4. These policy choices on behalf of social control over social assistance are informed in both direct and indirect ways by racism. The distorted popular imagery surrounding both welfare and crime conveys racist stereotypes that mobilize harsh public sentiment against people of color specifically and against social assistance policies generally. Furthermore, racism is implicated in the very production of vulnerability to poverty via the many ways that educational systems and labor markets continue to operate with unequal opportunity and disparate impact.

5. Given su :h political economic dynamics, it is predictable that grandparents cf color who are struggling economically end up becoming disproportionately represented among grandparent caregivers of children of incarcerated parents.

Of course, none of the foregoing dynamics is inevitable. At any juncture the nation could choose a political course that offers more equitable access to education and jobs and that focuses on collective welfare rather than individualized punishment and group scapegoating. This is not to pretend that mobilizing political will for a different course would be easy. But it is to suggest that apart from such a course, we will continue to see families broken apart by imprisonment and grandparents burdened beyond their means, even if not beyond their willingness to assume larger family responsibilities than they anticipated.

References

Adalist-Estrin, A. (1986). Parenting from behind bars. *Family Resources Coalition Report, 5,* 12–13.

American Correctional Association. (1990). *The female offender: What does the future hold?* Washington, DC: St. Mary Press.

Barnhill, S. K. (1994). *Three generations at risk: Imprisoned women, their children, and grandmother caregivers.* Generations, 20, 39–40.

Barry, E. (1995). Legal issues for prisons with children. In Gabel, K., & Johnson, D. (Eds.), *Children of incarcerated parents* (pp. 147–166). New York: Lexington Books.

Baunach, P. J. (1985). *Mothers in prison.* New Brunswick: Transaction Books.

Beck, J., & Gillard, D. (1995). *Prisoners in 1994.* Washington, DC: U.S. Department of Justice.

Bloom, B., & Steinhart, D. (1993). *Why punish the children? A reappraisal of the children of incarcerated mothers in America.* San Francisco: National Council on Crime and Delinquency.

Burton, L., & Bengtson, V. L. (1985). Black grandmothers: Issues of timing and continuity of roles, In V. L. Bengtson, & J. F. Robertson (Eds.), *Grandparenthood* (pp. 61–77). Beverly Hills: Sage.

Camp, G., & Camp, C. (1996). *The corrections yearbook 1995: Adult corrections.* South Salem, NY: Criminal Justice Institute.

Chappell, N. L. (1990). Aging and social care. In R. H. Binstock, & L. K. George, (Eds.), *Handbook of aging and the social sciences* (3rd ed., pp. 438–454). New York: Academic Press.

Donziger, S. (1996). *The real war on crime.* New York: Harper Collins.

Dressel, P. L., & Barnhill, S. K. (1994). Reframing gerontological thought and practice: The case of grandmothers with daughters in prison. *The Gerontologists,* 34, 685–691.

Dressel, P. L., & Kelley, S. (1996). *Grandparent caregivers: Expanding the agenda.* Paper presented at the annual meeting of the Gerontological Society of America, Washington, D.C.

Egley, C. C. (1992). Outcome of pregnancy during imprisonment. *Journal of Traumatic Stress,* 37, 131–134.

Fritsch, T. A., & Burkhead, J. D. (1982). Behavioral reactions of children to parental absence due to imprisonment. *Family Relations,* 30, 83–88.

Fuller-Thomson, E., Minkler, M., & Driver, D. (1997). A profile of grandparents raising grandchildren in the United States. *The Gerontologist,* 37, 406–411.

Greenfield, L. A., & Minor-Harper, S. (1991). *Women in prison.* Washington, DC: Bureau of Justice Statistics.

Hairston, C. F. (1995). Fathers in prison. In K. Gabel, & D. Johnson (Eds.), *Children of incarcerated parents* (pp. 31–40). New York: Lexington Books.

Johnson, D. (1991). *Jailed mothers.* Pasadena: Pacific Oaks Center for Children of Incarcerated Parents.

Johnson, D. (1992). *Children of offenders.* Pasadena: Pacific Oaks Center for Children of Incarcerated Parents.

Johnson, D. (1993). *Intergenerational incarceration.* Pasadena: Pacific Oaks Center for Children of Incarcerated Parents.

Johnson, D. (1995a). Intervention. In K. Gabel, & D. Johnson (Eds.), *Children of incarcerated parents* (pp. 199–236). New York: Lexington Books.

Johnson, D. (1995b). Effects of parental incarceration. In K. Gabel, & D. Johnson (Eds.), *Children of incarcerated parents* (pp. 59–88). New York: Lexington Books.

Johnson, D., & Gabel, K. (1995). Incarcerated Parents. In K. Gabel, & D. Johnson (Eds.), *Children of incarcerated parents* (pp. 3–20). New York: Lexington Books.

Kampfner, C. J. (1995). Post-traumatic stress reactions in children of imprisoned mothers. In K. Gabel, & D. Johnson (Eds.), *Children of incarcerated parents* (pp. 89–100) New York: Lexington Books.

Kessler, R. C., Price, R. H., & Wortman, C. B. (1985). Social factors in psychopathology: Stress, social support, and coping process. *Annual Review of Psychology, 36,* 531–572.

Koban, L. (1983). Parents in prison: A comparative analysis of the effects of incarceration on the families of men and women. *Research in Law, Deviance, and Social Control, 5,* 171–183.

McCall, C. J., Casteel, J., & Shaw, N. C. (1985). Pregnancy in prison: A needs assessment of prenatal outcome in three California penal institutions (Contract #84-84085). Sacramento: Department of Health Services.

McGowan, B. G., & Blumenthal, K. L. (1978). *Why punish the children?* Hackensack, NJ: National Council on Crime and Delinquency.

Minkler, M., & Roe, K. M. (1993). *Grandmothers as caregivers: Raising children of the crack cocaine epidemic.* Newbury Park: Sage.

Reed, D. F., & Reed, E. L. (1997). Children of incarcerated parents. *Social Justice, 24,* 152–169.

Scharlach, A. E., & Boyd, S. (1989). Caregiving and employment: Results of an employee survey. *The Gerontologist, 29,* 382–387.

Smith, G. (1995). Practical Considerations Regarding Termination of Incarcerated Parents' Rights. In K. Gabel, & D. Johnson (Eds.), *Children of incarcerated parents* (pp. 183–195). New York: Lexington Books.

United States Bureau of the Census. (1990). *Current population reports: Marital status and living arrangements* (Series P-20, No. 450). Washington, DC: U.S. Government Printing Office.

United States Department of Justice. (1994). *Women in prison* (Special Report, No. NCJ-145321). Washington, DC: Bureau of Justice Statistics.

Zalba, S. (1964). *Women prisoners and their families.* California: Department of Social Welfare and Department of Corrections.

Chapter 12

Profile of Contemporary Grandparenting in African-American Families

Diane R. Brown and Joan Mars

Surrogate parenting by grandparents and other kin is a well-established pattern in African-American families where grandparents and older family members assume parenting responsibilities for children whose parents are temporarily or permanently unable to do so (Burton, 1996; Strom et al., 1996; Wilson, 1986). The kinship care traditions within African-American families are unique in that they reflect complex cultural, environmental and institutional factors that define Black family life in America. The purpose of this chapter is to provide a profile of contemporary African-American grandparents and other kin who are engaged in surrogate parenting for a grandchild or similar child; to describe the circumstances under which surrogate parenting takes place and to examine the sources of stress and social support experienced by African-American grandparents.

This research was funded by the AARP Andrus Foundation. The authors wish to thank the following research assistants for their help in preparing this paper: Angela Boyce and Lina Beydoun.

The historical importance of kinship networks in African-American families predates its expansion and development as an adaptive response to Black family disintegration occasioned by slavery, and can be traced to West African family traditions which favored the extended family model (Scannapieco & Jackson 1996; Yusane, 1990). Surrogate parenting among African-American families is part of a system of kin and quasi-kinship networks that distinguish the Black family as an institution defined not only by blood ties but also by a complex system of relationships based on spatial proximity, shared values and functional affiliations that are continually evolving over time (Allen, 1995; Billingsley, 1993; Stack, 1974). These extended family networks have included a "kin help system" of social support and mutual assistance encompassing intergenerational ties that involve various forms of caregiving (Wilson, 1986). Although current studies of intergenerational caregiving have tended to focus solely on grandparenting (Aldous, 1995; Dowdell, 1995; Jendrek, 1994; Minkler, 1994), they tend to exclude consideration of common practices among African-American extended families, whereby surrogate parenting is provided by a broader range of caregivers including aunts, uncles, cousins, great grandparents and pseudokin.

In recent years, surrogate parenting by grandparents and other kin has received greater attention from social scientists and gerontologists because of the expanded array of circumstances under which the surrogate parenting is occurring. As an example, research has historically documented intergenerational surrogate parenting in response to out-of-wedlock births, separation and divorce, unemployment, poverty, economic problems and other family crises (Billingsley, 1968; 1993; Martin & Martin 1978; Shimkin, Shimkin, & Frate, Stack, 1974; 1978). More recently, factors, such as parental drug and alcohol abuse, violence and homicide, incarceration, HIV/AIDS, and teen pregnancy, have contributed to circumstances where biological parents are unable, unwilling or limited in their ability to care for their children. In some instances, these children are taken into the foster care system, but in many other cases, African-American grandparents, other relatives, and pseudo-kin assume the full-time child care responsibilities.

Socio-Demographic Context of Surrogate Parenting

The circumstances of surrogate parenting in African-American families is apt to differ from those of their White counterparts not only because of cultural differences but also because the sociodemographic circumstances of midlife and older African-American differ in significant ways from their White counterparts. This is of considerable importance because these sociodemographic differences have ramifications for their ability to assume parenting responsibilities for their grandchildren and for the resources they bring to their surrogate parenting responsibilities.

African-American grandparents are more likely than comparable Whites to have lower incomes and live in poverty (Mannheimer, 1994). Given fewer economic resources, many mid-life and older African-Americans find employment a necessity. Data show that older Black females aged 65 years and older are more likely to work than their White counterparts (U.S. Department of Labor, 1985 update). Further, older African-American women are likely to be working despite conditions of poor health and family responsibilities (Brown, 1988). They also have lower levels of education, fewer skilled and professional jobs, lower salaries, and more frequent periods of unemployment (Brown, 1988).

Racial differences in sociodemographic circumstances also occur with regard to marital status and living arrangements. Among African-Americans 65 years of age and older, the ratio of men to women is lower than in the White population. In addition, older African-Americans are less likely to be married and to remarry, if widowed or divorced (Mannheimer, 1994). Consequently, midlife and older African-American women are more likely to be nonmarried and to be householders than are their White counterparts (Brown, 1988). Regarding living arrangements, older African Americans are slightly more likely than older Whites to live in larger households and households consisting of multiple generations (Brown & Monye, 1995). Sharing a household with an adult child is a common living arrangement for many older African Americans.

Significant differences exist also in terms of health status. African Americans have poorer health status than similar Whites as evidenced in greater rates of morbidity and mortality (Centers for Disease Control, 1997). The social stresses associated with lifelong poverty and low income, in conjunction with experiences of racial or ethnic discrimination contribute to poorer health across the age span. Among older African Americans 65 to 74 years of age, the rates of diabetes, hypertension, and cardiovascular disease exceed those of their White counterparts (Centers for Disease Control, 1997). Further, not only do older African Americans have shorter life expectancies, but they also have greater functional disability during their later years (Mannheimer, 1994). Given the overall poorer health status of minorities and the likelihood of other chronic conditions, African-American grandparents and other older kin who are assuming the primary care for grandchildren are likely to do so despite circumstances of poor health.

Impact of Surrogate Parenting

To examine the impact of surrogate parenting on the health and well-being of grandparents, social scientists have borrowed heavily from studies on caregiving for ailing elders. For example, findings from research on elder caregiving document that caregiving can be burdensome and stressful and can result in considerable distress or depression for the grandparents (Brody, 1985; Scharlack & Boyd, 1989). Conversely, researchers applying this same stress and coping framework to the study of grandparents raising grandchildren have reported inconsistent findings regarding the impact of caregiving on the health and well-being of the caregiver. Burton and Dilworth-Anderson (1991) found that providing the primary care for a grandchild was not a particularly desired role for the contemporary African-American grandmother.

Moreover, in a subsequent analysis, Burton (1995) indicated that caring for grandchildren was associated with more psychological, physical and economic costs, even though parenting grandchildren was generally viewed as an emotionally rewarding experience. Jendrek (1993), using data from a predominantly White sample, also noted both positive and negative effects of parenting grandchildren with more strain occurring in three-generation households. In a study that focused on surrogate parenting in African-American families in response to the crack cocaine epidemic, Minkler, Roe, and Price (1992) reported that slightly more than a third (36.6%) experienced deterioration in their emotional health since they began caregiving. Nonetheless, for many respondents (45%) their health did not impede them from doing what they needed to do.

Families and Other Sources of Support

Although there are many stresses associated with surrogate parenting, there is also evidence that grandparents and other kin have access to sources of assistance and social support. The importance of family bonds as sources of social support among African-Americans has been well documented (Billingsley, 1993; Ellison, 1990; Gary et. al., 1989; Martin & Martin 1983; Scannapieco & Jackson, 1996; Stack, 1974; Wilson, 1986). Informal social support networks provide instrumental and emotional support for families during times of chronic and acute illness (Taylor, 1988).

Older African-American women, in particular, are more likely than similar Whites to call on friends, neighbors and coworkers for informal help, especially if they are not married. Involvement in church and religious activities also serves as a well established source of social support for African-Americans (Frazier, 1974; Lincoln et al., 1990; Randolph et al., 1994; Smith, 1994; Taylor & Chatters, 1988). Further, church members play an important role in the informal support networks of many older African-Americans, in which support includes financial assistance, household services, transportation, and meals as well as emotional support from visitation and companionship (Taylor & Chatters, 1988).

Methods

Data from our study of surrogate parenting among African-American grandparents corroborate many of the circumstances documented in the literature as well as provide additional insights into contemporary situations. The data were gathered through interviews with 140 African-Americans, 38 years of age and older, who had primarily parenting responsibility for a school-aged child for whom they were not the biological parent. Selection of respondents was based on a stratified proportional random sampling strategy using the school-aged population of a major eastern city (Brown & Monye, 1995). Interviews were conducted with the caregiver identified by the child's school. For the purposes of this analysis, the grandchild is referred to as the sample child.

The demographic characteristics of the grandparents are illustrated in Table 12.1. As would be expected from the literature, most of the respondents were female 131 (93.5%), although nine (6.5%) were male. The average age was 55.0 years, with ages ranging from 38 to 80. Although 37.1% of the grandparents had less than a high school education, most had at least a high school education. Approximately, one quarter of the grandparents (25.9%) had one or more years of college education and a smaller number (4.3%) had attended graduate school. Slightly more than half of the grandparents (58.6%) were not employed at the time of the survey mainly because of retirement or health reasons. Exactly a quarter of the grandparents (25.0%) were married, whereas the remaining were divorced or separated (36.4%), widowed (26.4%) or were never married (12.1%).

Forty percent of the grandparents lived in single parent households, with the grandparent being the only adult in a household with one or more

TABLE 12.1 Demographic Characteristics of Grandparents

	N	%
Gender		
Male	9	6.4
Female	131	93.6
Age (years)		
38–45	34	24.3
46–55	39	27.9
56–65	41	29.3
66–80	26	18.6
Education		
8 years or less	14	10.0
9 to 11 years	38	27.1
High school graduate	46	32.9
Some college	36	25.9
Graduate school	6	4.3
Employment		
Employed	58	41.4
Not employed	82	58.6
Household income		
Less than $6,000	15	11.7
$6–11,000	33	25.8
$12–24,999	26	40.3
$25,000+	54	42.2
Household structure		
Single parent	56	40.0
Single parent augmented	51	36.4
Nuclear	19	13.6
Nuclear augmented	14	10.0
Number of persons in household		
Two	1	.7
Three	24	17.1
Four	28	20.0
Five	49	35.0
Six	16	11.4
Seven or more	22	15.7

TABLE 12.1 *(continued)*

Number of children in household		
One	2	1.4
Two	56	40.0
Three	37	26.4
Four	33	23.6
Five	4	2.9
Six	4	2.9
Seven or more	4	2.9
Marital status		
Married	35	25.0
Divorced	27	19.3
Separated	24	17.1
Windowed	37	26.4
Never Married	17	12.1

children 18 years of age or younger. Another 36.4% were in augmented single parent households consisting of the grandparent, at least one other nonspousal adult (usually one or more of the caregiver's adult children), along with one or more minor children. At the same time, 14.6% of the grandparents were in nuclear family households, encompassing married grandparents with one or more minor children. Another 10% were in nuclear augmented households with married grandparents, another adult (usually grandparent's child), and one or more children. On average, there were 3.1 minor children per household (SD = 1.3), with an average household size of five persons.

Findings

Caregiving Circumstances

Most of the grandparents (71.3%) were taking care of a grandchild—primarily a daughter's child; others were assuming care for other kin such as a nephew, niece, or great-grandchild (17.4%) and nonkin (11.3%). Table 12.2 provides an indication of reasons given by grandparents for

TABLE 12.2 Reasons Why Parents Were Not Primary Grandparents

Reasons	Father N	Father %	Mother N	Mother %
Deceased	12	8.6	18	12.9
Health problem	2	1.4	8	5.7
Incarceration	21	15.0	4	2.9
Financial/poverty	13	9.3	15	10.7
Child abuse	2	1.4	5	3.6
Drug addiction	12	8.6	57	40.7
Teen pregnancy	3	2.1	5	3.6
Extended family setting	2	1.4	7	5.0
Abandonment	27	19.3	11	7.9
Out of town residence	6	4.3	1	.7
Unknown identity or whereabouts	40	28.6	9	6.4

why biological parents were not providing primary caregiving responsibility. The reasons vary depending on the gender of the parent. In the case of the father, 8.6% were deceased. However, for about 30%, the grandparents did not know the reasons or else did not know the father's identity or whereabouts. For nearly one fifth (19.3%), the father had abandoned the child.

Specifically, grandparents indicated that the father had either failed to take responsibility for the child, had denied paternity or had merely never shown any interest in assuming the parenting responsibilities. For example, grandparents described the child's father as "unstable" and "irresponsible" or stated that the father "can hardly take care of himself." In 15.0% of the cases, the sample child's father was incarcerated. Financial reasons or poverty were given to explain the lack of parenting responsibility for 9.3% of fathers; and drug abuse was given as the reason for 8.6%. To be noted, grandparents were asked to provide only one reason, so it is possible that the fathers may have relinquished their parenting responsibilities for more than one reason (e.g., drug use *and* abandonment).

Drug addiction was the most frequently mentioned reason (40.7%) for the sample child's mother not parenting the child. Another 12.9% of the mothers were deceased, whereas 10.7% were too poor to care for the child, and 7.9% had abandoned the child. In only a few cases (6.4%), the grandparent did not know the reason, the identity, or the whereabouts of the mother. Another 5.7% of the mothers had health problems including HIV/AIDS and could not care for the child.

Evidence of strong family bonds was also seen in responses to questions about reasons for assuming care of the grandchild. Grandparents were specifically asked, "Why did you take on regular parental care of this child?" The open-ended responses were grouped into two major categories: familial responsibilities and "other." Most of the grandparents (89.3%) indicated that they were parenting the child because of kinship.

The grandparents varied in how they perceived the circumstances leading to their assuming care. The largest percentage (31.4) indicated that the child was not being cared for, was being neglected, abused, or was abandoned—most often because the mother was on drugs. Another 18.6% stated specifically that they provided care because the child was "family". In most of these cases, the mother had died and there was no one else to care for the child. Other grandparents (14.3%) expressed a positive sense of loving the child and wanting to improve the child's life, to provide the love and care the child deserved, and to ensure the child's well-being and safety. Another 13.6% said that they began caring for the child to provide assistance to the child's mother, many of whom were trying to go to school, worked long hours during the week, were unemployed or financially incapable, or were ill. To be noted, a small percentage (2.9%) stated that they had no choice, the child was "pushed" on them. Avoidance of having the child placed in foster care or protective services was given as a reason by 8.6% of grandparents. The "other reason" category (8.6%) included grandparents who for the most part were not family members; most of whom were family friends or "fictive" kin.

Approximately half of the grandparents (49.2%) had a legal framework for providing care for the child; this included: custody (17.1%); guardianship (21.4%); adoption (2.1%); and foster care (8.6%). However, conversely, about 50% of the grandparents were providing care without legal responsibility for the child. Approximately one quarter of the grandparents (27.9%) stated that they are serving as a substitute parent for the sample child, without a legal relationship. The remaining grandparents (22.9%) claimed that they were informally serving as a parent. Many of these indicated that they "were just taking care of the child"; others stated that the child had informally been adopted. Another stated that the daughter had notarized a form providing for temporary custody, whereas several stated that they were assisting the mother or substituting for the mother. For most, it appeared as if this might be a temporary relationship, but, in a few cases, grandparents stated that the parent had relinquished custody until further notice.

At the time the study was conducted, grandparents reported having assumed parental care of the child from as early as birth right up to as recent as one month prior to the study. The mean length of time for care-giving was 5.5 years (SD = 3.7). It is very important to note that nearly half (45.7%) of the grandparents were also caring for other children in the household in addition to the sample child. As noted earlier, the average number of children per household was 3.1.

Social Support and Informal Sources of Assistance

Several measures were included to obtain an indication of the extent to which grandparents participated in social support network where informal assistance was received from friends and family. Overall, the grandparents appeared to have a substantial network of family members and friends on whom they could potentially call on for social support. This was evidenced in response to the question "how many total relatives, who you see or talk with regularly, who live nearby," responses ranged from none to more than 100. The average number was 13.1 nearby relatives (SD = 18.2), although 40.7% of the grandparents had five or fewer relatives in the area. In general, most grandparents felt close to other members of their family.

In terms of receiving assistance from family members, grandparents were asked a general question about the frequency in which they received help from family members. Nearly half (47.9%) of the grandparents stated that family members very often helped out; 52.1% received assistance "never" or "not too often." Family members were the most frequently used source of baby-sitting for the sample child (37.1%), although 34.3% of grandparents used a family center, 15.7% used a friend/neighbor, and 2.8% used a teenager or other person. However, 10.0% indicated that "no one" was used to provide baby-sitting. Most grandparents (92.8%) indicated that they "never" or "not often" paid anyone for baby-sitting. Only 4.3% very often paid someone to take care of sample child when the grandparent had something to do.

Grandparents were also asked to indicate the total number of nearby friends whom they see or talk with regularly. The mean number of friends was 8.6 (SD = 14.5), the median was 4. Only 5.7% had no friends nearby. Nearly half (46.8%) stated that their friends fairly often or very often helped out. In addition, grandparents were asked, "is there anyone to whom you can really open up about your most private feelings without having to hold back?" Most (87.1%) said "yes." The average number of confidantes was 1.1 (SD = .34).

Grandparents were queried about other potential sources of social support such as church and participation in community organizations. Membership in community organizations primarily centered on involvement in church or religious organizations, although 48.6% of grandparents were involved in the PTA, and 18.0% were members of civic groups. Overall, the religious involvement appeared to be an important source of social support for grandparents. More than half (52.1%) attended church at least once a week or more, and 27.9% attended at least a few times a month.

Sources of Stress

Although most of the grandparents reported the availability of sources of social support, many also indicated sources of strain and concern. For example, grandparents contributed substantially to the financial support of the child. Approximately, two thirds of grandparents were receiving government financial assistance for raising the child, primarily from AFDC and Social Security. However, this assistance did not cover most of the costs of raising the child. On the average, government assistance provided only one fourth of the costs for the child. The remaining financial support came primarily from the grandparent. For the one third who received no governmental assistance, most of these grandparents were providing 100% of the costs of supporting the child. Only a few received financial assistance from one of the child's parents or another family member.

When asked what concerned the grandparent most about his or her ability to raise the sample child, grandparents provided a range of responses. The most frequently mentioned response (27.1%) pertained to their own health. Grandparents said, "I am getting too old and I have health problems," "living long enough to see (child) care for himself," "my immobility—I'm disabled and cannot get to the school unless someone takes me," and "my health is not as good as it used to be." Another 16.4% expressed concern about being able to provide good education, discipline, guidance and parenting for the child. For example, grandparents said they were concerned about seeing that she "gets a proper education," "being a good role model," "I may not be able to control him," and "I don't know if I am doing it right."

Grandparents (15.7%) were concerned about the stress that they experienced; many giving this response indicated that they were concerned about their ability to have the patience, energy and strength needed to continue raising the child. Concerns were also mentioned related to providing a safe home and neighborhood environment (7.9%), and being able to meet the special emotional and/or physical needs of the sample child (2.9%). Other responses (6.4%) covered worries related to interference from the child's mother and having sufficient financial resources. One grandparent stated, "as a single parent I am concerned about lack of support and resources available to me because I am not his biological parent."

Conclusions

Overall, this study provides further documentation of the intergenerational caregiving that historically has occurred in African-American families where older family members step in to care for children whose parents are temporarily or permanently unable to do so. In a contemporary urban setting, the findings from this population-based sample of urban midlife and older African-Americans indicate that most of these individuals are female, single householders, averaging 55 years of age. Some were employed and the majority had at least a high school education.

Intergenerational caregiving or surrogate parenting in African-American families occurs under a variety of circumstances. Although parental substance abuse has emerged as a major reason for grandparents engaging in surrogate parenting, it is by far not the only reason. Historically, as well as contemporaneously, reasons for surrogate parenting range from the death of the child's parent(s) to incarceration, poverty, illness, immaturity, teen pregnancy, and employment or education of child's parent in a distant location.

Whatever the reason for surrogate parenting, many midlife and older African-Americans are assuming surrogate parenting responsibilities for their children's children as well as the children of other kin and nonkin. Findings from this study pointed to the importance of kinship bonds in African-American families, as most of the grandparents were caring for a relative's child. Further, in most cases, these surrogate parents are caring for multiple grandchildren.

However, despite the additional caregiving responsibilities, grandparents expressed a strong sentiment to nurture and enhance the child's well-being, and to provide opportunities for growth and development. Because of familial obligations, most wanted to avoid having the child placed in foster care system or child protective services. However, only about half of the grandparents in this study had a legally determined relationship with the child in their care. Concomitantly, informal surrogate parenting characterized the caregiving circumstances of 50% of the grandparents in the study.

It is evident from the findings that most African-American grandparents who are engaged in surrogate parenting face struggles with their circumstances. In particular, inadequate financial resources to cover the cost of raising the child were a source of stress and strain for grandparents. Only a few received financial help from the child's parents or other family members. Even for those receiving some governmental financial assistance, such assistance on the average covered about one fourth of the costs of raising the child.

In addition to the inadequacy of material support, caregivers were also concerned about their perceived inability to provide a safe environment for the child, as well as proper education, and social and emotional support necessary for appropriate child development. Conversely, most caregivers appeared to have a substantial network of family members and friends on whom they could call for help and assistance. In addition, involvement in church or religious organizations and membership in community organizations were also important sources of social support and assistance for the caregivers.

In conclusion, findings from this study point to the enduring importance of intergenerational ties in African-American families. Surrogate parenting continues to be an important and complex tradition that provides for the care of children who are kin and nonkin. However, although the positive aspects of surrogate parenting and intergenerational familial support in African-American families are to be applauded, social scientists, social policymakers and practitioners need to vigilant regarding circumstances of stress and strain, particularly in low-income families where surrogate parenting may not be conducive to the well-being of the child or the grandparent caregiver.

References

Aldous, J. (1995). New view of grandparents in intergenerational context. *Journal of Family Issues, 16*, 104–122.

Allen, W. R. (1995). African-American family life in societal context: Crisis and hope. *Sociological Forum, 10*, 569–592).

Billingsley, A. (1968). Black families in White America. Englewood Cliffs, NJ: Prentice Hall.

Billingsley, A. (1993). *Climbing Jacob's ladder: The enduring legacy of African-American families*. New York: Simon & Schuster.

Brody, E. M. (1985). Parent care as a normative family stress. *The Gerontologist*, 25, 19–29.

Brown, D. R. (1988). *Employment and health status among older Black women: Implications for their economic status*. Wellesley, MA: Center for Research on Women.

Brown, D. R., & Monye, D. B. (1995). *Midlife and older African-Americans as intergenerational caregivers of school-aged children*. Final Report to AARP Andrus Foundation.

Burton, L. M. (1996). Age norms, the timing of family role transitions, and inter-generational caregiving among aging African-American women. *The Gerontologist*, 36, 199–208.

Burton, L. M. (1995). Context and surrogate parenting among contemporary grandparents. *Marriage and Family Review*, 20, 349–366.

Burton, L. M. (1992). Black grandparents rearing children of drug-addicted parents: Stressors, outcomes, and social service needs. *The Gerontologist*, 32 (6), 744–751.

Burton, L. M., & Dilworth-Anderson, P. (1991). The intergenerational family roles of aged Black Americans. *Marriage and Family Review*, 1–2, 311–330.

Centers for Disease Control and Prevention. (1994). *AIDS surveillance report: Cumulative AIDS cases through September 30, 1994*. Atlanta: Author.

Dowdell, E. B. (1995). Caregiver burden: Grandparents raising their high risk grandchildren. *Journal of Psychosocial Nursing*, 33, 27–30.

Ellison, C. G. (1990). Family ties, friendships, and subjective well-being among Black Americans. *Journal of Marriage and the Family*, 52, 298–310.

Gary, L. E., Brown, D. R., Milburn, N. G., Ahmed, F., & Booth, J. (1989). Depression in Black American adults: Findings from the Norfolk Area Health Study. Washington, DC: Howard University.

Frazier, E. F. (1974). *The Negro church in America*. New York: Schocken Books.

Jendrek, M. D. (1993). Grandparents who parent their grandchildren: Effects on lifestyle. *Journal of Marriage and the Family*, 55, 609–621.

Frazier, E. F. (1994). Grandparents who parent their grandchildren: Circumstances and decisions. *The Gerontologist*, 34, 206–216.

Lincoln, C. E., & Mamiya, L. H. (1990). *The black church in the African-American experience*. Durham, NC: Duke University Press.

Mannheimer, R. (1994). *Older persons almanac*. Detroit: Gale Research.

Martin, E., & Martin J. (1978). *The Black extended family*. Chicago: University of Chicago Press.

Minkler, M. (1994). Grandparents as parents: The American experience. *Aging International*, 3, 24–28.

Minkler, M., Roe, K. M., & Price, M. (1992). The physical and emotional health of grandmothers raising grandchildren in the crack cocaine epidemic. *The Gerontologist*, 32, 752–761.

Pruchno, R. A., & Johnson, K. W. (1996). Research on grandparenting: Current studies and future needs. *Generations*, *20*, 65–70.

Scannapieco, M., & Jackson, S. (1996). Kinship care: The African-American response to family preservation. *Social Work*, *41*, 190–196.

Smith, J. M. (1994). Function and supportive roles of church and religion. In J. S. Jackson, L. M. Chatters, & R. J.Taylor (Eds.), *Aging in Black America* (pp. 101–123). Newbury Park, CA: Sage.

Randolph, S. M., Billingsley, A., & Caldwell, C. H. (1994). Studying Black churches and family support in the context of HIV/AIDS. *National Journal of Sociology*, *8*, 109–130.

Scharlach, A., & Boyd, S. L. (1989). Caregiving and emiployment: Results of an employee survey. *The Gerontologist*, *29*, 382–387.

Shimkin, D., Shimkin, E., & Frate, D. (1978). The extended family in Black societies. Chicago: Aldine.

Stack, C. (1974). All our kin: Strategies for survival in black community. New York: Harper.

Strom, R., Strom, S., Collinsworth, P., Strom, P., & Griswold, D. (1996). Intergenerational relationships in Black families. *International Journal of Sociology of the Family*, *26*, 129–141.

Taylor, R. J. (1988). Aging and supportive relationships. In J. S. Jackson (Ed.), *The Black elderly*. New York: Springer.

Taylor, R. J., & Chatters, L. (1988). Church members as a source of informal support. *Review of Religious Research*, *30*, 432–438.

Wilson, M. N. (1986). The Black extended family: An analytical consideration. *Developmental Psychology*, *22*, 246–258.

Yusane, A. Y. (1990). Cultural, political, and economic universals in West Africa in synthesis. In M. K. Asante, & K. W. Asante (Eds.), *African culture: The rhythms of unity* (pp. 39–70). Trenton, NJ: Africa World.

Chapter 13

Culture and Caregiving: A Study of Latino Grandparents

Carole B. Cox, Lisette Resto Brooks, and Carmen Valcarcel

Latino grandparents are one of the groups in which raising grandchildren has become increasingly common. Data from the U.S. Census indicate that almost 6% of Hispanic children are living with their grandparents or other relatives (Saluter, 1992), whereas Chafie's (1994) national study of skipped-generation families showed Latinos composing 10% of relative caregivers. With the rapid increase in the Latino population in the United States and the expansion of elderly persons within this population, particular attention must be given to the issues confronting those who find themselves responsible for their grandchildren.

Two of the most prominent social problems contributing to this phenomenon are AIDS and substance abuse, which are disproportionately represented among Latino populations (Soriano, 1993). These problems, coupled with traditional cultural values, contribute to the propensity of grandparents to become responsible for raising their grandchildren when their children are absent. However, as they strive to meet the demands of both their family and their grandchildren, they find themselves encountering new and unexpected challenges. Adjusting to the new situation and role is difficult and often very stressful.

This chapter discusses the many factors influencing and affecting grandparent caregiving among Latinos. In particular, it examines aspects of Latino culture and tradition which may be influential in shaping the responses and behaviors of grandparents raising grandchildren. Ethnicity takes shape and is transmitted through families and through generations, and thus to better understand the responses of any ethnic group, it is essential to understand their perceptions of their roles and society. The chapter also describes a community program designed to strengthen and enable Latino grandparents. Case examples of program particpants are used to illustrate the ways in which culture may influence the interactions and behaviors of Latino grandparents.

Demographic Profile

Hispanics are the fastest-growing group in the elderly population, projected to double from 3.6% of the total elderly population in 1990 to 6.3% in 2010 and 11.7% in 2050 (U.S. Bureau of the Census, 1986). Data from the Census also reveal that Cubans tend to be the eldest among the subgroups with a median age of 41.4 years; Puerto Ricans, at 26.8 years, and Mexican American, at 26.8 years, are considerably younger.

Most Hispanic Americans were born in the United States. However, whereas most of the general population of elderly, 88%, were born in the United States, only 58% of the Hispanic elderly were nativeborn. Not surprisingly, only a slight majority of elderly Hispanics, 60.7%, claim to be proficient in English (The Commonwealth Fund Commission, 1989). In addition, the population has the lowest median number of school years completed, 7.5, in comparison with 8.4 years for elderly Blacks and 12.2 for elderly Whites.

Hispanic elderly have high rates of poverty with median incomes only slightly above the poverty level (U.S. Bureau of the Census, 1990). In 1989, 20.6% of the population was in poverty with the rate even higher, 26.3%, for those aged 65 to 74 years. As found among the Black elderly, women are more likely to be poor than their male counterparts. Moreover, Hispanic elders are less likely to receive Social Security benefits than either non-Hispanic whites or African Americans (U.S. Department of HHS, 1990). Consequently, this population of older persons is more likely than other groups to depend on public assistance.

Given their poor economic status, it is not surprising that older Hispanics report poorer health than other groups of elderly. They have higher rates of disability and more days of restricted activities than either older Whites or Blacks but at the same time make fewer physician visits (Select Committee on Aging, 1989). As they are less likely to have Social Security, they also have a much lower rate of Medicare coverage than other older groups. Consequently, they are more likely to receive Medicaid. The lack of health insurance not only affects the older population. Hispanic children are less likely than other groups to be covered by private insurance (Children's Defense Fund, 1994).

The impact of poverty and poor physical health impact on psychological well-being is indicated in a study of older immigrants from Mexico, Cuba, and Puerto Rico (Krause & Goldenhar, 1992). As a group, these immigrants tend to have strong Hispanic identities and low levels of education and to be less acculturated than other groups. The interrelationships of these factors were related to increased financial strain and social isolation and linked to psychological distress. Others (Andrews, Lyons, & Rowland, 1992) have also found poor health status, lower education, and lower-paying jobs related to older Hispanics having lower levels of life satisfaction than other groups of elderly. Moreover, among all Hispanic subgroups, Puerto Ricans appear to be the most psychologically distressed (Guranaccia, Good, & Kleinman, 1989).

Compounding the stress facing older Hispanics is the worry they frequently experience regarding their immigration status and their eligibility for services. The 1996 changes in welfare legislation added to their anxiety about seeking assistance because of the ambiguity associated with their immigration status as well as changes in requirements. The 5-year limit on welfare payments is a major source of anxiety, particularly for those not eligible for SSI. Concerns over eligibility for programs, such as SSI, Medicaid, and Food Stamps have been intensified by worries that their immigration status in the United States could be jeopardized because of a lack of proper documentation.

Both cultural and social forces have contributed to the family being the primary source of help, specifically the spouse or adult child, for older Hispanics. A national survey of older Hispanics (The Commonwealth Fund Commision, 1989) found the population more likely than other groups of elderly to live with their adult children. More than three fourths of Hispanic elderly live with their family compared with two thirds of non-Hispanic white or black elderly. Although many live with their children to receive assistance, it is important to also recognize that the relationship with adult children is reciprocal as these older persons are the primary sources of help to their children and grandchildren.

Familism

Latino culture has a strong basis in familism that stresses the needs of the family and the group rather than the individual with a preference for assistance from within the family. Older persons are frequently relied on to assist with child care and thus are likely to be called on to assume primary responsibility for raising grandchildren when parents are incapacitated or absent. Not accepting their care or turning to formal agencies for assistance may be perceived as not adhering to traditional values and expectations.

Within the family, Latino elderly play important roles in the socialization of children, providing emotional support, particularly in times of need and crisis, and providing meaning and direction to family members (Sotomayor, 1988). These traits are viewed as consistent among all Latino subgroups as they reflect shared values and traditions including a reliance on family ties, a strong sense of community, and religion.

The traditional culture emphasizes the role of mother as central for women as it is through this role that a woman realizes herself and derives her greatest life satisfactions. Interdependence within the family and strong norms of reciprocity remain salient. Adult children are expected to care for their aging parents in exchange for the support that parents have given. In addition, as reported by Sanchez-Ayendez in her study of elderly Puerto Rican women, women are expected to provide help to their children and grandchildren (Sanchez-Ayendez, 1995). Doing so remains a source of emotional satisfaction as parental obligations continue to be fulfilled.

Hispanic grandparents' involvement in intact families has been explored in several studies. Interviews with Hispanic grandparents, primarily Puerto Rican, in New York City found that they often retired and moved closer to their children. These grandparents saw themselves as teachers of traditions, actively helping to maintain family life, in periods of transition (Raphael, 1988).

Sanchez-Ayendez's (1988) study of older Puerto Rican women in the United States suggests that their involvement and contributions to the family are characterized by feelings of "respeto" (respect or respect to authority figures) and "personalismo" (high importance to interpersonal relationships). These values shape the supportive exchanges, expectations, and attitudes of older women in their familial relationships. However, as grandparents assume the parenting role for their grandchildren, they foster a "skipped generation" of parents in that their own children may not be accessible to provide care for them. While one norm is fulfilled, another is at risk of being broken.

Grandparents Raising Grandchildren

Insight and understanding of the circumstances and issues affecting Latino grandparents raising grandchildren is critical for the development of appropriate policies and services. One effort to obtain this information was through a series of focus groups with Latino grandparents conducted by the Grandparent Information Center of the American Association of Retired Persons (AARP, 1997). Participants in the groups reported that the two major problems affecting them were physical and psychological limitations and limited incomes.

The grandparents received support from their families and were interested in agency help only as it could give them direction in dealing with specific problems. Such help was greatly needed because of their limited knowledge of English. At the same time, the focus group participants tended to be wary of support groups in which personal problems would be shared. However, they were interested in informative groups with speakers who would also be able to make referrals.

A study of Latino grandparents, primarily Puerto Ricans, in New York City found that the reasons for their assumption of the parenting role, their role obligations, and the costs and benefits involved, were similar to those of African-American grandparents (Burnette, 1996). Thus, substance abuse, HIV/AIDS, and incarceration were primary reasons in both groups with each experiencing a strong sense of family loyalty and responsibility.

The Latino grandparents in Burnette's study had low levels of education and income with most, 81%, having incomes below the poverty threshold. Although they had lived in the United States for an average of 35 years, their proficiency in speaking English was low. Most had chronic health conditions, and nearly half had symptoms of mild depression. The majority needed information and support services related to child rearing, with the greatest barrier to service use being a lack of knowledge. The grandmothers expressed a strong interest in having available resources in Spanish that could assist them in caring for their grandchildren.

The following section of this chapter reports on a program developed in New York City for Latino grandparents raising grandchildren.

Descriptions of two of the grandmothers attending the program are given to illustrate the issues affecting this population of custodial grandparents and the ways in which culture and social institutions affect their roles.

Description of the Program

In 1995, The Children's Aid Society Community Schools in the Washington Heights area of New York City found themselves dealing with a growing phenomena of kinship caregivers who were primarily Latino grandparents (an estimated 40% of the student population). The dominant factors creating these new families included substance abuse, working parents who needed the grandparents to provide care both during the day and evening, parental desertion, incarceration and HIV/AIDS.

The stresses of coping with intergenerational parenting were compounded among these grandparents by high poverty rates, premature death and incarceration of their children, unemployment, and language barriers. Further unsettling to their situations is the fact that often children and grandchildren move back and forth between Puerto Rico or the Dominican Republic and New York. This shifting of homes further complicates relationships and the adjustment of both generations. In addition, many of the grandparents had left the role of caregiver for one of advisor. They viewed themselves as providing the next generation with wisdom, guidance, and emotional support rather than daily care.

Because of the growing population of custodial grandparents, the Children's Aid Society began piloting in 1995 a Kinship Parenting Education and Support Program. The Program focused on meeting the overwhelming needs of Latino intergenerational families and the lack of parenting support and services for kinship caregivers raising a second generation of children. The initial outreach efforts involved reaching out to families of the children already within the immediate community surrounding the school. Based on the needs of the grandparents, the educational currriculum addressed the following issues.

• Problems as well as joys of parenthood
• Stages of child development
• Discipline and responsibilities of parenthood
• Strengthening relationships/communication
• Child care issues
• Entitlement, such as welfare, Medicaid, and so on

The program offered parent workshops in 16-week cycles with certificates presented to all participants who finished the course. All of the workshops were taught in Spanish by Latino workers. As well as providing information, the objective of the workshops was to encourage caregivers to discuss issues in an open and confidential forum. The sessions provided the opportunity for socialization, minimized feelings of isolation, and developed a network of support among peers. Throughout the program, basic parenting skills, child development milestones, and caregiver-child interactions were emphasized. In addition, the grandparents were given access to a video and educational materials in a library established for the group.

As the program grew, it became obvious that many of the grandparents were dealing with serious health ailments and disabilities, and thus the program was modified to meet their needs. For example, the program offered homebound grandparents parenting and educational workshops in their homes. Home visits also provided an opportunity to see the family in their natural environment, assess needs, provide support, and minimize feelings of isolation. These visits also served to connect the grandparents to the school as the social worker was able to explain directly various programs, such as after-school activities and the parent-teachers association. These links provided the "personalisimo" needed to bring the grandparents into the formal system.

The curriculum was revised as more was learned about intergenerational struggles and individual needs of families. The program offered two cycles: the first focused on parenting education; and the second focused on the individual, cultural values and traditions, and the relationship with the child and his or her school environment. Guest speakers offered workshops on topics, such as domestic violence, nutrition, entitlement, special education, and Alzheimer's disease. In addition, existing and available resources within the school were made available to the grandparents.

The program also evolved into a psychoeducational group for grandparents in which they were given the opportunity to reflect on their generation, their changing role in the family, and their influence on the life of their grandchildren within a safe, supporting, and nurturing environment. A recurring theme in the group discussions was the grandparent's overwhelming sense of grief and loss. Many felt that their own parenting mistakes led to their children's deaths, imprisonment, or illness. At times, the grandparent's ability to respond in the groups was compromised by these feelings. A major focus and goal of the support group was to deal with these feelings by continually reinforcing the positive and significant contributions they had made to their families and their communities.

The group discussions continually underscored the role played by the church and religion in these lives. Almost all of the grandparents were deeply religious, viewing the church as a major source of support. Balancing the members' religiosity with a need to become more proactive regarding seeking and using other services was a constant challenge for the group leader.

The program continues to confront the ongoing need for concrete services, advocacy, and linking participants with available resources including medical, mental health, and dental services. A large percentage of the grandparents migrated to the United States and had not applied for citizenship or become proficient in English. The language barrier remains a major obstacle for those in need of social services. Many are monolingual, which creates a greater sense of isolation, reduces accessibility to services, and hinders their ability to navigate systems and advocate for themselves. Having workers of Latino descent who speak the language and share and understand the culture has been a major support to the group.

At the end of the year, a celebration is held for the grandparents on their accomplishments in the program and their own personal achievements. This offers support and acknowledges their difficult tasks as caregivers. The program has been helpful in changing the attitudes of grandparents, encouraging them to become active in their grandchild's school and neighborhood, and comfortable in exploring their issues with their peers. In particular, it has enabled grandparents to adapt their own cultural experiences and customs to the mores of their new society. This involves changing their discipline techniques, developing effective communication skills, and understanding the peer and societal pressures of their grandchildren.

Each of the grandparents is dealing with a unique set of circumstances, although they all share a familiar background of immigration, poverty, and stressors associated with raising grandchildren. The following case vignettes illustrate the types of issues and problems faced by the Latino grandparents.

Ms. Diego is a 56-year-old Puerto Rican woman who moved to New York in 1990. She has a 2-year college education and worked for 15 years as a secretary. Ms. Diego is raising her two grandchildren, a 12-year-old boy and a 16-year-old adolescent girl. She is also taking care of her 76-year-old husband who has terminal prostate cancer.

Ms. Diego was brought to the grandmothers' support group by another member. She joined the group because she wanted to expand her social life and meet other grandmothers who were raising children.

In the beginning, Ms. Diego appeared cautious about disclosing any concerns or problems. Though friendly, she played more of an active listener role, until she felt safer and learned to trust the other group members. Because of her perceived emotional strength, she became a source of support for other grandmothers. Her willingness to share parts of herself with the group was also noticed. She was able to express feelings of vulnerability and acknowledge feeling overwhelmed from taking care of two grandchildren and a sick husband.

At one point, Ms. Diego invited the whole group to her home. It was there in the warmth of her living room and surrounded by group members that she disclosed an intimate and heretofore unmentioned aspect of her life. Several months after she had become a group member (at the end of the school year), she approached the group's clinician to ask for an individual session. Ms. Diego expressed concern about her grandson who was having adjustment problems in school and also seemed unruly at home.

Ms. Diego explained that her grandchildren's father (her son) was in the military based in California. He had divorced the children's mother, and subsequently the mother was given custody. While the mother was raising her two children, she became a drug addict. When the daughter was 13 years old and the son was 8 years old, she could no longer cope with her maternal duties as her drug problem had became out of control. The mother left her 8-year-old son with Ms. Diego's sister in Puerto Rico, and Ms. Diego kept the granddaughter. Because the boy was exhibiting behavioral problems, he was seen by a psychiatrist. When Ms. Diego's sister could no longer take care of the boy, he came to live with her.

Ms. Diego's grandson was assessed as depressed. Low self-esteem and a weak sense of self seemed to be operating as a result of feeling abandoned by his biological parents. According to Ms. Diego, her grandson announced that soon he will be moving with his mother. However, his mother has not been able to maintain minimal communication with him, although she does communicate with her daughter by phone and allows her daughter to visit. This has been a source of rivalry and envy between the two siblings.

The grandmother acknowledged that the grandson felt rejected by his father because he remarried and was raising his other children. His major support to his son tended to be material rather than emotional. The grandson's conflicts were acted out through challenging and defiant behavior toward Ms. Diego, intensified by demands for expensive toys that she could not meet.

Mrs. Diego reported that she felt very stressed and that her health had deteriorated. She developed high blood pressure, and her osteoarthritis became worse. She worried that her diabetes would also be negatively affected.

Discussion

Ms. Diego was seen for individual counseling on a weekly basis to help her to cope better with the problems with her grandchildren. The counselor continued to validate her strengths and the stability she offered her grandson. She was also shown ways in which whe could enhance her parenting skills while still maintaining her cultural preferences. As Ms. Diego became familiar with her grandchildren's psychodevelopmental stages, she became less anxious about interpreting their rebelliousness as pathological. She was also helped to establish firm and clear boundaries with both children. In addition, Ms. Diego began to learn to respond empathetically in her verbal interaction with both grandchildren.

Issues of family "secrets" were explored in connection to the children's mother's whereabouts as these secrets created a situation in which both grandchildren were left longing for an absent mother. Ms. Diego was also encouraged to become less involved in some areas of her grandchildren's lives and to pay more attention to her own needs, especially her health needs.

When Ms. Diego brought in her grandson for counseling, she emphasized that he had a very negative attitude toward any kind of therapy. In exploring this issue with Ms. Diego, it became evident that she shared these same reservations. She was concerned about confidentiality and felt shameful of disclosing family "problems" to an outsider. This attitudes reflected a Latino cultural expectation that women should be self-sufficient and must not show vulnerability by disclosing family problems outside the home environment. The issue of confidentiality was discussed, and she was reassured that all conversations would remain private, and her personal stories would not be discussed in the group unless she decided to share them.

The cultural trait, personalism, which emphasizes intimate and close relationships, was reflected in the group itself. As the group participants shared similar issues and concerns, it was perceived as being an informal rather than formal system, with each grandmother able to empathetically respond to each others needs. Consequently, the group offered a sense of affiliation and belonging and a safe place in which Mrs. Diego could discuss her problems. It became an extended family. At the same time, the group provided a means of being connected to the larger community.

The importance of *familism*, giving priority to the family over the individual, is clearly reflected in the behavior of Mrs. Diego. Not only did she give central importance to caring for her family, she was reluctant to use any outside assistance. When the worker suggested a possible home attendant for her husband to relieve her of some of her responsibilities and stress, Ms. Diego immediately stated that her husband "likes me to take care of all his health matters." Even though the strain of providing his care was becoming severely taxing, the need to feel self-sufficient took precedence over obtaining any relief.

Familism also prevented her from taking a firm stand in the conflict between her son and granddaughter as she feared offending either one or both of them and thus hoped to protect the unit. Consequently, she became exhausted in trying to support each without offending either one.

This second vignette further illustrates the issues faced by Latino grandparents:

> Ms. Santos is a 66-year-old, dark-skinned Dominican female who became a documented U.S. resident in 1986. Although able to read a little English, she had difficulty in speaking or writing it. Mrs. Santos was dependent on SSI and lived in a one-bedroom apartment with her grandchildren.
>
> She had raised her five children in the Dominican Republic and was brought to New York by her daughter so that she could take care of her three grandchildren while her daughter worked. Subsequently, her daughter died of AIDS contracted through her husband who was a drug addict. This daughter had also been a victim of domestic violence which was often witnessed by the two oldest children.
>
> Ms. Santos was given legal custody of the two girls ages 7 and 4, and her sister was granted custody of the boy (age 10) and took him to live with her and her husband in Puerto Rico. The boy was deeply traumatized by the violence at home and subsequently by his mother's death. While living in Puerto Rico, he started exhibiting inappropriate behavior, such as petty stealing and destructive acts. Because both of his guardians worked and they feared he would hurt himself, they decided to send him to New York and place him in a juvenile state facility in New Jersey.
>
> Ms. Santo's granddaughters were attending one of the Children's Aid Society's Community Schools. It was there that a CAS worker invited Ms. Santos to the grandmother's support group in which she became a regular participant.
>
> The support group became an avenue for Ms. Santos to become involved with her granddaughters' education. She was also able to meet other grandmothers who were also grieving the loss of a son or daughter. The support group provided her with a needed space in which she could express her rage and begin to forgive.
>
> By learning to participate in school activities and becoming more involved in her granddaughters' education, she began to find the challenge of raising her grandchildren more enjoyable and gratifying. Her grandchildren were enrolled in different programs offered by the community school, such as the extended day program, summer camp, educational field trips, cultural celebrations, and counseling and health services. These services helped maintain the family stability by addressing their physical, emotional, and social needs.
>
> Assisted by the family worker, Ms. Santos was able to locate the facility where her grandson was placed and re-establish contact with him. (She

had lost contact with him on account of her inability to communicate with the authorities in English.) To initiate weekend visits, Ms. Santos needed to get an extra bed (they required him to have his own bed). Through the resources available to her through the community school, she was able to purchase a folding bed and clothing for her grandson.

However, for the granddaughters the road to healing was still very bumpy. The death of both parents early in their development resulted in severe emotional problems. The youngest girl expressed suicidal thoughts, such as "I want to go with my mother." This sentiments were difficult for Ms. Santos to understand. But, as she discussed them with the worker and in the group, she realized the child's need for counseling and finally agreed to a referral for professional help.

Discussion

Interventions through the school assisted Ms. Santos in learning to better cope with her granddaughters' feelings of rejection, abandonment (by their mother) and rage toward their father for "causing their mother's death." As difficult as it was, Ms. Santos was encouraged to be a container for her granddaughters' feelings.

Intergenerational differences resulted in conflicts with her grandchildren. Ms. Santos adhered to a traditional belief regarding a woman's behavior. "Una mujer se tiene que dar su lugar" (A woman has to behave properly, with modesty). Not surprisingly, her granddaughters, growing up in New York, did not share these values, and consequently conflict ensued. In junior high school, despite counseling and Ms. Santo's attempt to establish firm authority, they started to stay out late and experiment with sex resulting in further family dissension. From the perspective of Mrs. Santos, the grandchildren were not displaying proper respect as they failed to adhere to her code of appropriate behavior.

Familism is strongly reflected in the situation of Mrs. Santos who came to this country as a result of her daughter's need for child care and who continued to place her grandchildren's needs above her own. She maintained a strong sense of obligation to provide care, and her sense of duty to her family took precedence over her own needs. However, by participating in the group, she was able to learn to deal with the stressors associated with raising her grandchildren. In her own view, the group was a major source of support while it also taught her to develop more understanding and to be less judgmental regarding her grandchildren.

Conclusion

Ethnicity and culture remain salient factors in American society, helping to shape and influence individuals' perceptions of themselves, their roles, and their interactions with society. As can be seen in the vignettes of grandparents presented here, culture, particularly the salient value of familism, continues to influence the ways in which Latino grandparents accept and enact their roles. Adherence to traditional values gives priority to the family over the individual, and, although such feelings are supportive and sustaining of the family unit, they may sorely undermine individual well-being.

Latino grandparents raising grandchildren are fulfilling traditional expectations and obligations, but, at the same time, they are in need of support and assistance. Low incomes, an absence of resources, lack of proficiency in English, and little knowledge of existing services affect both their ability to parent their grandchildren and their own well-being.

The situations of these grandparents are further complicated by the fact that they, similar to other groups of custodial grandparents, are often attempting to cope with the loss of their own child as well as deal with the grief of their grandchild. Yet, at the same time, a propensity to keep feelings and secrets within the family can deter them from seeking professional help.

In addition, many Latino grandparents find themselves raising their grandchildren in a vastly different society and cultural milieu from that in which they raised their own children. They may neither understand or accept the demands of their acculturated grandchildren, causing further friction and stress within the family.

Programs and services that recognize the special needs of these grandparents and are sensitive to their values and traditions can be major sources of support. As they design interventions to assist them, service providers must assure that they are in accord with the group's culture and responses. Understanding the ways in which groups perceive their roles, their expectations of themselves and their grandchildren, and their perceptions of services is fundamental to effective involvement.

As well as understanding key values that may shape behaviors, it is also essential to understand the experiences that this population may have had with social institutions. As with any ethnic group, previous patterns of indifference or discrimination, poor or inadequate services, and providers who did not speak the language or were insensitive to cultural values can instill feelings of distrust. At the same time, a lack of familiarity with programs can further deter service use. Overcoming these barriers is essential if services are to be accepted.

The parenting education and support group offers an example of how a program may be developed to meet the many needs of the population. Beginning with information and education, the group was able to develop into a support group in which problems and concerns were shared. By incorporating the feelings of personalismo among its participants, it could begin to address many of the emotional issues they faced. With the service offered in Spanish by workers of the same culture, the group was able to link the grandparents to both the school and other community resources.

Hispanics are the fastest-growing minority group in the United States. Within the population, the elderly continue to play major roles within the family. As the data indicate, increasing numbers are also becoming responsible for raising their grandchildren. Recognizing and meeting the needs of this population of grandparents is essential if they are to fulfill their demanding roles effectively. Without assistance and support, both they and the generation they seek to raise are in jeopardy.

References

Andrews, J., Lyons, B., & Rowland, D. (1992). Life satisfaction and peace of mind: A comparative analysis of elderly Hispanic and other elderly American. *Clinical Gerontologist*, *11*, 21–42.

Burnette, D. (1996). *Assessing strength and needs of grandparent caregivers in inner-city latino families* (Final Report to the AARP Andrus Foundation). Washington, DC: American Association of Retired Persons.

Chalfie, D. (1994). Going it alone: A closer look at grandparents parenting grandchildren. Washington, DC: American Association of Retired Persons.

Childrens Defense Fund. (1994). *The health insurance crisis for America's children*. Washington, DC: Author.

Guarnaccia, P., Good, B., & Kleinman, A. (1990). A critical review of epidemiological studies of Puerto Rican mental health. *American Journal of Psychiatry*, *137*, 1449–1456.

Krause, N., & Goldenhar, L. (1992). Acculturation and psychological distress in three groups of elderly Hispanics. *Journal of Gerontology*, *47* (Suppl.), S270–S288.

Raphael, E. (1988). Grandparents: A study of their role in Hispanic families. *Physical and Occupational Theapy in Geriatrics*, *6*, 31–62.

Sanchez-Ayendez, M. (1988). Elderly Puerto Ricans in the United States. In S. Applewhite (Ed.), *Hispanic elderly in Transition: Theory, research, and practice* (pp. 17–31). Westport, CT: Greenwood.

Sanchez-Ayendez, M. (1994). Elderly Puerto Rican women: Value orientations and adjustments to aging. In M. Sotomayor (Ed.), *In triple jeopardy: Aged Hispanic women: Insights and experiences*. Washington, DC: National Hispanic Council on Aging.

Sotomayor, M. (1994). Aged Hispanic women: The external circumstances of their lives. In M. Sotomayor (Ed.), *In triple jeopardy: Aged Hispanic women: Insights and experiences*. Washington, DC: National Hispanic Council on Aging.

Sotomayor, M., & Applewhite, S. (1988) The Hispanic elderly and the extended multigenerational family. In S. Applewhite (Ed.), Hispanic elderly in transition: Theory, research, and practice (pp. 121–133). Westport: Greenwood.

The Commonwealth Fund Commission on Elderly People Living Alone. (1989). *Poverty and poor health among elderly Hispanic Americans*. Baltimore: Author.

U.S. Bureau of the Census. (1986). *Projection of the Hispanic population: 1983 to 2080* (Current Population Reports, Series P-25, No. 995). Washington, DC: U.S Government Printing Office.

U.S. Department of Health and Human Services, Social Security Administration. (1990). *Income of the population 55 or older, 1988*, (No. 13-11871). Washington, DC: U.S. Government Printing Office.

SECTION V

Services and Interventions

Chapter 14

Support Groups in the Lives of Grandmothers Raising Grandchildren

Carol S. Cohen and Rolanda Pyle

> I found a place where I could find support—with mothers like me that can understand my hurt.
>
> —Member, Grandmothers as
> Mothers Again Support Group, Brooklyn

The act of giving and receiving help from people that truly understand your troubles and joys is one of life's most powerful experiences. For grandmothers raising their grandchildren, support groups provide an arena in which they can be with others "in the same boat." They join other grandmothers in the role of second-time parent through terrible events in the lives of their families including violence, incarceration, and debilitating illness. Often these women are isolated from their former social networks. Many live with guilt and shame and can find the burden of explaining themselves to others insurmountable. They may face subtle and overt rebuke for their being "out of sync" with generational patterns. A support group is one place in which there is little need for explanation, where members share special knowledge and sisterhood derived from shared experience.

Therefore, it is not surprising that grandmothers raising grandchildren credit support group membership as their most valued resource (Minkler & Roe, 1993). Previous chapters have discussed the many issues surrounding grandparent caregivers including their diversity and needs and their mental and physical challenges. Grandmothers raising grandchildren must deal with an accumulation of demands for money, time, and realignment of family relationships, within the context of an ambiguous role that may or may not have legal status. Support groups do not in themselves solve all problems nor meet all grandmothers' needs. However, support groups can provide an oasis from the day-to-day struggle, a place to gather strength to reenter the world.

Development of Support Groups for Grandmothers Raising Grandchildren

---

Although the concept of self-help and social support groups has been traced to pre-industrial civilizations, its contemporary popularity dates to the 1960s. (Gartner and Reissman, 1984)

The self-help support group gained special prominence in the area of caregiving for the elderly, especially with caregivers of persons with Alzheimer's disease. Grandparent caregivers, however, are a more recently identified population.

Awareness and interest in grandparents raising grandchildren reached the national consciousness in the 1990s, with stories such as: "Grandparents, the Silent Saviors," on the cover of *U.S. News and World Report* (December, 1991). The joint publication of Grandparents as Parents of Last Resort, by New York City's Department of Health and Department of Aging in 1991, focused the social service community's attention on growing numbers of grandparent caregivers and their children (Brovard & Joslin, 1991). Further, the 1993 formation of both the Brookdale Grandparent Caregiver Information Project in California (Driver, 1993), and the Grandparent Information Center, funded by AARP (1993) resulted in increased focus and assistance to grandparents raising grandchildren. Grandmothers raising grandchildren continue to attract public attention including a recent report on National Public Radio (1998) that talked with several grandparents in the empowerment project discussed elsewhere in this book.

Operating outside the professional community, the early 1990s saw the birth of self-directed support groups by grandparents. Self-help support groups enabled grandparent caregivers to have somewhere to turn in times of crisis and on an "as-needed" basis, along with a regular timetable. Grandparent caregivers believed that they possessed the necessary expertise to organize themselves and held many solutions to their own problems. Group meetings became a conduit for the exchange of this knowledge and personal experience. Barbara Kirkland, the founder of "Grandparents United," reported that self-help groups for grandparents serve the purposes of eliminating isolation, gaining perspective, and developing a sense of empowerment (Kirkland, 1992).

In Minkler and Roe's landmark study (1993), African-American grandmothers stated that being among people with similar problems and life situations "relieves a lot of stress" because the members "understand and relate to what you are saying, and you do not have to feel bad or embarrassed about it." The second reason support groups were highly valued by their members was the instrumental assistance provided. Initially, support groups were started to provide informational and emotional support. However, many groups have since expanded their base to include more tangible assistance, like emergency aid, food, housing assistance, respite care, grandchildren's support groups, empowerment training, and in-depth counseling to both grandparents and grandchildren.

Allied with the overall "grandparent rights" movement, many groups have also broadened their horizons and focus on advocacy efforts, engaging grandparents in legislative and policy issues, coming together with other groups, and coordinating their efforts to fight for broader system changes. In New York City, for example, the Kin Care Task Force has advocated for the legislation that would enable expanding grandparents' legal rights to care for grandchildren (New York State Senate, 1998). The legislation was first proposed by the New York City Department of the Aging to amend the General Obligations law so that grandparents and other nonparents who are raising grandchildren can obtain authorization from the parent, legal guardian, or custodian to make certain decisions on behalf of children in their care. These decisions include nonemergency medical and dental treatment, enrollment in school, and participation in school, all currently restricted solely to parents and legal guardians.

Seen as a key resource, the Grandparent Resource Center, founded in 1994 by the New York City Department of the Aging, has collected and disseminated information useful for grandparents and social agencies, and has convened conferences and coalitions of service providers. Their first publication was the curriculum guide *Grandparents Raising Grandchildren: A Series of Workshops to Help You COPE*, developed in 1996 with the support from the New York State Office for the Aging (Grandpareant Resource Center, 1996). It consists of a plan for six workshops, starting with the most user-friendly topics (such as steps to follow for making good connections with the agencies that can help) and leading to more sensitive areas (such as dealing with the biological parent). The book has been used extensively by support group facilitators who have suggested other topics they considered of crucial importance for discussion in the support group workshops. In 1998, the Department for the Aging developed new workshops to add to this curriculum including: "Kinship Foster Care, Maintaining Relationships with Families and Friends"; "Staying Healthy, Fit, and Sane While Raising Your Grandchildren;" and "Transitions: Grandchildren Going Out or Moving Back With Their Biological Parents."

With growing resources and public attention, the number of support group programs for grandparents raising grandchildren have greatly increased (Minkler & Roe, 1996). However, to meet the needs of the increasing numbers of custodial grandparents, even more programs are needed. The remainder of this chapter focuses on key parameters of support groups for grandparents raising grandchildren to support this expansion.

Characteristics of Support Groups

Support groups share common purposes. Preeminent among these is the provision of social support through the mutual assistance of group members. In describing the purposes of support groups, Schopler and Galinsky (1993) identify the expansion of social resources, knowledge relevant to members' situation, relief and reassurance, and enhanced coping skills as primary. These purposes are realized through the mutual aid of members— the person-to-person exchange of reassurance, information, and resources. As Hirayama and Hirayama suggest, the power of a group is its potential to serve as a "reservoir of power resources where individual participants can get help and receive support" (1986, p. 124).

The interactive nature of the stressors on grandmothers raising grandchildren can have a negative effect both on grandmothers and grandchildren. Morevoer, the literature has shown that grandmothers raising grandchildren often experience problems of social isolation and decreased socialization. Their new caregiving responsibilities may mean less time with other family members or friends and may also restrict participation in church and other important social organizations. Therefore, support groups for grandmothers raising grandchildren have been organized across the country to help grandmothers cope with their new role demands.

Because social support is typically a mediator of stress, groups allow grandmothers an opportunity to discuss immediate concerns, past mistakes, and set future goals. Possibly the most important aspect of grandparent support groups is the encouragement and camaraderie among participants. Members often develop strong emotional ties that extend outside the group.

Although a wide variety of support groups share common purposes, their leadership, composition, operating structures, and activities are quite varied. Using Roselle Kurland's model of group planning (1978), the following sections focus on such variations in greater depth.

Support Group Leadership

Although it is not the only way to distinguish one from another, support groups are commonly categorized as either "self-help" or "professionally led." It is unfortunate that these labels can lead one to view self-help groups as "leaderless" because grandmothers themselves take direct responsibility for facilitating the group. Similarly, members' leadership activities can be overlooked when professionals are the facilitators.

This section focuses primarily on the formal leadership of support groups, as "people in designated positions who are expected to accept special responsibility in the group by virtue of their positions" (Hartford, 1971, p. 213). However, organizers of support groups must also consider the informal leadership that emerges regardless of the formal structure. For example, grandparent caregivers, who have not yet joined a support group, are more apt to make the connection if another grandparent is the contact person or group leader, suggesting that grandparents be encouraged to take leadership roles in the area of recruitment and orientation whether or not they are the formal leaders of the group (Cohen, 1995).

Choices about who should lead a particular support group reflect the vision and values of the originating program or founder. Such decisions may be based on established agency practice, ideas about group process, or expediency. One leadership arrangement is not "better" than another; rather, each brings potential benefits and challenges. Organizers should choose leadership arrangements most useful for the members that are consistent with the group's auspice. Further, they must be prepared to explore shifting the formal leadership structure as the group evolves.

Self-Help

In self-help groups, grandmothers take the lead in starting their own groups. The agenda of a grandparent-led group tends to flow directly from what the participants articulate as their needs. The members plan and execute their own activities and recruit their own members. A grandparent-led group can live beyond the founder's leadership when it develops the leadership capacities of its members and can continue functioning longer than groups that are completely dependent on outside leadership. The independence of a self-help group can help it survive changes in the social service climate, such as changes in funding and service priorities.

A challenge for grandparent-led groups is that they cannot rely on a professional leader with expertise in group facilitation who can help the group weather a difficult period in its development. In addition, groups that are grandparent led sometimes lack the resources and connections necessary to get concrete and therapeutic help for their members. These challenges can be addressed through linkages with social service institutions and coalitions with other support group programs.

Professional Facilitation

Many organizations that launch grandparent support groups assign a staff member to lead the group. The group leader is often a professional social worker, psychologist, or nurse but is sometimes a staff member without professional credentials. Therefore, the term professional is used loosely to identify a leader from outside the group. Ideally, leaders are chosen for expertise in group facilitation. Many professional leaders have established contact with grandparent caregivers through other agency programs and bring an understanding of their struggles. Professional leaders generally are not themselves grandparents raising grandchildren, but such an arrangement is not precluded.

Professional leadership increases the chance the group will fulfill the agency's purpose in sponsoring the group. This arrangement enables the agency to maintain tight control over the group and its activities. Conversely, true professional leaders should consider members' needs as primary and ensure that they are not compromised by the agency. A clear, mutually agreed contract among group members, leaders, and sponsoring agency is critical in avoiding conflicts of interest and unethical practice.

Professional leadership can be one of the fastest methods of helping members to interact and commit to the group because of the skills and resources of the worker. Just as in the case of self-help groups, professional leaders must pay attention to encouraging leadership by members if the group is to flourish. The mutual aid of members to each other must be seen as the primary vehicle for support rather than assistance coming from the leader to the members (Kurland & Salmon, 1992). Often, in a professionally run group, when the leader leaves the group falls apart because members may be reluctant to develop relationships with a new leader. However, when the relationships among the members are valued, groups can accommodate changes in leaders and leadership structures more easily.

Mixed Leadership Models

Many groups have chosen a middle ground and have found that co-leadership can maximize the advantages and alleviate some problems found in either a professionally led or grandparent-led group. Although the delegation of responsibility can vary, many co-led groups depend on the professional for information, resources, and meeting arrangements and on the grandparent leader for mutual support and understanding. In co-led groups, the professional's role can be to provide direction and to move the group toward self-help. The professional leader ensures that the group moves in the agency's direction and brings the needed resources to the table. The grandparent leader ensures that the group mirrors what the participants need and makes initial contracts with potential members. The grandparent leader most often takes the role of mobilizing others in the group to publicize the meetings. The professional can also model sensitive, empathic practice to the group and encourage these attitudes in others. Coleadership by professionals and grandmothers provides a balance and helps the group leaders cope with member issues and crises. Concerns for the leaders include turf conflicts, professional and grandparent leader resistance, and other group dynamics.

Training and Support for Leaders

Identifying a gap in the ongoing training and support for group leaders, the Grandparent Resource Center of the New York City Department of Aging implemented a Grandparent Support Group Facilitator's Network, through which grandparent support group leaders exchange ideas, share information, collaborate on events, and receive training. Examples of training topics include group work skills, emotional needs of grandmothers, mutual aid and self-help in support groups, legal authority and financial entitlement, and elder abuse. This support group network birthed the idea of a training curriculum for grandparent support group leaders that provides sample workshops with topics that can be addressed at support group meetings. Support group leaders affectionately call the network "a support group for support group leaders" providing a model that can be replicated in other areas.

Composition of Support Group Membership

In this context, composition refers to the number and characteristics of members that participate in the group. Organizers will need to consider the impact of a wide variety of individual characteristics of potential members, and make decisions about the level of homogeneity and heterogeneity that will best serve the group. Taken together, grandparents raising grandchildren are an extremely diverse population. However, their shared characteristic of caring for their children's children because of family crises provides a great deal of commonality, suggesting that these groups can accommodate a great deal of heterogeneity in other areas (Cohen, 1997).

Agency context and the founder's vision will have a great impact on how groups are composed. Other issues may also affect composition, such as the need to speak a common language in the group and the ability to travel to meetings. The areas of composition highlighted in the following section are not comprehensive but serve as models of the way individual characteristics are considered in the process of planning the group.

Geographic Considerations

Support group organizers must consider the areas in which the participants live, the location of the meeting place, as well as the distances members must travel. For example, grandmothers who identify strongly with a particular area and neighborhood may not venture outside for services. Conversely, some grandparents do not want to attend support group meetings in their "home base" because they do not want neighbors to find out about them.

In rural areas, grandparents may be forced to travel long distances to participate in support groups, whereas grandparents in urban areas may have a choice of locations, either in or outside their neighborhood. For many grandparents, the effort of travel, adequacy of transportation, and financial cost are issues that could prevent support group participation. Expanding technologies, such as the Internet and teleconferencing, provide intriguing opportunities to bridge distances and bring more grandparents into both "real" and "virtual" support groups.

Legal Status of Grandparents

Organizers should consider the impact of composing groups with heterogeneity or homogeneity around the issue of legal status between grandparent and grandchild. Sometimes, this issue is settled by a sponsoring agency, as in the case of support groups organized by foster care agencies. These groups tend to be limited to participant in the agency programs, such as families served in "kinship" programs in which grandparents are legal guardians as foster parents. In some cases, support groups are linked with mandated training for grandparents as a condition of continuation in that status. In other cases, groups are composed of grandparents without legal status. Such groups may invite legal advisors to the group to enhance members' individual and collective advocacy activities.

Alternately, many groups include members with a wide range of legal statuses and encourage members to help each other negotiate a variety of guardianship issues that affect the members. Clearly, there is not only one way to deal with this issue. Like other elements of composition, one must consider the impact of legal status of members on group cohesion and support.

Age of Grandchildren

The question of whether membership in a particular grandparent support group should be limited by the age of the grandchildren is of interest when opportunities for forming multiple groups is possible. For example, grandparents raising teens may become frustrated in a group with grandparents raising younger children, feeling that the others have not even scratched the surface of the problems associated with reparenting. In addition, these caregivers have, in most instances, already gone through the infant, toddler, and preschool stages and would often prefer theses stages to the demanding adolescent stage. Instead of learning about immunizations, they may need guidance about how to prevent their grandchild from dropping out of school.

Although age-specific groups merit consideration, many support groups include members with grandchildren of all ages. This is important for grandmothers caring for more than one child but also can have benefits for the group. Grandparents of adolescents can provide a wealth of knowledge and support to the grandparents who are just beginning and can be a source of sharing. In addition, it must be remembered that most members have gone through these stages with their own children. Thus, discussions of adolescence may be important for grandparents caring for toddlers as well because it provides an opportunity to discuss their own parenting practices and their feelings about their effectiveness.

Special Populations

Although grandparent caregiving can transcend cultural, racial, and socioeconomic boundaries, the care provided to the grandchild may be further complicated by special conditions. For example, the family dynamics associated with substance abuse and parental incarceration have a bearing not only on the provision of care to the child, but on the caregivers' emotional state as well. When substance abuse is involved, a discussion of codependency and its affect on family dynamics might be fruitful, and when parental incarceration is the reason for kinship care, the issue of recidivism needs to be addressed.

Often grandchildren have special needs related to drug exposure, a challenging physical condition (such as developmental disabilities), or a life-threatening illness, such as AIDS. Further, in cases of a parent with AIDS, families are strongly affected by social stigma and at the end of life, by the pre-morterm and postmortem bereavement associated with a terminal illness. A specialized support group can effectively address these issues where all members can feel free to participate. Although homogeneity regarding children's conditions is not mandatory, groups in which some members, or only one member, face challenges that cannot be appreciated and brought into the group experience will fall short of reaching its potential. Thus, group leaders must consider how each member's caregiving experiences will enrich rather than divide the group.

Operating Structures of Support Groups

The structural components of support groups refer to all of the arrangements concerning the operation of the group. These include temporal arrangements, such as the duration, frequency, and time of meetings. The physical arrangements of the group (place, room, transportation, etc.) and the group's rules and policies are considered part of the group's structure as well.

One aspect of group structure that should be present in all grandparent support groups is a process that supports decision making by members. The actual decisions of groups may not be the same, nor the particular methods of reaching them (i.e., voting, consensus, etc.), but in each group, members should be encouraged to assume the maximum level of self-determination that will serve their needs and encourage empowerment.

Just as in the case of composition and leadership, structural elements are often determined by the agency or environmental context of the program. In such cases, the support group's organizer must consider the impact of the imposed structural elements on the group. When choices of arrangements are more open, the organizer has the opportunity to weigh the consequences of one course of action over another. In either case, the conscious consideration of the impact of structural elements on the work of the support group is critical in fostering program success.

Time and Place

Grandparent support groups meet in senior centers, libraries, churches, child welfare agencies, public schools, health, social service, and mental health or other agencies. Groups can also meet in a grandparent's home. Some groups have donated space, whereas other groups rent their space. Scheduling is important, and it can be difficult to balance the scheduling demands of members, workers, and other constituents needing space.

Many groups meet during the day while grandchildren are in school. However, because many grandparents work, other groups meet either in the evenings or on the weekends. For those who work during the day, taking time out for an evening meeting may be difficult, and child care may be a problem. Groups that are able to have meetings during the day, evenings, or weekends can satisfy the needs of grandparents who wish to attend.

In choosing a place to hold support group meeting, it is important to chose a place that is nonthreatening to grandparent families. For example, one support group began meeting in a mental health clinic, only to discover that attendance was very low. The leader discovered that although they wanted to be a part of the group, grandparents did not want to come to the clinic. The group meeting place was changed to a local high school, where the attendance and participation immediately grew.

Frequency of Meetings and Membership Restrictions

The frequency of support group meetings depends on the host agency or the group members. Some groups meet every week, others biweekly, and still others once a month. Group members are more concerned, however, with the consistency of group meetings rather than the number of times the group meets. Frequency of group meetings is also governed by the type of group. If the group is open-ended, it may meet less over a longer span of time. Open-ended support groups usually allow new members to join at any time and allow old members to come and go as they please. Time-limited groups are more focused on an interval meeting schedule. For example, some groups meet for 12-week sessions and others for 4-month sessions. These groups are often psychoeducational in nature and do not allow new members to join after the second or third week. Participation in a group that follows a structured curriculum is often followed with membership in a more flexible, support-oriented group. The number of group session is usually determined by the group focus and the agency mission.

Contact Outside Group Meetings

Grandparents have said that support group meetings dramatically increased their perceived ability to cope and provided a real sense that they were not alone. Members of support groups bond and often continue their relationships, networking outside official meetings through phone calls, and home visits. Grandparents often benefit from the alliances formed outside the actual meeting. These alliances lead to emotional support during stressful times or to concrete activities, such as accompanying one another to medical and a social service appointments or attendance at social events. Seasoned members are often more than willing to give back to someone in a worse predicament. Group leaders in the "Grandparent Support Group Facilitators Network" report that their groups have unofficial grandparent mentors (New York City Department of the Aging, 1998). These mentors are grandparents who have taken on the role of being in charge of new members who are "coming up the ropes," to facilitate their integration into the group.

Child Care

Child care is often the reason cited for not attending support group meetings. Most grandparents can neither afford baby-sitters nor do they have family members or friends to watch their grandchildren. Many groups, therefore, schedule their meeting during the school year, taking off the summer months while others provide child care especially for preschool children and infants. Often, supplies like books, games and activities for the children are needed. Child care often brings two new issues to the group—additional space and a responsible person to look after the children. Some groups have volunteers to watch the children. In child welfare agencies, volunteers may have to go through a screening process to ensure that they have no child abuse or criminal records.

Some groups try to resolve the child care problem by having meetings with both grandparents and grandchildren present. The problem with this approach is that children need attention and invariably distract the grandmothers during their meeting. Although improving the quality of grandmother and grandchild relationships is important, the support group is generally designed to meet the grandmothers', not children's, needs. Grandmothers consistently report that the support group fulfills its purposes by providing time away from their family responsibilities with the opportunity to focus on themselves and their concerns. Many support groups plan activities that include grandchildren and other family members, but these are seen as auxiliary rather than central to the groups' purposes.

Content and Activities of Support Groups

This section focuses on "what" the support group does and "how" it spend its time. Although most of the time in many grandparent support groups is spent talking about common caregiving issues and providing mutual assistance among members, some groups incorporate a wide variety of activities. When they are clearly linked to the purpose of the group, activities, such as outings, games, and parties, can enrich the life of a group. Groups establish rituals that help set the tone for the group and help build cohesion. For example, many groups begin or end their meeting with a prayer or affirmation, and others engage in role playing to prepare for a task they will undertake before the next meeting.

Some grandparent support groups use a formal style of meeting, using agendas and minutes. Others have a more informal approach, often opening with an icebreaker and then opening the floor to members to recap their week, highlighting issues, crises, and joys they encountered. Still others plan formal activities using specific topics previously agreed on, and some groups use a particular curriculum or training module. As indicated in the following sections, the primary consideration in choosing content for support groups is the degree to which particular activities will enable the members to reach their goals.

Food and Refreshments

Most grandparent support groups serve food or refreshments during or immediately following their meetings. Members of some groups take turns donating and preparing refreshments. Other groups collect dues to provide refreshments or sponsoring agencies provide refreshments for the meetings. Providing refreshments enhances both group attendance and participation and adds a comfortable flavor to the meetings. Many groups celebrate birthdays, special occasions, and holidays by having pot luck suppers or cultural dinners.

An example of how food enhances support group meetings can be found in a grandparent support group in East Harlem, New York, that meets in a convent. After each meeting, the grandparents socialize while eating homemade soup prepared by a nun in residence. The grandparents report that they not only look forward to their meetings but also to the delicious homemade soup. Sharing soup or "breaking bread" has symbolic meaning to many of the grandmothers and facilitates the building of group relationships through culturally syntonic activities.

Speakers

Many groups invite outside experts to address specific issues within the group. Some of these experts include mental health practitioners, health care specialists, attorneys, or representatives from aging, social service, or educational agencies. For example, groups have invited a nurse to talk the importance of mammography and breast checkups during Breast Health Awareness Month. Grandparent groups often look within their own group for expertise on a particular topic as well. Many grandparents have extensive work histories and knowledge of systems from their own personal experiences or from workshops they have attended. Generally, grandparents are more than willing to share their knowledge with their colleagues. It can also boost the group's morale to have one of their own speak to a particular issue.

Recreational Activities for Grandparents and Joint Activities With Grandchildren

---

Grandparent caregivers are isolated from peers because of child rearing responsibilities that may mean less time with friends, family members, and colleagues. Caregiving also constricts participation in social organizations, church, and other activities important to the grandparent. Some support groups spend time discussing ways of reconnecting with existing social networks. However, many programs have initiated social and recreational activities that help fill this void through programs that meet the particular needs and scheduling constraints of the members. For example, many groups solicit donated tickets from theaters and other organizations to give grandparents a night out on the town. Other groups have planned activities for both grandparents and grandchildren to socialize together at events, such as the circus, picnics, and holiday parties. Grandparents who often don't have the money to pay for recreational activities for their grandchildren welcome these opportunities.

In planning collateral programs, it is important to listen to the members desires and be careful that the outside activities are consistent with the group's purpose. For example, when the suggestion to design an outing for grandmothers and grandchildren came up in one particular group, the members ultimately decided not to spend their time planning such an event. In the course of their discussion, and despite their initial enthusiasm for an intergenerational event, they reminded each other that they cherished the support group because it gave them time away from their charges (beloved as they might be). This group decided on a trip "downtown," an outing exclusively for the members. Conversely, other groups have chosen intergenerational activities as an important outlet for normalizing their grandchildren's situation of living with a grandparent. In both examples, social support continues to the central focus of the members, and much of the planning of auxiliary activities occurs during meetings, as part of the common decision-making and mutual aid process.

Respite Components

Respite programs are designed to give grandmothers some "time off" from child care responsibilities and can be developed in a variety of ways. For example, in 1994, a grandparent program in Brooklyn featured an intergenerational respite component. In conjunction with the New York City Department for the Aging's Intergenerational Program, high school students from a neighborhood school provided child care during biweekly grandparent support group meetings. On alternate weeks, grandparents would bring their grandchildren to the agency and leave them with the teenagers who provided respite for a few hours. As a result, the caregivers were able to keep appointments, visit friends, run errands, or just relax. The preschool-age grandchildren had the opportunity to learn and socialize with other children. Each high school student was assigned one family and worked individually with a particular child and grandparent, creating a multigenerational relationship.

Another example of a respite component is the Grandparent Support Project, an early project of the Grandparent Resource Center at New York City Department for the Aging. The Project took a community-based approach to recruitment, training, and supervision of older volunteers. The senior volunteers provided care, companionship, and escort services to grandparent families in their homes. The volunteers were recruited from the neighborhoods in which the grandparent families lived and were trained and matched with families. A case manager worked along with the families to ensure they received necessary services. Again, the collaborative component of the program, which included the grandparents in its implementation, was closely allied with the purpose of increasing support.

Additional models of respite include programs outside the community. In one example, both grandparents and grandchildren attended a weekend retreat, in which the adults and children participated in separate activities. Grandchildren were independently supervised and were able to meet others in similar family circumstances. In another example, children were provided with scholarships, making it possible for them to attend summer sleep-away camp. In such arrangements, the grandchildren may be mixed with the general camping population or may be a part of special activities for children being raised by grandparents.

Although respite components are not in themselves support group activities, the members can collectively engage in planning these programs and assessing their implementation as part of their group meetings. Thus, they receive a dual benefit. In addition to needed relief from child care responsibilities, grandmothers build their confidence and support each other by joining in the planning and evaluation process.

Conclusion

Support groups are a low-cost, yet highly effective intervention approach for grandmothers raising their grandchildren. Grandparent support groups serve both emotional and instrument functions, providing an opportunity for grandparents to give voice to their feelings and frustrations as well as enabling the exchange of information and resources. As found in the literature, support groups take a wide variety of forms. They differ from each other on the basis of their leadership arrangements, membership composition, organizational structure, and activities inside and outside the group.

The unifying theme among the diversity of grandparent support groups is their common purpose to support members through the collective struggle of reparenting. It is the experience of mutual aid, in which members engage in the process of giving and receiving help, that provides a support group's greatest benefit. Therefore, the variety of arrangements and activities available in the development of support groups should be evaluated as to their potential for maximizing this mutual-aid phenomenon. The value of support groups can be understood from the words of members who report: "I don't want to make the same mistakes with my granddaughter as I did with my girls;" "I'm not isolated anymore"; and "When I give help, I feel better". Clearly, these groups are powerful vehicles for their grandparent members and the grandchildren they raise.

References

American Association of Retired Persons. (1993). *Grandparents raising their grandchildren*. Washington, DC: AARP Grandparent Information Center.

Brouard, A., & Joslin, D. (1991). *Grandparents as parents of last resort: A survey of three department of health child health clinics*. New York: City of New York Department of Health and Department for the Aging.

Cohen, C. S. (1995). Making it happen: From great idea to successful support group program. *Social Work with Groups, 18,* 67–80.

Cohen, C. S. (1997). The impact of culture in social work practice with groups: The grandmothers as mothers again case study. In E. P. Congress (Ed.), *Multicultural perspectives in working with families* (pp. 311–331). New York: Springer.

Driver, D. (1993, February). *Brookdale grandparent caregiver information project newsletter*. New York: Brookdale Foundation.

Gartner, A., & Reissman, F. (1984). *The self-help resolution*. New York: Human Services Press.

Grandparent Resource Center. (1996). *For grandparents raising grandchildren: A series of workshops to help you COPE*. New York: New York City Department for the Aging.

Grandparent Resource Center. (1998). *For grandparents raising grandchildren: More help for you and your family*. New York: New York City Department for the Aging.

Hartford, M. (1971). *Groups in social work*. New York: Columbia University Press.

Hirayama, H., & Hirayama, K. (1986). Empowerment through group participation: Process and goal. In M. Parnes (Ed.), *Innovations in social group work: Feedback from practice to theory: Proceedings of the annual group work symposium* (pp. 119–132). Binghamton, NY: Haworth Press.

Kaye, L. (1997). *Self-help support groups for older women: Rebuilding elder networks through personal empowerment.* Washington, DC: Taylor & Francis.

Kirkland, B. (1992, February). Definition of a self-help group. *Grandparents United Newsletter,* p. 1.

Kurland, R. (1978). Planning: The neglected component of group development. *Social Work with Groups, 1,* 173–178.

Kurland, R., & Salmon, R. (1992). Group work vs. casework in a group: Principles and implications for teaching and practice. *Social Work with Groups, 15,* 3–14.

Landers, S. (1992, March). "Second-time-around-families" find aid. *NASW News,* p. 5.

Minkler, M., & Roe, K. M. (1993). *Grandmothers as caregivers.* Newbury Park, CA: Sage.

Minkler, M., & Roe, K. M. (1996). Grandparents as surrogate parents. *Generations, 20,* 34–36.

New York State. (1998). *New York State Assembly Bill A3917-C & Senate Bill S4264-C.* New York: New York State Assembly & Senate.

Schopler, J. H., & Galinsky, M. J. (1993). Support groups as open systems: A model for practice and research. *Health and Social Work, 18,* 195–207.

U.S. Bureau of the Census. (1991). *Current population reports: Marital status and living arrangements* (Series P-20, No. 450). Washington, DC: Government Printing Office.

U.S. News and World Report. (1991, December). *Grandparents, the silent saviors,* pp. 80–89.

Chapter 15

Empowering Grandparents Raising Grandchildren

Carole B. Cox

W hen offering assistance to either individuals or groups, there is an inherent danger of focusing exclusively on their needs and problems, over-looking gheir innate strengths. Yet, it is these inner strengths that should be developed and encouraged. Empowerment training strives to accomplish this goal.

As noted throughout this book, grandparents raising grandchildren encounter often overwhelming issues for which they are poorly prepared and which can sorely tax their coping skills. They have extensive needs for assistance and supports in many areas of their life, ranging from finances to parenting skills. However, the very fact that they have assumed responsibility for their grandchildren in itself conveys inherent strength and resilience. These grandparents, rather than being perceived as victims of their families or society, should be perceived as heroes in that they are willing to accepted the challenge of a new role and responsibility.

In this regard, empowerment-oriented strategies that seek to develop self-reliance and the ability for self-help are particularly suited to these

This project was supported by a grant from the New York Community Trust.

grandparents. Rather than just offering assistance, empowerment aims to encourage self-efficacy building on individuals' innate strengths. Among the many definitions of empowerment are the ability to influence people, organizations, and the environment affecting one's life (Cochran, 1987; Hasenfeld, 1987); gaining, developing, seizing, enabling, or giving power (Staples, 1990); and attaining control over one's life and democratic participation in the community (Berger & Neuhaus, 1977; Katz, 1984).

Gutierrez and Ortega (1991) describe the personal level of empowerment as concerned with the individual's feelings of power and self-efficacy, whereas the interpersonal level is concerned with an individual's ability to influence others. Solomon's (1976) concept of powerlessness is closely tied to these definitions as negative self-evaluations impede effective actions. Economic insecurity, absence of access to information, lack of training in abstract and critical thought, and physical and emotional stress contribute to feelings of powerlessness (Cox, 1988). Practical knowledge, information, real competencies, concrete skills, material resources, genuine opportunities, and tangible results are necessary factors by which empowerment is developed and sustained (Staples, 1990). Learning to reach out to the community and larger system that impinges on one's life is an important step in reinforcing new attitudes, self-evaluations, and personal power.

Once having accepted to role of parenting grandparent, grandparents, as has been discussed in earlier chapters, may become overwhelmed by the problems of their children, grandchildren, and the social milieu in which they live. Being thrust into a situation for which they had little preparation, assuming a new role out of a sense of loyalty and responsibility rather than choice, having to formulate that role with few guidelines, and having to suddenly cope with the demands of a grandchild as well as the systems with which the grandchild interacts can undermine their sense of power or control. Such feelings of powerlessness are intensified when physical and social resources are limited, the situation of many custodial grandparents.

Empowerment Process

In the empowerment process, the practitioner does not act as the expert or as the provider of power to the powerless older person. As discussed by Cox and Parsons (1994) the process involves four key elements: (a) Attitude, values, and beliefs—developing a sense of self-efficacy, belief in self-worth, and an internal locus of control; (b) validation of collective experiences—recognizing that experiences are shared rather than individual so that self-blame is decreased; (c) knowledge and skills for critical thinking—learning to think critically about problems and the factors contributing to them; and (d) action—Learning to develop action strategies that influence others and work toward goals.

Strategies to foster empowerment are commonly practiced with groups. Within the group, participants are able to share concerns, learn from each other, and practice specific techniques. As participants become comfortable with these techniques, they are encouraged to use them in other settings. Role playing and the use of videos can help in reinforcing new behaviors. The role of the group leader is that of a facilitator who recognizes that the participants are the experts and that they learn best from each other and from understanding that their problems are not unique. At the same time, to be most effective, empowerment requires participants to acquire information and knowledge that can assist them in developing their skills and resolving their problems.

Empowering Grandparents

The project described here sought to empower a group of African-American grandparents raising grandchildren in the Greater Harlem Community of New York City. The group represents only a small fraction of such grandparents in New York, where 12.4% of the city's children are being cared for by other relatives, primarily grandparents (U.S. Bureau of the Census, 1990). Harlem is an area that has been heavily impacted by AIDS with women in Harlem having the highest incidence and mortality from HIV/AIDS of any area in the City (Health Systems Agency of New York, 1992). As a result of both AIDS and substance abuse, grandparents frequently assume responsibility for their grandchildren.

The grandparents selected for the training were all members of a grandparents support group sponsored by a local nonprofit organization. The group was established in 1994 and had grown to approximately 40 members. The group met monthly usually under the guidance of a social worker who acted as facilitator. As well as offering support, many of the participants had become active in local government projects. Several had participated on a city task force concerned with the issues faced by parenting grandparents and the development of more resources.

Given this involvement, the members of the support group were responsive to the idea of empowerment training, which they saw as another means of helping them to achieve their own goals and objectives. Fifteen participants were selected for the training based on the length of time they were in the group, their interest in the program, and their commitment to attending the classes.

Project Objectives

The objectives of the project were to strengthen the parenting skills of the grandparents and to increase their effectiveness in the community as advocates for themselves and for other grandparents raising grandchildren. These objectives were seen as interrelated. Enhancing personal skills and abilities were necessary for subsequent efforts at interpersonal and social change.

Description of Participants

Although the program was open to both men and women, only grandmothers participated. According to the participants, it was difficult to recruit grandfathers into their programs as they were either working or felt uneasy attending a group composed predominantly of women.

Fifteen grandmothers began the training with 14 completing the program. One grandparent was forced to stop because of poor health. The grandmothers ranged between the ages of 50 and 75 years, with a mean age of 64 years. The average number of grandchildren cared for was two. Two of the grandmothers were married, with the others divorced or widowed. Three of the participants continued to work, with two working as home attendants and one employed in catering. One grandmother was attending classes at a community college. Previous to their retirements, the grandmothers had worked in nursing, clerical positions, day work, and administration. Almost all were active in their churches, with several involved in local politics.

Substance abuse and HIV/AIDS were the primary reasons for raising the grandchildren, and, for eight of the grandparents, the children had died, either because of drugs or AIDS. Almost all of the grandparents were raising their daughters' children. Most of the group had legal guardianship of the grandchildren and had sought guardianship to prevent the children from going into foster care. One quarter of the group received SSI with the participants average income being approximately $13,500 per year. Almost half of the grandchildren, 40%, received Medicaid. Several of the grandparents had received food stamps but had had the benefit stopped or sharply reduced as a result of changes in the eligibility criteria following reductions in the program.

Many of the grandparents assumed the parenting role after a crisis in the lives of their own children. In one instance, a daughter had been murdered, and others had been incarcerated or had abandoned the children. Consequently, there was often little time to adjust to the role of parenting grandparent. Four of the grandmothers had had little contact with the grandchild before becoming the caregiver.

Further complicating adjustment was the fact that three of the grandmothers had not really raised their own children who had been cared for by relatives in the South. The grandparents did not begin raising their children until they were adolescents. Now, responsible for their grandchildren, they were unsure of their parenting skills and anxious over their ability to cope. These uncertainties were heightened by feelings of guilt over their own children and the ways in which their lives had evolved.

Health problems were common among the grandparents, including diabetes, heart problems, cataracts, asthma, and arthritis. At the same time, only two of the participants felt that their health interfered with their ability to provide care. However, the relevance of health to role enactment is vividly depicted in the case of one grandmother, hospitalized for heart problems. At discharge, she was refused temporary home care as she had a 16-year-old granddaughter living with her whom the agency felt could assist her. In addition, she was told that if she was not able to manage, her grandchildren could be removed from her care. It is important to add that this "empowered" grandmother took this threat to the deputy chief of the department, demanded her rights, and was provided with a temporary home attendant.

Issues Confronting the Participants

Concerns about the future of the grandchildren were prominent. Most worried about who would care for the grandchildren if they were no longer able as well as what would happen if the parent demanded custody. Thus, as difficult as it was to adapt to the parenting role, fears that the children would be taken away were also common. In one instance, the daughter of one of the grandmother's completed a drug rehabilitation program and regained custody of the grandchildren who the grandmother had raised for 5 years. The grandmother had to contend with this loss as well as anxiety over the security of the grandchildren.

Issues related to legal rights and available benefits permeated the lives of the grandparents. Having limited incomes with many dependent on public benefits, changes and reductions in programs had a direct impact on them and their ability to provide for their grandchildren. Several were not clear regarding either their eligibility for services or that of their grandchildren. Conversely, although some members of the group felt at the mercy of the system, other grandmothers had successfully challenged denials for services and had benefits reinstated. These participants were eager to share their strategies for successfully dealing with agencies.

Communicating with their grandchildren, dealing with behavior problems, and developing relationships were also common areas of concern. Grandparents were particularly worried about how to deal with adolescent peer groups and grandchildren's demands for greater freedom. Setting limits without severing their relationships with their grandchildren was a difficult task.

In addition, most felt anxious about sexual activity and drugs and ways to assure that their grandchildren did not become involved. They also worried about HIV/AIDS and how to protect their grandchildren. For those whose children had been addicts or were HIV infected, these subjects were particularly painful to discuss. At least one of the grandparents had never shared with her grandchildren the fact that their parent had AIDS. This painful "secret" thwarted communication and continued to affect their relationship.

Development of the Curriculum

This discussion with the grandparents helped to shape the curriculum as it highlighted their immediate concerns and areas where empowerment training could be particularly important. The curriculum was designed specifically for the group. As well as helping them to deal with their own grandchildren, it involved material on reaching out to others, an important facet of the empowerment training. The program included the following 12 classes:

- Introduction to Empowerment
- The Importance of Self-Esteem
- Communicating With Grandchildren
- Dealing With Loss and Grief
- Helping Grandchildren Deal With Loss
- Dealing With Behavior Problems
- Talking to Grandchildren About Sex, HIV/AIDS, and Drugs
- Legal and Entitlement Issues

- Developing Advocacy Skills
- Negotiating Systems
- Getting Your Message Across
- Review

The complete curriculum was given to each participant including an outline for each class with session objectives; lecture notes; reference materials; and, when appropriate, brochures. The classes were 3 hours each and were given at the university with transportation provided. This setting was an important part of the empowerment training as it helped to familiarize the participants with environments outside of their community. In addition, attending classes at a large university was in itself an "empowering" experience.

The sessions were held twice a week, and participation was mandatory. If participants missed as session, they remained responsible for learning the material. With two sessions missed, the person was dropped from the training. As a means of reinforcing the learning and also as a means of increasing grandmothers' comfort in making presentations, members in the group were responsible for sharing the material of the missed session with the absent grandparent. This technique was very effective as participants became eager to show what they had learned.

At the end of each class, the grandparents completed a brief evaluation describing how much they felt they had learned and what was most and least important. Unlike many students, the group tended to write that "everything was important" and that what they really wanted was more time.

The support group that the participants continued to attend was an important adjunct to the training. Having it readily available meant that within the classes, the grandparents could focus on the curriculum. Personal experiences and problems were frequently raised during the classes, and, if these began to dominate the discussion or if they required specific counseling, they could be referred to the support group.

Each class involved a variety of teaching techniques, and lecture was kept to a minimum. With the goal being empowerment, it is important that the facilitator not be perceived as the expert (Gutierrez, 1990; Lowy & O'Connor; 1986). Although the classes focused on specific material to be learned, the grandparents were expected to be active participants, and discussion was encouraged. At the same time, as the group was eager to share their thoughts, the challenge to the facilitator was to limit the discussion so that the presentation could precede.

Role playing was used in each class. As most of the grandmothers were unfamiliar with the technique, it was at first greeted with some trepidation. But, as the grandmother's became comfortable with it, they became increasingly enthusiastic and less self-conscious. It was particularly helpful in assisting the grandparents in dealing with sensitive and difficult situations. As an example, role plays of talking to grandchildren about sex and HIV helped the grandparents to feel comfortable in the actual discussion. Role playing within the group reduced the tension around issues as the grandparents acted out both their own roles and that of their grandchildren.

Role playing was also a critical part of learning how to navigate the service system. Participants rehearsed strategies for dealing with rude or unhelpful agency staff and techniques that could help to assure that their demands were met. These techniques were used both on the telephone and in personal contacts. Moreover, by assuming the role of the agency worker, the grandmothers received additional insight into the stresses that the workers may be encountering. The secure atmosphere within the group was supportive in trying out the new behaviors. The expertise of several of the grandparents who had successfully dealt with agency staff was helpful in reinforcing the learning.

After studying the factors involved in effective presentations, each participant was required to give a short talk to the group on one of the topics covered in class. This activity, although dreaded by several of the grandmothers, was actually one of the most enjoyable. The experience helped them to overcome fears of public speaking as they spoke on subjects in which they were interested to others in the same situation. The participants critiqued each other's presentation, describing what was particularly strong and where improvement was needed.

The grandparents were given homework assignments in which they had to use the material learned in class at home and to report on the experience to the group. In one instance, Mrs. G., a 75-year-old grandmother, reported her discussion on the use of condoms with her 17-year-old grandson, telling him to be sure to use them, to be sure that they were latex, and to be sure not to keep them in his back pocket where the heat could damage them. She reported that after his initial shock, he told her she was really pretty cool!

At the completion of the 12 sessions, a graduation ceremony was held at the university to which the grandparents brought their grandchildren, relatives, and friends. The event was a further reinforcement of the training as well as formal recognition of the accomplishment of the grandparents. Presentations were made by the dean of the school and representatives of community agencies and foundations involved with grandparents. As the grandmother participants received their diplomas, they were accompanied onto the stage by their grandchildren. The graduation in itself was empowering, as it was the first college graduation that most of the grandchildren had attended, and in this instance, it was for their grandmothers. The event publicly validated the groups' efforts and achievement. Reinforcing its significance was the fact that a reporter from National Public Radio who had interviewed the group attended the graduation. The entire empowerment program, including interviews with the grandmothers, was later described in detail on national radio.

Examples of the Classes

The following are examples of two of the classes with a summary of the background material, objectives, content, and class activities.

Helping Children Build Self-Esteem

Background

Self-esteem is the value that we place on ourselves. Children treated with love, respect, and guidance learn that they are valuable people and begin to develop high levels of self-esteem. On the other hand, children who have been neglected, abused, ignored, or abandoned grow up believing that they have little value or worth and are at risk of having low self-esteem. It is these children who are particularly vulnerable to being influenced by others, those who they see as powerful and important, and those who they wish to be like.

Objectives.

The following objectves were identified:

1. Participants will describe three reasons why self-esteem is important.
2. Participants will discuss why their grandchildren may have problems with self-esteem.
3. Participants will discuss at least four ways of promoting their grandchildren's self-esteem.

Content

The material in the class centered around the importance of self-esteem and described the reasons why grandchildren being raised by their grandparents are vulnerable to having low self-esteem. It addressed issues of rejection, abandonment, and trust and the impact that they have on the grandparent-grandchild relationship. The class emphasized the importance of making the child feel secure, of understanding the "testing" that a child may do, and the need for consistency and structure in the home.

The material in the class discussed ways to promote self-esteem. Grandparents were taught the importance of giving compliments, showing children that they were proud of them, listening, responding to broken rules, spending time with their grandchildren, and hugging.

Class Activities

The class activities reinforced the learning by giving the grandparents the opportunity to experiment with behaviors tied to self-esteem. In one situation, participants had to demonstrate their actions and comments to a young grandchild who had just spilled the milk. In another activity, a grandmother talked with a granddaughter who felt very unhappy with her looks.

To reinforce the learning, at the end of the class, the grandparents were asked to summarize the material, and what they felt was critical to their own situations. At the beginning of the next class, each of the participants had to report how they had used one of the techniques at home and what the results were. This type of immediate application was an important part of the learning process as grandparents could discuss what they had tried, what worked, and what didn't work. At the same time, feedback from the group helped in reinforcing the learning.

Developing Advocacy Skills

Background

Advocacy involves all of the activities that one may do to make needs known and to obtain changes in policies and services so that these needs may be met. Advocacy may also involve reaching other grandparents to inform them about services and benefits. Thus, advocacy strategies may be used to increase members in grandparent support groups for as the group becomes more numerous, it becomes more powerful. Advocacy is closely related to power and power depends on your knowledge of the issues and ability to influence others. By learning to advocate for yourself, you begin to take control of your own life.

Objectives

At the end of this session, participants will be able to do the following:

1. Discuss several types of community outreach activities.
2. Describe effective ways of contacting community leaders who have access to needed information or resources.
3. Effectively telephone and write letters to government officials regarding their needs or concerns.

Content

This class discusses approaches toward advocacy beginning with deciding what is needed, who must be contacted to meet that need, and what is desired from the contact. The material stresses the importance of having clear objectives so that strategies to reach them can be developed. If the objective is to expand the support group, a strategy may be to distribute brochures at schools or other places where grandparents may be present. If the aim is to educate community leaders about service needs, a strategy may be to talk at a local community meeting or even have an open house to which key officials are invited.

Participants were taught how to locate and contact those persons and community leaders who were influential in the development of policies and programs. The class stressed the need for being specific in describing problems or conditions and having material organized. The power that grandparents can have was discussed and highlighted by one of the grandmothers who had obtained changes in her local parent-teacher association so that it would be more accessible to grandparents.

Activities

In class the grandmothers demonstrated how they might start a conversation with other grandparents in the community to inform them about their program and other services. They also demonstrated how they would telephone a local official to inform him about a need for services or changes in a specific policy. A role play was enacted of giving a talk at a public hearing regarding the effect of benefit reductions on the ability to care for their grandchildren.

Within the group, the grandparents demonstrated how they would attempt to reach and talk with an agency worker regarding an application for benefits that had been denied. As several had experienced this situation, they were eager to experiment with new techniques. Learning how to present oneself to the agency, how to be assertive without becoming angry, and how to demand speaking with a supervisor thoroughly engaged the group members while also permitting them to try out new techniques.

Each class was based on developing knowledge, skills, and behaviors to increase grandparents' effectiveness. The classes demanded a great deal of interaction among the participants as they worked to apply the material to their own lives. These interactions also invoked much reflection as the participants were asked to question and critique themselves continually. This type of active learning was seen as critical to the grandmother's understanding and application of the material.

Project Outcomes

With the completion of the training, the grandparents began their ongoing task of reaching other grandparents in the community. They were responsible for giving presentations to groups at schools, senior centers, churches, tenant associations, and in other settings that they felt appropriate. As discussed earlier, these presentations were viewed as a part of the empowerment process as they provided the format for reinforcing their own self-efficacy.

The grandparents made these presentations in groups of two or three, with each deciding on her own specific topic. Often, they engaged in role plays with one playing the role of the grandchild or a worker and the other demonstrating correct and incorrect ways of interacting.

One of the most exciting presentations was one given to a group of Latino grandparents. Three of the African-American grandparents made presentations through an interpreter about communication, self-esteem, and services. The common needs of the grandparents and the eagerness of the two groups, one to receive the information and the other to provide it, overcame all cultural and language barriers as an immediate and intense rapport developed. The presenters were invited back to give further presentations. The response of the Latino group generated their own demand for similar empowerment training.

The presentations also revealed several areas where further preparation was needed. These included having very clear directions to programs and having sufficient background information on the audience. Although these requirements had been discussed in class, the significance was not clearly understood until the grandparents began their presentations. As an example, it took more than two hours for the presenters to reach one site as they were not clear about the location. In other situations, the grandparents had prepared to discuss legal issues associated with raising grandchildren, but no one in the group was actually raising a grandchild. Fortunately, one of the presenters was prepared to discuss communication and self-esteem, a subject that was of interest to the group.

As the presenters began going out into the community, they also became increasingly cognizant of the importance of being well informed on the site for the presentation. They learned that presentations at nutrition programs must be given within a specific period as participants tend to leave directly after lunch. Presentations at senior centers require adequate publicity and promotion to assure sufficient attendance. Conversely, presentations at grandparent support groups are likely to involve lengthy discussion as those attending are anxious for information and education.

The presentations also indicated areas in which further training was necessary. As the facilitator accompanied the grandmothers to their initial talk, areas needing subsequent training were identified. Although the grandparents had been anxious and often very nervous about speaking, once they began, they found it difficult to end. In one presentation, "in closing" was repeated several times, with the closing itself taking more than 20 minutes. There was a pressing need for more practice in closing presentations, including limiting questions. Conversely, the enjoyment they discovered in making the presentations and the enthusiasm with which they were received underscored the effectiveness of the empowerment training.

As well as making presentations, the group also became engaged in outreach in the community. They developed brochures and flyers about their support group, which they distributed in schools, churches, and physician's offices. Several approached older persons on the street who appeared to be grandparents with grandchildren to discuss their program and invite them to participate. In addition, they attended local community meetings and began making their needs widely known. In one instance, several attended a forum at a local college being presented by social service agency directors regarding changes in agency priorities. Given the opportunity to speak, the grandparents questioned these directors, demanding to be placed on agency advisory boards so that they could have direct involvement in policy.

Implications and Recommendations

The results of this empowerment training project indicate that even though grandparents raising grandchildren have a plethora of needs that can appear to be overwhelming, they also have formidable strengths and resiliency that must not be underestimated. Building on these strengths through empowerment training is one strategy for assisting them in coping with their own immediate problems as well as providing a means for them to help others.

The grandparents in this project benefited from having an ongoing support group in which personal issues raised in the training could be discussed in depth. Subjects, such as loss and grief, engender many highly charged emotions that need to be addressed but that cannot be adequately dealt with in the training. By assuring that counseling and support are available to participants, the training is able to remain focused. It is not clear that the training would have been as successful without this parallel support group.

However, even with the support group, group leaders are likely to find that participants have a tendency to want to relate their own experiences during the training. Facilitators must be sensitive to both individual and group needs. If personal experiences begin to dominate the discussions, the session can easily be diverted from its objectives. Not only does this disrupt the training, but it also affects the interest of the other participants. A common comment in the session evaluations was that participants felt too much time was devoted to listening to one person's personal story.

As with many other organizations, a core group of grandparents emerged who took on the responsibility for keeping the group engaged and maintaining its momentum. In addition, having a facilitator available who can continue to provide support and guidance without undermining the self-efficacy of the group is also important as help is likely to be needed in activities, such as scheduling events and locating resources.

The results of the empowerment training also suggest that grandparents may play significant roles as peer educators. Other groups of older persons warmly responded to hearing from persons who shared the same experiences and with whom they could easily identify. The grandparents are able to offer examples from their own lives that parallel those of their audience and are valuable in establishing rapport. Consequently, most presentations have ended with invitations to return.

Finally, this program underscores the eagerness of grandparents to learn and to obtain information that can improve their skills. Empowerment training assists participants as it imparts new knowledge and ways of thinking that impact on their roles as grandparents and members of society. By applying the learning to their own situations and interactions with their grandchildren, relatives, and services and by reaching out to others, these grandparents are taking control of their lives and shaping their own roles.

References

Berger, P., & Neuhaus, R. (1977). *To empower people: The role of mediating structures in public policy.* Washington, DC: American Enterprise Institute for Public Policy Research.

Cochran, M. (1987). Empowering families: An alternative to the deficit model. In K. Hurrelman, F. Kaufmann & R. Losel (Eds.), *Social intervention: Potential and constraints* (pp. 105–119). Berlin: Walter de Bruyter.

Cox, E. (1988). Empowerment interventions in aging. *Social Work With Groups, 11,* 111–125.

Cox, E., & Parsons, R. (1994). *Empowerment-oriented social work practice with the elderly.* Pacific Grove: Brooks/Cole.

Gutierrez, L. (1990). Working with women of color: An empowerment perspective. *Social Work, 35,* 149–154.

Gutierrez, L., & Ortega, R. (1991). Developing methods to empower Latinos: The importance of groups. *Social Work With Groups, 14,* 23–43.

Hasenfeld, Y. (1987). Power in social work practice. *Social Service Review, 61,* 467–483.

Health Systems Agency of New York City. (1992). *HIV/AIDS Strategic Plan: Vol. 2. HIV/AIDS Data Book.* New York: Author.

Katz, R. (1984). Empowerment synergy: Expanding the community's healing resources. *Prevention in Human Services, 3,* 9–36.

Lowy, L., & O'Connor, D. (1986). *Why Education in the Later Years?* Lexington: Lexington Books.

Solomon, B. (1976). *Black empowerment: Social work in oppressed communities.* New York: Columbia University Press.

Staples, L. (1990). Powerful ideas about empowerment. *Administration in Social Work, 14,* 29–42.

U.S. Bureau of the Census. (1990). *Census of Population and housing summary.* Washington, DC: Author.

Chapter 16

Grandparents and Schools: Issues and Potential Challenges

Nina M. Silverstein and Laila Vehvilainen

Over the past decade, an increasing number of researchers have explored the needs and experiences of the burgeoning population of custodial grandparents. However, an underreported area of the prior research is the grandparent caregivers' interactions with the school systems responsible for their grandchildren's education. Schools have changed a great deal since their own children were in school, not only in terms of the curriculum offered but also their milieu. Increased incidence of the use of drugs and alcohol and in-school violence present new challenges and stressers to grandparents who are parenting again. Further, many grandparents may not be aware

An earlier version of this chapter entitled, "Beyond the Bake Sale: Grandparents Raising School-Age Grandchildren," was presented at the 50th annual scientific meeting of the Gerontological Society of America, November 1997, Cincinatti.

The data for this chapter are drawn from a project report entitled, "Raising Awareness About Grandparents Raising Grandchildren in Massachusetts" by N. M. Silverstein, and L.Vehvilainen, University of Massachusetts-Boston Gerontology Institute and Center, 1998.

of in-school resources available to them, such as special education or counseling, nor have they taken steps to work with the schools to make their needs known.

The purpose of this chapter is threefold: (a) to summarize the findings of a descriptive study conducted at the University of Massachusetts–Boston of grandparents raising grandchildren, (b) to highlight the findings of the study examining the grandparents' interactions with schools and address areas that merit further research, and (c) to discuss relevant findings and offer strategies that would assist and enhance the grandparents' involvement with schools. It is hoped that the data presented in this chapter will stimulate discussion of the issues; exploration of how schools are currently responding to the needs of grandchildren who are being raised by their grandparents; and reflection on future initiatives.

Prior research has found that children who are being raising by grandparents are at a high risk for emotional and developmental disorders (Beardslee, Bempora, Keller, & Klerman, 1983) . In comparison with children raised in traditional families, those raised by grandparents are more likely to repeat a grade and to have lower academic performance (Solomon & Marx, 1995).

The Situation in Massachusetts

Currently, there is not any one public or private agency responsible for addressing the needs of grandparents who are raising their grandchildren. This family structure does not neatly "fit" in our current organizational systems. Although the State Unit on Aging, the Executive Office of Elder Affairs in Massachusetts, has provided a sympathetic ear and has devoted some attention and resources to understanding the needs of grandparent caregivers, the reality is that many of the grandparents are under age 60 and are not considered the "legitimate" constituency of this agency.

The concern of grandparent families and other kin is an intergenerational issue that warrants collaboration between state agencies, the aging network, and the child welfare network. In Massachusetts, there are examples of several state agencies whose collaborative efforts have brought attention to the needs of grandparent-headed families. The Massachusetts Executive Office of Elder Affairs has established the Massachusetts Grandparent Resource Network, which offers a forum to discuss issues and share information.

In addition, the Massachusetts Executive Office of Elder Affairs and the Massachusetts Executive Office of Health and Human Services demonstrated their collaboration through the development of *a Resource Guide for Massachusetts Grandparents Raising Their Grandchildren* and regional *Wellness Days*. Moreover, the Department of Social Services Kinship Program is in place in every regional office to give more emphasis and support to kin placement, most of which are grandparent placements. The Department of Mental Retardation is also starting to facilitate grandparent support groups to the growing numbers of grandfamilies they serve.

Finally, a very promising initiative that will begin to address the need for supportive housing environments is the GrandFamilies House demonstration in Dorchester, Massachusetts. This is one encouraging example of a public/private partnership addressing the special housing challenges of grandparent caregivers. With the first grandparent moving in with her grandchildren in October 1998, the GrandFamilies House will eventually provide 26 grandparent caregivers in Massachusetts who have Section 8 housing certificates with housing in the new site. The housing was designed specifically for grandparents who are raising their grandchildren. The funds for the housing were raised by Boston Aging Concerns Young and Old United, Inc. (BAC-YOU) who will manage the building. Educational, recreational, and support services will be offered on site through the YWCA.

Study Methodology and Key Findings

A descriptive study of 134 grandparents raising grandchildren in Massachusetts serves as the cornerstone for discussing relevant issues and challenges in this chapter. Although this began as a study of grandparents raising school-age children, it soon became apparent that to begin to understand their relationships to schools it was first necessary to have a fuller picture of these families. Educators talk of "readiness" to learn. The profile of this sample may help the teacher begin to understand how this complicated family structure affects Johnny's readiness.

Methodology

The purpose of the study was to understand better the characteristics and needs of grandparents raising grandchildren in Massachusetts, particularly as they relate to school-age children. A sample of 177 grandparents in Massachusetts who were raising their grandchildren was identified through a snowball sampling technique. Ultimately, 134 grandparents were interviewed by telephone. The sample recruitment strategy included announcements in print media and on cable television, the distribution of flyers to grandparent support groups, and dissemination of flyers through Councils on Aging. In addition, several school district superintendents included the study announcement in their school bulletins. Referrals made by grandparents who completed the telephone interviews also generated additional study participants.

An action-research methodology was used. This type of research model partners the university researcher with community leaders or agency representatives to address an issue of public concern (Bass & Silverstein, 1996). To receive guidance about survey content development and other aspects of the study design and sample recruitment, an advisory board was assembled. The community partners who the advisory board comprised were representatives from the Massachusetts Executive Office of Elder Affairs (State Unit on Aging), grandparent support group leaders, the Massachusetts Department of Mental Health, a school guidance counselor, housing and elder advocates, and grandparent caregivers. The interviews were conducted by 53 students participating in the Frank J. Manning Certificate in Gerontology program in the College of Public and Community Service at the University of Massachusetts–Boston. The length of the interview ranged from 15 to 90 minutes, with the average being 38 minutes.

Grandparent Caregiver Characteristics

Because of the descriptive nature of the study, findings are not generalizable beyond the 134 grandparent caregivers in the study (see Table 16.1). Nevertheless, the demographic profile of the grandparents in the study was similar to that reported in other studies of grandparents who raise grandchildren. Most of the grandparent caregivers in this study were women (86%), and 61% were married (consistent with the 63% national figure previously reported by Pruchno & Johnson, 1996). The average age of the grandparents surveyed was 60 years and ranged in age from 41 to 83 years, which is slightly higher than the ages, 55 to 57, previously reported in the literature (Chalfie, 1994; Kornhaber, 1996). Thirty-two percent of the respondents in the sample were older than the age of 65 years. Most of the grandparents were White (74%), with an average age of 61 years. Black grandparents (23%) had an average age of 59 years. Almost all the grandparents were born in the United States (95%). With 20% having completed 4 or more years of college, this sample of grandparents was more educated than samples in other studies (Chalfie, 1994).

TABLE 16.1 Demographic Profile (N = 134)

Description	Number or %
Number of children currently raising	2 children (mean) 1 to 7 children (range)
Currently living with grandchildren	90%
Lived with grandchildren within the past year	10%
Duration	5 years (median) Less than one month to 21 years (range)
Age of child	33%<1 year; 6 years (mean); SD = 5.7
Current situation	73% Permanent 16% Temporary 11% Unknown
Legal custody	63% Have legal custody
Parentage of child[a]	74% Daughter's child 26% Son's child
Parental involvement with child	35% Both parents 38% Mother only 9% Father only 18% No involvement

[a] Two percent of the respondents were raising children of both sons and daughters. Four percent were also raising great-grandchildren.

The median household income reported was about $22,000—higher than reported in other studies of grandparent caregivers (Chalfie, 1994) but comparable with that of other households in Massachussetts headed by people aged 65 to 74 years (Gerontology Institute, 1992). The median reported household income for White grandparents was $30,000 versus a median of $15,000 for the Black grandparents.

More than half (56%) of the grandparents said that there had been a change in their household income since they began raising the children.

For most, 63%, their household income had decreased. More than a third of the grandparents agreed that they "worried about making ends meet." In part, the decrease in income can be explained by the change of employment. Before raising their grandchildren, 43% of the grandparents in this study were employed full time, and 12% were working part time. After assuming care of the grandchildren, only 18% were employed full time, whereas 21% were now working part time.

In terms of housing, more than two thirds (69%) of the grandparents in this study owned their homes, and 31% rented. Thus, the proportion of homeowners is comparable with that of the state, where in 1990, 68% of people age 65 or older lived in owner-occupied housing compared with 78% that has been reported nationwide (Gerontology Institute, 1992, p. 26). Of those who rented, 21% or eight grandparents were in rent-controlled apartments. Sixty percent of the renters were in apartments, 37% in single family homes and 5% in retirement or elderly housing units. A quarter of the grandparents surveyed had to move when the children came to live with them. An additional 23% renovated their homes to accommodate the children.

Caregiving Situation and Experience

More than 40% of the grandparents reported that they "worried a lot" about raising their grandchildren. Often that worry translated into: "Who will care for them when I am gone?" More than a quarter, 27%, of the grandparents admitted that they did feel "a lot" of burden in their caregiving role. Additional stressors included conflict with the biological parents, unpleasant interactions with the Department of Social Services, and concerns about the future and the physical demands associated with child rearing. They also expressed frustration at not being able to do what they had planned to do when they retired: "We do not have enough time together with our spouses," or "We are exhausted most of the time." Many were also providing care to other family members.

Conversely, most (87%) of the grandparents expressed "a lot" of satisfaction and pleasure from raising their grandchildren. Grandparents expressed enjoyment in watching their grandchildren grow into confident young adults, in being able to provide them with a safe and nurturing environment, and in being around them as they learned new skills or played. One grandparent said that the experience of raising children made them (the grandparents) feel young and gave them a new perspective on life: "so much wonder seeing things through the child's eyes. He is creative and challenges me to do things I never thought I could."

The grandparents were raising an average of two children, and most were caring for the children of a daughter (74%). The average age of the children was 6 years (SD = 5.7) with one third of the children less than 1 year old. Half of the children had been in their grandparents' care for 5 or more years. On average, the child was less than 1 year old when he or she first came to live with their grandparent.

Usually, there was more than one reason that the children were in their grandparents' care. The most commonly cited reasons were child neglect (50%), followed by substance abuse (49%), parent(s) unable to afford to raise their child (39%), the parent(s) were too young (32%), parent moved away (24%), and parent ill or disabled (23%). Grandparents who noted substance abuse also tended to also report child neglect ($r =. 40, p< .05$), a finding consistent with other studies of this population (Minkler, Roe, & Price, 1992) in which child neglect was a by-product of the biological parents' substance abuse.

When asked how the decision was made to place the children in their care, almost half (47%) of the grandparents said that there was a family discussion that included the biological parent(s). Thirty-eight percent said that there had been a family discussion that did not include the biological parent(s). Fifteen percent of grandparents responded that "there was no discussion, it just happened." It is important to mention that in at least one situation when a grandmother was asked the reason she was caring for her grandchild, she responded, "I was told by the judge that I had no choice." In fact, 39% of the grandparents said that there had been a court agreement placing the children in their care. An additional third of the grandparents reported that the arrangement was the result of a Department of Social Services agreement.

Most (73%) of the grandparents perceived their arrangement as permanent, whereas 16% thought it was temporary and 11% did not know (see Table 16.1). Almost two thirds (63%) of the grandparents reported that they had legal custody of their grandchildren. More than half (54%) of the grandparents with legal custody reported that they had a guardianship arrangement, whereas 10% had temporary legal custody, 10% had adopted the grandchildren, and 5% were foster parents.

More than a third, 38%, of the grandparents reported that only the mother was involved with the children with nearly as many, 35%, stating that both parents were involved. Few persons, 18%, reported that there was no parental involvement from either the mother or the father. One grandmother stated that the most difficult part of raising her grandchild was that "he always asks where is mother is and (she) has a hard time making the child understand that the parent's leaving is not his fault."

Health of Grandchild and Grandparent Caregiver

More than a third (35%) of the grandparents reported that at least one of the grandchildren in their care had health problems. The grandparents cited asthma and chronic ear infections (otitis media) as the most common health problems encountered by the children. A prevalence rate of 10% to 20% is reported for all children nationwide for asthma (PEDBASE, 1998). Ear infections rank second to the common cold as the most common health problem in preschool children. Almost all (98%) of the grandparents reported that the children had a primary care physician whom they had visited within the past year (96%). More than a quarter (27%), however, had an emergency room or urgent care center visit within the past 6 months.

Jendrek (1992) reported grandparents experiencing difficulty obtaining health insurance for the grandchildren in their care since private insurance policies do not cover grandchildren or the grandparents do not qualify for Medicaid. In the current study, almost all (96%) of the grandchildren were covered by health insurance, with most (65%) being covered by Medicaid (or Mass Health as it is named in Massachusetts). Thirty-two percent had private insurance coverage, with 10% reporting being part of a HMO plan. Ninety percent of the grandparents reported that they had health insurance for themselves.

More than a third of the grandparents, 38%, identified chronic health problems that limit their activity. Arthritis was the most frequently cited health problem cited followed by hearing problems and mobility impairments. A quarter of the grandparents reported that their health was "worse" now than before they began caring for their grandchildren Very few, 9%, claimed to be frequently depressed during the past month.

Community Service Utilization and Unmet Needs Service Use

In the current study, 42% of the grandparents participated in grandparent support groups, which is a relatively high percentage compared with several recent studies. In an ongoing national study of 453 grandmothers who are raising a grandchild by Pruchno et al. (1997), only 11% of the grandmothers reported belonging to a support group, yet 85% of the respondents would like to belong to one. The disparity with national data may be at least partially explained by the fact that recruitment flyers were distributed to support group leaders to share in their groups. Most (85%) of the grandparents who attended support groups found the meetings to be "very helpful." Support group members were more likely to use community services and are less likely to report feeling depressed.

The most frequently used services were counseling for both the grandchild (80%) and the grandparent (36%), followed by clothing allowance (32%) and subsidized childcare (28%). Among services that grandparents would like to have were respite including baby-sitting, after-school programs, and affordable day care. There was also a need for more local grandparent support groups, financial aid, food stamps, and legal services. Grandparents who reported that they would like additional services were more likely to report less overall satisfaction with their caregiving situation than grandparents who did not perceive the need for additional services ($r = -41$, $p<.05$). The following barriers to services were described: a lack of information about available services, not meeting eligibility criteria, service is not affordable, service is not available, service is not accessible, on wait list for services.

Grandparents and Schools

Although the findings in this study revealed that most of grandparents were actively involved with their grandchildrens' schools, several areas for further exploration were identified. The specific areas of grandparent involvement with schools that were examined were overall satisfaction with schools, grandchild's adjustment and use of counseling services, help with homework, contact with teachers, use of before- school or after-school programs, and participation in school activities. Eighty percent of the school-age children were attending public schools, and 20% were in private schools. The average grade level for the school-age children was fourth grade. Eleven percent of the children under the age of 5 were enrolled in preschool programs, such as Headstart or other early childhood education programs.

Most of the grandparents surveyed took an active role in their grandchildren's education and had, on the whole, reported a positive experience with the grandchildren's schools. Most (75%) of the grandparents surveyed were very satisfied with the schools that the children were attending. Though not statistically significant, older grandparents tended to express greater satisfaction than younger grandparents. The comments to open-ended questions suggested that the older cohort was still operating under a reluctance to question authority, expressing a "teacher must be right" sentiment.

Moreover, most grandparents reported that they were involved with school activities. Most of the grandparents attended school events (78%) and had contact with the children's teachers (84%). However, it is not known whether "contact" was of a positive or negative nature. That is, was their contact in the course of regularly scheduled parent/teacher conferences, or were the grandparents called in for problem behavior? A limitation of this study is that the survey did not include a follow-up question to determine the reason for teacher contact, which could have provided further insight into the teacher/grandparent/child relationship.

Most (79%) of the grandparents did help with homework, and most (77%) felt comfortable with this task. Math homework was considered to be the most difficult subject for the grandparents in assisting the children. Eighty-six percent of the grandparents who reported that they helped with homework mentioned having difficulties with assisting with math homework. Other subjects that were considered difficult were language arts (32%) and science (27%).

The survey results revealed several areas that invite further exploration. Almost a third (32%) of the grandparents reported that the children needed to change schools when they moved in with their grandparents. This raises the question as to the impact that changing schools had on the well-being of the child, that is, whether relocation negatively or positively influenced the school adjustment and academic performance. Another area that merits further attention is the use and need of counseling services. More than half (55%) of the grandparents reported that the children received counseling. Thirteen percent received counseling in school, 33% were in counseling programs outside of school, and 8% had both in-school and out-of-school counseling.

Further analysis also revealed a significant relationship between substance abuse on the part of the parents and the use of counseling services by the child (chi sq were [1] = 23.1, $p<.001$). However, the survey did not provide information about the actual reasons that the children were receiving counseling services, nor did it address whether those who may have emotional or behavioral problems actually had access to those services.

Almost half, 42%, of the grandparents reported that at least one of the grandchildren in their household had "special needs"—learning disability, attention deficit disorder/Attention Deficient Hyperactivity Disorder, depression, or developmentally delayed difficulties. However, because of the phrasing of the question: "Does your grandchild(ren) have any special needs?" and its subjective interpretation, it may be that a portion of the grandchildren who were identified as "special needs" may not be enrolled in special education programs. Although not directly comparable, it is interesting to note that in Massachusetts, 16.5% of school-age children enrolled in public schools are in special education programs (Massachusetts Department of Education, 1995), whereas nationally the figure is 12% (U.S. Department of Education, 1995).

Typically, child care programs, such as before- and after-school programs, are developed to accommodate working caregivers and may or may not be offered within the individual school or school system. The grandparents were asked about the availability of these programs and their use of them. A quarter of the grandparents noted that the schools their children attend had before-school programs, and almost a third (32%) of these grandparents used these before-school programs. Most schools, 60%, had after-school programs, and almost half (45%) of the grandparents, for whom after-care was available, used the program. Grandparents who used before-school programs were likely to use after-school programs as well ($r = .60$, $p<.05$).

Most of the children were involved with after-school activities. The activities most frequently cited included after-school sports; religious education; music, dance, or drama classes; and boy/girl scouts

---

Discussion and Implications

It is hoped that the study findings will serve as a starting point for discussing critical issues facing grandparents who are raising their grandchildren. There is no doubt that school faculty and administration are challenged to respond to the needs of complicated family structures of which grandparent caregivers are just one example. Grandparents who are raising grandchildren may be confronted with a host of potential obstacles on several different levels when relating to schools. Some school districts are legally unable to sign a child's permission slip for a field trip. On a personal level, the grandparent may feel uncomfortable interacting with teachers for fear of being stigmatized ("Apparently they failed with their children") or not feeling comfortable with helping children with homework.

Another important consideration that pervades the relationship with the school is that this group of children is reported to be at higher risk for developmental delays and behavioral problems. This means that the grandparent must not only interact and dialogue with the teachers and administrators, but also be knowledgeable about special education programs and counseling services.

These data, as well as the reactions by the project advisory board to the findings, provide some insight into the grandparent caregiving experience in Massachusetts. Although on the whole, the results of this survey describe a sample of grandparents that had frequent interaction with their grandchildrens' schools and were active participants in the grandchildrens' education, that may be more reflective of the sample bias of self-selection than representative of most grandparent caregivers. Further, characteristics of this sample, such as higher education, greater participation in support groups, and greater percentage with legal custody of grandchildren may also account for their increased interaction and involvement with schools.

Though caution must be exercised in generalizing the findings to all grandparent caregivers because of the nonprobability selection of the sample and the limited sample size, several areas merit further discussion. Both these and specific strategies follow that may be applicable to schools to help support grandparents raising grandchildren.

Increase Outreach From Schools to Grandparents

Teachers, guidance counselors, and school nurses may provide great support to the grandparent and child. School assessments and referrals also may inform the grandparents of federal and state programs and services for which they may be eligible. In addition, workshops on curriculum (particularly math) and "help with homework" strategies may benefit some grandparent caregivers as indicated by the survey results. An example of a school-based initiative in Massachusetts is the *Kinship Family Resource Center* in Fitchburg, Massachusetts, where a school guidance counselor has taken the lead in providing support to grandparent caregivers and their grandchildren and acts as a liaison with community services providers. As a result, grandparent caregivers have been identified within the school system, and targeted support has been developed for them. For example, a school counselor can provide referrals for health and social services, such as counseling to help cope with emotional and psychological problems.

Sensitize Educators About Grandparent Caregiver Needs and Concerns

School personnel often are the first "alert" to a child's behavior, health, and learning problems and, therefore, should be aware of the child's familial circumstances. The project advisory board offered several actions that may be considered to narrow the perceived gap between the educator and the grandparent caregiver. Potential actions to be taken include adding the topics of "grandparents as parents" or "grandparents as partners in education" to in-service training or continuing education seminars for teachers. In addition, as substance abuse by the biological parents was the major reason for these grandparents assuming care of their grandchildren, school counselors and teachers might benefit from drug and alcohol education.

School boards or administrators might also appoint grandparent caregiver representatives to parent-teacher councils and encourage grandparent membership in parent-teacher associations. Deborah Doucette-Dudman, author of Raising Our Children's Children, has offered several workshops to both grandparents and professionals in Massachusetts that focus on issues that "hamper kinship care within a family." Her workshops deal with such concerns as relating to a troubled birth parent, reaching consensus when grandparents do not agree, and advising on legal and financial concerns regarding kinship care.

Explore Access to Respite Care

Almost half of the grandparents surveyed identified respite as an additional support service that they would like to receive. Schools could prepare information or fact sheets about before- and after-school programs, and other "respite care" programs for children. In this study, 19% of the grandparents were also caregivers for an ill or disabled spouse, parent, or other relative in addition to the grandchildren. These "multiple" caregivers are likely to be in greater need of respite services as are those claiming that "no one" helps them care for the children.

Provide Information on Grandparent
Caregiver Support Groups

Schools could provide information about grandparent caregiver support groups or if the grandparent population is large enough start a school-based one. Councils on Aging could be approached to partner, facilitate, or host support groups. A potential outcome is that grandparents who attend support groups may be better informed about available resources to address their needs and the needs of their grandchildren. Most (85%) of the grandparents in this study who attended the meetings found them to be very helpful in terms of coping and learning about community services. Support groups can also help grandparents address strategies for planning for the future care of the children.

In Fitchburg, Massachusetts, for example, a school-based support group was founded and currently, there are also plans to start a new support group for grandchildren to address and discuss issues such as their grandparents' aging and feelings toward their biological parents. In addition, support groups can serve an advocacy function by providing a link for sharing information between policy makers, service providers, and the grandparents.

In summary, the grandparents in this study are playing vital and active roles in their grandchildren's lives and in their schools. Further study will help to better define the nature of these school relationships and to strengthen it. Encouraging grandparent involvement in the education system will serve to benefit not only the grandparents but also the schools, communities, and children whom they serve.

References

Bass, S. A., & Silverstein, N. M. (1996). Action-research: A practical model to link teaching, research and community service. *Metropolitan Universities, 7,* 85–94.

Beardslee, W. R., Bempora, J, Keller, M. B., & Klerman, G. (1983). Children of parents with major affective disorders: A review. *American Journal of Psychiatry, 240,* 825–832.

Boston Aging Concerns Young and Old United, Inc. (1997). *Annual report.* 67 Newbury Street, Boston, MA 02116.

Burton, L. M. (1992). Black grandparents rearing children of drug-addicted parents: Stressors, outcomes, and social needs. *The Gerontologist, 32,* 744–751.

Chalfie, D. (1994). *Going it alone: A closer look at grandparents parenting grandchildren,* Washington, DC: AARP Women's Initiative..

Department of Education. http://nces.ed.gov. U.S. Department of Education National Center for Education Statistics.

Doucette-Dudman, D. (1996). *Raising our children's children.* Minneapolis, MN: Fairview Press.

Dressel, P. L., & Barnhill, S. K. (1994). Reframing gerontological thought and practice: The case of grandmothers with daughters in prison. *The Gerontologist, 34,* 685–691.

Gerontology Institute. (1992). *The older population in Massachusetts 1980–1990.* University of Massachusetts-Boston.

Jendrek, M. (1994). Grandparents who parent their grandchildren: Circumstances and decisions. *The Gerontologist, 34,* 206–216.

Joslin, D., & Brouard, A. (1995). The prevalence of grandmothers as primary caregivers in a poor pediatric population. *Journal of Community Health, 20,* 383–400.

KidSource OnLine. (1998). Questions and answers about otitis media, hearing and language development. http://www.kidsource.com/asha/otitis.html.

Kornhaber, A. (1996). *Contemporary grandparenting.* Thousand Oaks, CA: Sage.

Minkler M, et al. (1997, September). Depression in grandparents raising grandchildren: Results of a national longitudinal study. *Archives of Family Medicine, 6,* 445–452

Minkler, M., Roe, K. M., & Price, M. (1992). The physical and emotional health of grandmothers raising grandchildren in the crack cocaine epidemic. *The Gerontologist, 32,* 752–761.

Minkler, M., & Roe, K. M. (1996, spring). Grandparents as surrogate parents. *Generations,* 34–38.

PEDBASE. (1998). Facts about asthma. http://www.icondata.com/health/pedbase/files/asthma-a.html.

Pinson-Millburn, N. M., Fabian, E. S., Schlossberg, N. K., & Pyle, M. (1996, July–August). Grandparents raising grandchildren. *Journal of Counseling & Development, 74,* 548–554

Pruchno, R. A., & Johnson, K. W. (1996, spring). Research on grandparenting: Review of current studies and future needs. *Generations,* 65–70.

Roe, K. M., Minkler, M., & Saunders, F. F. (1995). Combining research, advocacy, and education: The methods of the Grandparent Caregiver Study. *Health Education Quarterly, 22,* 458–475.

Solomon, J., & Marx, J. (1995). "To Grandmother's house we go": Health and school adjustment of children raised solely by grandparents. *The Gerontologist, 35,* 386–394.

U.S. Bureau of the Census. (1997, March). *Population Survey* (Working paper, Series No. 26). Washington, DC: US Government Printing Office.

Chapter 17

Community Interventions to Support Grandparent Caregivers: Lessons Learned From the Field

Kathleen M. Roe

The last 10 years have witnessed the emergence of a creative and resourceful array of supportive interventions for grandparent-headed families in communities across the United States. From support groups in small town kitchens in the late 1980s to late 1990s online chat rooms, interventions for parenting grandparents have grown with both the phenomenon and the times. This chapter outlines the evolution of community-based interventions, drawing lessons from the field and inspiration from programs in support of families in which children go to grandmother's house—and stay.

First-Generation Programs:
Support Groups to Comprehensive Services

Most interventions begin with a support group. The first groups were started in the late 1980s, frequently by grandparents suddenly raising grandchildren. Some of the earliest groups began in small rural communities, facilitated by a parenting grandparent reaching out to others. In larger cities, groups were convened in churches, schools, hospitals, or senior centers, facilitated by a volunteer health or social service worker who had noted the increasing number of young children in the care of older clients or community members. With names, such as ROCK (Raising Our Children's Kids), GAIN (Grandparents Are Indeed Needed) and GOLD (Grandparents Offering Love and Direction), and more recently Family Circles and RAPN (Relatives as Parents Network), more than 300 support groups were operating across the country by 1993 (Minkler & Roe, 1993, 1996), growing to more than 500 by 1998 (Aging Alert, 1998).

Informal assessments repeatedly indicate that grandparent caregivers' top concerns are legal issues regarding custody, financial support (including affordable housing for their extended family), social services (particularly health care and counseling), and dealing with the schools and their grandchildren's education. Support groups are ideally suited to offer beginning assistance in each of these areas, with the added and sometimes surprise benefit of peer and reciprocal support. Some groups are facilitated by professionals, such as social workers or community psychologists. Some are run and facilitated entirely by grandparent caregivers themselves. Other groups, such as the one supported by South Coast Head Start in Coos Bay, Oregon, partner a grandparent caregiver with a professional facilitator for group leadership.

The collective experience of the many groups around the country strongly suggests that support groups face common challenges rooted in the psychosocial complexity of reconfigured intergenerational families (Minkler, Driver, & Roe (1995). Children in the care of their grandparents range in age from infants through older teens. Many have special medical, psychological, or educational needs. Grandparent care givers themselves may range in age from early 30s to early 80s. The families face competing and changing demands for care givers' attention, energy, and resources.

Some of the small early support groups, such as those affiliated with Grandparents Raising Grandchildren of Colleyville, Texas, shared resources and information as a network of chapters joined together under a common mission statement, whereas other groups spring up almost spontaneously as purely local endeavors. An earlier chapter has discussed both the structure and dynamics of these groups and the factors contributing to their survival. However, the collected anecdotal experience of support groups over the past decade clearly indicates that without the commitment of consistent external support in the way in which it is most needed by the local group, most support groups come and go as caregiver and community interests are exhausted or engaged (Minkler & Roe, 1996, Roe & Minkler, 1998).

Over the past decade, support groups have become more sophisticated in their understanding of what children and grandparents need. In Rochester, New York, the Skip Program of the Southwest Family Resource Center has partnered with the Monroe County Office of Aging and Kids Adjusting Through Support (KATS), a nationally recognized organization that develops support groups for children who have experienced the loss of a parent through death, incarceration, illness, or foster care placement. This first collaboration between KATS and grandparent caregivers acknowledges the different ways in which parents and children may experience the loss of the family member who may still be alive but is unable to parent. Grandparents and grandchildren meet weekly for 10 weeks in parallel group sessions for support, relaxation, and fun. Through the facilitation of the KATS staff, both grandparents and grandchildren learn to face, grieve, and then embrace the loss that has brought them together.

Support groups reach out to others in the community who may need basic information about local resources. For example, the Relatives as Parents Program of the Westchester County Office for the Aging in New York State has developed Resources-at-a-Glance cards with national, state, regional, and local contact numbers for assistance with child care, legal and financial concerns, grandparents' rights, health care and the local support groups. Thousands of the cards have been distributed throughout the county at post offices, banks, libraries, health care facilities, and other community sites. Some years earlier, Celestine Greene, the founder of an early support group in Oakland, California identified the need for a hotline for isolated relative care givers. Staffed by peer volunteers from local support groups, the Grandparents as Second Parents "warmline" received more than 1,000 calls in its first 6 months of operation and has been replicated by support groups across the country and in different languages.

Comprehensive Services

The visibility and success of many of the early support groups, and the growing recognition of both the number and needs of grandparents raising grandchildren, led to the development of more comprehensive programs in the mid-1990s. Among the first to receive multiyear funding was Project GUIDE in Detroit, which developed intergenerational programs for families and neighborhoods devastated by substance abuse. Project

GUIDE's comprehensive approach to caregiver support, and its emphasis on African-American pride, family esteem, and mutual assistance, encouraged the growth of other expanded efforts.

Around the same time, comprehensive services for grandparents raising the children of their incarcerated children were being developed in Boston, Atlanta, and San Francisco, offering legal services, transportation for visitations, and respite for exhausted caregivers. More recently, Project Healthy Grandparents in Atlanta received 5-year federal funding to develop a comprehensive service program with an emphasis on family autonomy and participant leadership. Integrated interventions are provided by a team of social workers, nurses, attorneys, and tutors, who come directly to the grandparents' home. Project staff counsel and make referrals for public assistance benefits, mental health services, health care, early childhood education, and housing. In addition, parenting classes and monthly support group meetings are provided for grandparents, along with transportation and child care (Kelley, Yorker, & Whitley, 1998). These multifaceted programs modeled new funding possibilities, creative resource development, and integrated service delivery. They also demonstrated both the need and potential for coordinated system response, thereby leading to the next generation of supportive interventions for grandparents raising grandchildren.

Second-Generation Programs: Systems and Policy Advocacy and Response

---

The first nationwide assessment of community-based programs to assist grandparent caregivers, supported by the Brookdale Foundation Group, identified a new kind of intervention being developed by the mid-1990s (Minkler & Roe, 1996). Inspired by the growing advocacy of coalitions, such as ROCKING, Inc., a Pennsylvania-based organization providing assistance to dozens of support groups around the country, and the Wisconsin-based National Coalition of Grandparents, local and regional groups began to call for system and policy changes necessary to better support grandparents raising grandchildren. The 1991 "Washington Summit" on Grandparent Caregiving was an historic first step, as 10 leaders of the emerging grandparent caregiver movement converged on the nation's capital to strategize together and lobby policy makers. The presence and priority of grandparent caregivers and their issues at the White House Conference on Aging just a few years later was testament to the increasing visibility and political organization of grandparent caregivers and their allies (Administration on Aging, 1995).

The growing scope of the Grandparent Caregiver Project in San Jose, California, provides a good example of second-generation thinking. In early 1992, the staff of Senior Services at Catholic Charities began to notice that children were increasingly present in the elder housing program, and Children's Services staff noted that more and more young children were being brought to day programs by older relatives. When the staff read a newspaper story about the challenges facing a local grandmother who had suddenly assumed responsibility for her grandchildren, they decided to explore the extent of grandparent caregiving in the area and the ability of county social services to respond.

The first activity was a countywide forum. Widely disseminated publicity and individual outreach brought together key representatives of health, education, social welfare, judicial, immigration, recreation, and aging policy and services, and grandparents. The next activities, running the continuum from support groups to policy advocacy, were planned as a result of that forum, with grandparent care givers in key leadership positions. Through a series of subsequent conferences, forums, working groups, and seminars, dialogue and cooperation began between service groups that usually work in isolation. Within just a few years, the family court system, social workers, the local Area on Aging, and the growing grandparent leadership had formed a partnership dedicated to integrated services in support of grandparent-headed families.

The biggest difference between the 1992 conference and the current activities, according to Marilou Christina of Catholic Charities, is the activism and leadership of the grandparents themselves. "When we held our first conference, the grandparents were timid rabbits, reluctant to confront the system, wanting to be heard, wanting to have hope. Now, they are confident in articulating their problems and posing system solutions" (Marilou Christina, Personal communication, April 1997). Among the systems solutions they have effected are a comprehensive resource center, greatly increased interagency collaboration, greater sensitivity to the caregiver issues within the child welfare and aging systems, and the creation of an advisory position for a grandparent caregiver within the family court district to advise the judge on caregiver custody issues.

Resource Centers

One of the most important supports for system and policy advocacy, as well as local program development, has become the resource center. Small resource centers, often just a phone and a filing cabinet in a grandparent's home, serve as clearinghouses for caregivers and professionals in need of assistance or referrals. Several professional or service organizations have developed print or on-line resource lists, such as the "Grandparenting File Contents" of the Generations United Library, Family Counseling Services' "Relatives Raising Children: Printed and Visual Resources", and the on-line directory developed by the national Network for Family Resiliency. The volume of resources, and the range of organizations developing resource dissemination methods, speaks both to the growing requests for assistance and the growing realization of the importance of support for grandparent-headed families from a wide range of organizations.

The New York City Resource Center, established in 1994 through the New York City Department for the Aging, is a leading example of a second-generation resource center. The Center's hotline is staffed by a resource specialist who helps with issues, such as emotional support for care givers; information and referrals regarding financial, legal, or health needs; respite services; and assistance navigating the social service systems. Other services offered by Resource Center staff include technical assistance to community-based organizations seeking to support grandparent-headed families, support group training, and parenting curricula. The Center is researching the effectiveness of having older volunteers and a social worker provide direct assistance to overburdened grandparent care givers. Volunteers, age 50 or older, are recruited from the neighborhoods in which grandparent-headed families live. The volunteers are trained and matched with individual families, providing emotional, informational, and reciprocal support in the local neighborhood as well as an active link to the larger network of supportive services.

The largest resource center to date is the Grandparent Information Center housed in the national headquarters of the 33 million member American Association of Retired Persons (AARP). Founded with a seed grant from the Brookdale Foundation in 1993, the center now operates on a large and stable budget with a varied program of caregiver and system supports (Aging Alert, 3/25/98). The Center receives 2,500 calls and letters annually from grandparents facing a range of social, legal, financial, medical, educational, and emotional challenges as primary caregivers. Individual communications allow Center staff to respond to individual family needs. Center staff maintain a computerized database of support groups and services and can make referrals in both English and Spanish. The center's newsletter, published three times per year, has a mailing list of over 13,000 relative caregivers and professionals. Recent articles have included

"Tips for Raising Your School-Aged Children", "The Impact of Violence on Children's Ability to Lear" , "Assistance to Grandparents Adopting Their Grandchildren", and " Subsidized Guardianship", the regular listing of conferences and publications, an annotated guide to grandparent caregiver web sites.

With its national reach, the Grandparent Information Center also serves as an important resource for data collection on the extent and experience of relative caregiving. The center conducts an annual survey of grandparent caregiver needs and concerns and has recently completed, as discussed earlier in this book, conducted focus groups with African-American and Hispanic grandparents. In accordance with AARP's broader mission, the center has also become an important center of information and organizing around key policy issues affecting grandparent care givers and their families. As a case in point, the center played a key role in gathering data, organizing public testimony, and educating the media about proposed and actual welfare policy changes and their implications for grandparent care givers and their families.

Seed Grants for Local and Statewide Programs

Another initiative reflecting the expanded approach of second-generation strategies is the Brookdale Foundation's Relatives as Second Parents (RAPP) Program. Since 1996, the Brookdale Foundation has been awarding seed grants to community and state agencies to promote the creation or expansion of services for parenting grandparents and other relatives. By 1998, the initiative had stimulated comprehensive programs in 48 local sites as well as 15 programs to help states transcend the boundaries of the traditional aging network and work collaboratively with other state agencies and local communities in support of relative caregivers.

The RAPP Program builds program planning and resource development capacity through both the state and local initiatives. Second-generation thinking is stimulated through the wording and requirements of the program's objectives for grantees. For example, the objectives of the local initiative are (a) to encourage cooperation and collaboration among various service systems; (b) to ensure the development, expansion, and future continuity of local services; and (c) to create replicable service models. Minigrants of $10,000 over a 2-year period, supported by extensive technical assistance, have been awarded in regional cohorts. The creativity and design of the local interventions reflect the differences and imaginative insights of the local grantees. In addition to hundreds of new support groups, the local programs have developed multisector coalitions; communitywide events; symposia; training programs; and, most important, institutionalized their programs within existing local agencies.

The even broader expectations of Brookdales's statewide initiative direct grantees: (a) to initiate five new relative support groups in different parts of the state under the sponsorship and support of local agencies that do not currently provide such services, (b) to develop a statewide network of local organizations that link current programs and interested agencies, provide guidance and information to local programs, and stimulate expanded services, and (c) to establish or expand an "intersystem task force" of state agencies related to the issues of relatives as surrogate parents (Brookdale, 1996). The funded states have addressed their mandate in different ways, such as statewide helplines; training for support group leaders; regional or state conferences; assembling "best practice" curricula and resource inventories; developing and distributing training materials; producing satellite teleconferences for professionals working with relative caregivers, and providing personal, ongoing technical assistance by state representatives to local programs.

Key to the initiative's success have been the foundation's commitment to the project; and the energy, vision, and hard work of the local and statewide participants. Also important has been Brookdale's innovative approach to ongoing, collaborative technical assistance. All RAPP grantees, current and emeritus, are invited to an annual RAPP Training Conference and supported by bimonthly conference calls and a quarterly newsletter. This kind of accessible technical assistance has helped build an increasingly independent network of second-generation service providers and service models, encouraged early problem solving, and enabled wide dissemination of lessons learned and successful strategies.

Policy Advocacy

One of the defining characteristics of second-generation programs is their extension to policy advocacy in support of grandparent caregivers and their families. Even relatively small, local programs may make this extension as staff and care givers take increasingly proactive stands on issues, such as equitable financial support, streamlined service systems, and community consideration of the special circumstances of grandparent-headed families. Larger programs have established coalitions with specific policy agendas and forums for policy development and advocacy. A case in point is Connecticut's coalition of grandparent support groups, children's advocacy and service organizations, and community-based HIV/AIDS service providers. The eclectic coalition was formed to work toward passage of a bill in the state legislature that would allow low-income care givers to receive a subsidy for the children in their care comparable with the one provided to foster parents. In California, the Bay Area Policy Roundtable on Grandparent Care givers similarly brings together legal experts, policy makers, and service providers to identify problems in legal and social services and to develop strategies for expanding resources and services statewide.

Another example of a program with the dual vision of local service and broader policy advocacy is the Grandparent Caregiver Advocacy Project, based in Oakland, California. The project grew from the work of the nationally recognized Services for Prisoners With Children as staff noted the particular burden on families in which an incarcerated mother's children were living with their grandparents. Local activities seek to preserve families by creating a comprehensive legal, social, and health service delivery model while promoting institutional change to support grandparent and relative care givers and the children in their homes. To that end, the Grandparent Caregiver Advocacy Project brings together agencies offering policy advocacy (Legal Services for Prisoners With Children), legal services (Legal Assistance for Seniors), case management services (Nurses in Action), and a grandparent support network (Grandparents as Second Parents). Families benefit from coordinated services and a single point of access. Providers benefit from regular dialogue and problem solving with colleagues from the other disciplines.

The project, however, reaches beyond local service delivery. The Kinship Advocacy Project, an activity of one of the collaborating agencies, works through the legal system for relatives struggling to hold families together. In addition to organizing workshops, adult education courses, and conferences regularly, the project publishes, disseminates, and regularly updates a manual for relative caregivers and their advocates. The manual, published jointly with the Grandparent Caregiver Law Center at the Brookdale Center on Aging at Hunter College in New York City, details grandparent rights, public benefits, court procedures, and statewide resources.

The first relative caregiver manuals were specific to the benefits and laws of New York and California. However, the enormous demand for information regarding other state policies led the Project staff to develop a guide that could be used by organizations in each state to develop state-specific manuals. The guide now provides templates for each state to use in researching and explaining its particular laws and bureaucracy related to the myriad issues confronting grandparents raising grandchildren. Each chapter provides a starting point of key questions, model answers, and relevant citations that will help others customize the guide for their own jurisdictions. Recently, the Grandparent Caregiver Project put the Resource Manual online, adding a regularly updated supplement indicating changes in the law, conversations with national leaders in the grandparent caregiver movement, first-person accounts of raising grandchildren, and links to related websites.

Future Directions

Although support groups remain the heart of most community-based programs, several promising new directions are emerging as care givers, their allies, and advocates build on what they have learned. Increasingly sophisticated media advocacy by care givers and their allies promises greater public awareness of the ways in which America's families are changing. New communications technologies create new possibilities for dialogue, education, and organizing. Although some groups are going high-tech, others are going back to basics, reconceptualizing the problem and supporting grandparent-headed families by relying on age-old community-building strategies to support and nourish healthy communities.

Media Advocacy

Caregivers and their allies have learned to work with the media to reach out to isolated care givers, disseminate resources, raise awareness, and show the strength of community collaboration and support. Several communities have developed programs to be aired on local cable TV channels, showing Grandparents Day Celebrations or support group meetings. Other communities are looking with interest at the series of short vignettes produced by the North Carolina's Charlotte-Mechlenberg Senior Center. The pieces, specifically developed for local television, demonstrate the widespread nature of grandparent caregiving and how it affects people in a variety of circumstances.

Future initiatives will focus on increasingly strategic media advocacy designed to frame stories and educate the public on the need for more supportive service and policy responses. Community-based advocates have learned that many of the substantive systems-level changes needed to support grandparent-headed families better will need broad-based support.

Relationships with local news reporters are enabling caregivers and their allies to have increasing input into the focus, structure, and timing of coverage of grandparent caregiver issues.

Another promising direction is the development of at least 10 professional videos on the subject of grandparents raising grandchildren. Early training videos, such as *Divided Loyalties* (Ortiz/Simon Productions) helped spread awareness of the issues facing grandparents and grandchildren as families reconfigure without the middle generation. Other productions, such as *A Gift for My Children* (Family Center of New York City), which addresses custody planning when a parent is dying of AIDS, serve to raise awareness among the many professionals who interact, often unknowingly, with grandparents raising grandchildren. A public television program, "Raising Grandkids: A Love Story," by award-winning documentary producer Lori Maas Vidlak and developed in partnership with the Nebraska ETV Network, premiered at the 1998 Great Plains Film Festival and was then broadcast on stations throughout the country on Grandparents Day. The quality of this program and the acclaim it has received provide a unique springboard for community organizing and outreach.

New Technologies

New communications technologies offer previously unimagined possibilities for intergenerational activities, service networking, information exchange, and program technology transfer. For example, The Parent Place of Springfield, Illinois, has developed an intergenerational computer lab for grandparents and the children in their care. Although the lab is designed for fun and co-learning, computer literacy tutors and Internet access also enhance the advocacy skills of care givers and their children (RAPP Bulletin, winter 1997). On the Internet, the number of caregiver web sites expands regularly, with links to other sites with information regarding health care, parenting, education, legal and financial support, and policy advocacy. Several sites offer details of model programs, curricula for educational seminars, evaluation materials, and funding leads.

Another promising technology is video conferencing, which allows care givers, service providers, researchers, advocates, and policy makers to communicate via satellite links in their local areas. This is particularly welcomed as most programs operate on small budgets, without travel funds for staff, grandparents, or volunteers. Conferences or formal presentations may be broadcast via simultaneous video conferencing, with opportunities for viewers to interact with other conferees through phone, Fax, or e-mail. Prerecorded conferences or forums can also be disseminated later, shown in individual locations or broadcast simultaneously at several sites through satellite links, creating an ever-growing network of interested and influential colleagues, allies, and advocates.

Healthy Families in Healthy Communities

One of the most promising future directions for programs in support of grandparents and their families, and an indication of the growing maturity of the grandparent caregiver movement, is the move toward framing the central issues as those of a healthy community rather than merely the problems of individual families. This new direction is illustrated by Boston's newly opened Grandfamilies House, a "supporting community" of grandparents raising their grandchildren mentioned earlier in the chapter by Silverstein and Vehvilainen.

The project, codeveloped through a joint partnership of Boston Aging Concerns–Young and Old United and the Women's Institute for Housing and Economic Development is the first housing in the nation specifically designed to meet the physical and social needs of grandfamilies. Boston Aging Concerns had worked since the early 1970s on housing crises of the elderly. However, in the early 1990s, like social service providers around the country, Housing Resource Services staff began to notice that an increasing number of elderly clients, presumed to be living alone, were, in fact, caring for young children full time (Nathan Green, personal communication, September 1998). The presence of young children in housing designated for elderly residents raised legal, health, and safety concerns. Indeed, many client families had been evicted when grandchildren were discovered and finding housing that was affordable, suitable for both seniors and children, safe, and accessible was nearly impossible.

The formal project began with a study of 50 grandparent-headed families, formation of an action-oriented advisory committee with grandparent representation, and an information-sharing conference. Housing emerged as the grandparents' top concern. But Boston Housing Concerns took a holistic approach, in which merely building housing was not enough. Their explicit goal was to build healthy communities of what they called "grandfamilies" including grandparents, children, and those supporting them. They began by building housing, designed for and by grandparent care givers and the children in their care.

The partnership bought an abandoned nursing home in Dorcester and quickly focused on the community and neighborhood organizing for support of the concept and the necessary rezoning. The building was completely renovated, adding a third story and basement and creating brand new units of two- to four-bedroom family apartments. The complex can accommodate 26 families and up to 60 children of all ages, plus the on-site resident services coordinator and 24-hour staff manager. The complex has a large child care area opening onto a playground that can be observed by grandparents from the bay windows of their apartments. Other evidence of the insight of grandparents in the building's design include child-safe electrical outlets, elevators with grab bars, and wide grandparent-friendly doors perfect for strollers and wheelchairs. Both structure and process support the creation and extension of a caring and supportive community, assisted by service providers but led by grandparents, the natural family leaders.

The Boston YWCA provides a continuum of intergenerational services right where the families live. Through its "Generations Learning Together" program, preschool and after-school programs focus on enhancing the math, science, and literacy skills of the residents. The program supports grandparents and children to support each other as both care givers and active learners. State-of-the-art computer workstations were donated by a major corporation. Homework assistance is provided and grandparents serve as teachers' aides. Teens have opportunities for involvement in the YWCA's Youth Voice Collaborative media programs. On-site programs for grandparents themselves include fitness classes, educational workshops, individual advice and counseling, support groups, and linkage with other services as requested by residents, such as child welfare and health screenings. A van is available for shopping, medical appointments, and family field trips. Coordination with other groups, such as the nearby Boys and Girls Club, helps reconnect grandparent care givers and their families with the broader community. GrandFamilies House redefines the common goal from meeting needs to building strengths and linking assets toward a healthy community for all.

Lessons Learned

Almost a decade after the first support groups in grandparents' homes, community-based interventions supporting-headed families are growing in vision, complexity, and outreach. Hard work and visionary leadership have resulted in a patchwork of programs sharing common commitments but reflecting local diversity and imagination. Stitched together for this analysis, their collective patterns offer an invaluable glimpse into what works and what is essential in efforts to support grandparent care givers and their families. Twelve such lessons are offered subsequently.

1. *The most effective programs involve grandparent caregivers in every aspect of program development.* Grandparents raising grandchildren are among the best experts. They have lived the many routes to their shared point, they know the most urgent needs and the most privately held fears, and they best understand the nested challenges of parenting again and under these circumstances. Their involvement in understanding local caregiving and shaping community response can be invaluable.

   There are many ways to involve grandparents in program design, implementation, and evaluation. Currently, grandparents serve on advisory committees, help with gathering information on the extent of grandparent caregiving in their neighborhoods or social networks, help plan and coordinate special events, form and sometimes lead support groups, write newsletter columns, conduct outreach, staff warmlines, and help evaluate programs. With support from professionals who know the relevant bureaucracies and service systems, and resources to make the work empowering rather than an additional burden, grandparents' unique insight into what will work and what is most important can be a key factor in wise use of limited resources and the development of relevant and effective programs.

2. *Outreach efforts must cast a wide and reinforcing net.* The deeper social forces contributing to the current phenomenon of grandparent caregiving (particularly substance abuse, HIV/AIDS, violence, and inadequate mental health services) continue unabated, leading increasing numbers of grandparents to face the personal crisis of assuming primary responsibility for grandchildren. Continuous waves of new caregivers require basic information and outreach, no matter how long or well established the community-based program. It also appears that most grandparents experience a sometimes prolonged period of crisis management and subsequent isolation as the assumption of caregiving unfolds (Roe & Minkler, 1996). Program staff report that they often reach out to the same people many times, with a range of possible activities, before caregivers realize that the offerings relate to them and are able to respond.

   Wisdom from the field also reinforces the need to cast a wide net in outreach activities. Staff report that it is not at all unusual for surveys or flyers to be disseminated to thousands of people, with a net return of just 40 to 50 respondents. Yet providers insist that the effort is essential, as the information gleaned from those 40 families may provide insight and leads crucial to an effective program and be uniquely tailored to local needs (Sybil Lampart-Dyke, personal communication, September 1998). Others stress that within those 40 homes may be caregivers reached for the very first time and often with the most desperate needs. Broad community visibility also provides an indirect link to isolated families. Indeed, despite successful outreach and a full array of ongoing activities, many local programs report that their first contact with new grandparents is often the result of a friend or family member passing on a human interest article from the newspaper or a pamphlet from an information table at a community event. Outreach thus needs to be broad, inclusive, and ongoing.

3. *Although the sophistication of programs, advocacy, and research is growing, the concerns of parenting grandparents remain basic.* Nearly a decade of supportive interventions has resulted in a national network of researchers, policy advocates, decision makers, and program staff knowledgeable and experienced in the complex phenomenon of grandparent caregiving. The professional learning curve has been steep, challenging, and rewarding, as evidenced by the growing literature, resources, program innovation and visibility. Yet the basic dynamics of family crisis or tragedy, the assumption of caring, and the life changes they entail remain poignantly the same. Although policy and provider coalitions grow in vision and ambition, staff uncover new programming possibilities, and scholars develop new research questions, the priority concerns of most grandparent care givers remain child care and respite, financial assistance, legal issues, health care, and support. Program elements need to incorporate new elements while remaining basic and responsive to what grandparents feel they need. The wisdom from the programs cautions us to notice and carefully balance the sometimes different pressures of advancing a field and meeting basic needs.

4. *Small outside seed grants can help local groups leverage greater support.* One of the most remarkable aspects of the community response to grandparents raising grandchildren is just how much has been accomplished with such modest funding. Seed grants have been crucial in this regard. Foundation seed grants to states and community-based agencies, such as the Brookdale RAPP (Relatives as Parents) Program, have spawned hundreds of mini-grants to neigh-

borhood organizations, support groups, and programs with original and innovative ideas for meeting the needs of grandparent-headed households. Projects, such as Parents Again in Rockford, Illinois, and the GrandCare Program in Charlotte, North Carolina, have leveraged modest funds to attract corporate, foundation, and government support for priority and integrated services, such as additional support groups, respite, and mediation. Isolated and chronically underserved communities, such as Bay Point in Northern California, have been able to draw attention to their needs by the presence of a foundation grant as small as $3,000, resulting from the legitimacy and recognition outside funding brought to previously discounted local concerns (Richard Clark, personal communication, January 1996). Key to the success of seed grant investments are carefully worded expectations for furture growth and maximum flexibility in local implementation.

5. *Local assets can stretch limited funds.* Another lesson demonstrated from the field is the rich network of in-kind resources available in many communities. Many local foundations have been responsive to requests for support of grandparents raising grandchildren, particularly Community Foundations and the United Way. Foundation resources have been used to expand or formalize pilot programs, secure staff for support groups or concurrent child care programs, explore respite options, and fund community forums.

Special events are an excellent way to raise awareness and mobilize community assets in support of grandparent care givers and their families. Local merchants have helped with fund raisers, publicizing events in their windows, selling tickets on site, donating prizes or favors, or providing refreshments. Local resources also support ongoing programs. For example, service organizations, such as the Knights of Columbus, Kiwanis, and Rotary have organized tutoring programs, sponsored educational seminars, and organized clothing or baby furniture banks. High school students and youth groups have provided homework assistance, painted wall murals, and helped with summer outings. Faith communities across the country have donated weekday space for respite, dedicated service programs to caregiver support, and facilitated widespread outreach through notices in church bulletins, newsletters, and mailings. Local chapters of the Bar Association provide invaluable pro bono legal assistance through legal clinics, support group presentations, and assessment and referral appointments. Local corporations have donated computer labs, office furniture, food, and financial planning services to caregiver families and new programs.

University students are a source of unique enthusiasm and expertise. Partnerships between local programs and a university department or training program offer a reciprocal relationship for everyone involved. For example, graduate social welfare students from Bradley University have partnered with the Central Illinois Agency on Aging in Peoria to do telephone outreach to grandparent care givers, basic counseling, and referral. Undergraduate Health Science students at San Jose State University in Northern California organized a gift drive that enabled more than 200 children to receive age-specific books and toys at a Christmas party for grandparent-headed families. Local assets, both people and material, can enliven a stretched budget and visibly show grandparents the appreciation and goodwill of their own communities.

6. *Programs must be supported by intersectoral, systems-level dialogue and coordination.* Grandparents raising grandchildren must often navigate distinctly different and sometimes contradictory social service systems. Working collaborations of aging and child welfare systems, schools and health care, legal and financial services can significantly streamline the process for grandparents, thereby easing one of the burdens of raising children in crisis. Support for grandparent-headed families necessarily crosses preexisting lines of bureaucracy, funding streams, community alliances, and trust. To be most effective, local programs must be surrounded by a supportive network of allies and proactive advocates with influence in the broader social systems in which they are embedded.

Special community events or initiatives often provide the vehicle for bringing systems together the first time. For example, the annual Massachusetts multiagency collaboration on Wellness Days for Grandparents led to much deeper dialogue about the inequities between types of caregiving support and strategies for change.

Intersectoral working groups can also stimulate the necessary dialogue between system players that may lead to the kind of reimagination necessary to better support families of all configurations. Standard representation in grandparent caregiver coalitions comes from representatives of the aging network, family and social services, education, and the criminal justice system. Additional representatives have come from community recreation, local philanthropy, housing, community policing, immigrant services, and local media. Field experience shows that effective coalitions can be formed relatively easily around initial data collection into the extent of grandparent caregiving in a given community, special event planning, or beginning service delivery. The key, however, is to nurture the group beyond the fun of preliminary activities to the more complex challenges of systems analysis and change. This developmental step is crucial, as intersectoral coalitions are uniquely able to reach through multiple levels of the social system and stimulate policy and service coordination for longer term support of grandparents raising grandchildren.

7. *Programs benefit from continued technical assistance.* Developing effective supportive interventions for grandparent caregivers is as new as the contemporary phenomenon itself. The complexity of the issues, the still modest resources, and the formative state of the art lead to a pressing need for information exchange, peer support, and expert technical advising. Professional conferences and symposia, such as Generations United's 1998 conference on "Grandparents and Other Relatives Raising Children", provide unique opportunities for information exchange and peer support.

The largest regular gathering of people involved in community interventions in support of grandparent care givers is the RAPP (Relatives as Parents Program) Training Conference sponsored by the Brookdale Foundation. The three-day annual conference, attended by 200 to 300 RAPP participants, brings together representatives from funded and emeritus programs throughout the country to discuss common concerns, creative solutions, and strategies for strengthening community-based supportive interventions for grandparent-headed families. The conference offers research and policy updates, evaluation training, and repeating concurrent sessions on issues ranging from creative outreach, sustaining support group membership, expanding a statewide coalition, and institutionalizing your program.

8. *Sustained funding is crucial to local program success.* The current group of programs nationwide represent a cohort ready for institutionalization. Developed with seed money, volunteer commitment, and limited budgets, provider burnout and the predictable maturation of original families and volunteers leave many programs at a crossroads. Programs that have not developed long-term support risk dissolution if key volunteers or a single coordinating staff person leave. Granting programs would do well to provide resources not only for program development but also for project maintenance and permanency planning.

9. *It is time for collaborative program evaluation.* Small programs, clearly the norm for caregiver interventions, have been understandably reluctant to dedicate limited resources to evaluation or research. Staff, funders, and grandparents themselves have also been sensitive to the fine line between discovering, understanding, and reporting on the nature of contemporary caregiving and invading the privacy of families in pain. However, many programs and funders now acknowledge that programs would benefit from information on the processes of successful programs, and the relationship between program activities and family outcomes. It is also becoming clear that the lack of evaluation data may hinder long-term funding opportunities and investment. Other fields have explored the possibilities of proactive, collaborative evaluation dedicated to program improvement and success (Coombe in Minkler). These innovations offer promising strategies for gathering the data and telling the stories of effective, and not so effective, community programs and learning from them all.

10. *Intergenerational programs mobilize the assets, strengths, and insights of care givers and the community.* The necessary marriage of the aging and children's support networks quickly brought intergenerational thinking to the forefront in community-based programs supporting grandparent-headed families. In some communities, special events and outings are designed specifically to bring young and old together. Other programs are based on communitywide intergenerational support. For example, in the Upper Cumberland area of Tennessee, Americorps volunteers play with children during grandparent support group meetings. In Rochester, New York, young men from a local church serve as mentors to adolescent boys being raised by their grandmothers. Even policy collaborations can be intergenerational, as exemplified by the Gray Panthers' early embrace of children's issues within grandparent-headed families as part of their own advocacy agenda.

11. *Grandparent caregivers make powerful advocates.* The early support groups necessarily focused on meeting grandparents' basic needs for legal and financial assistance, child care support, and the day-to-day crises of raising grandchildren. However, as groups and their supporting programs have matured, support groups have also become a point of empowerment for grandparents in other aspects of their community. The types of efforts that can encourage and sustain such empowerment has been examined in a preceding chapter. As described, grandarents have the ability to be strong advocates for their

own needs. Grandparent caregivers advise family court judges, local representatives, and state governors. Caregivers testify at public hearings, provide comment to Congress and state legislatures, speak at conferences and national professional meetings, and appear on local and national television. Indeed, the eloquent presence of grandparent care givers at the 1995 White House Conference on Aging was credited as one of the reasons that their core issues were treated with such priority.

12. *The importance of framing the story.* Grandparents are often the pillars of their families and communities. As they provide stability to their grandchildren, they represent strong role models to younger families and contribute to the health of the larger community (Boston Mini-Village reference). Media accounts and social service reports often tell the stories of grandparent-headed families as examples of dysfunction, chaos, and failure. Yet the same stories can be framed as witness to moral integrity, family ties, love, and belief in the future. A decade of community experience now indicates that, after a while, some grandparents may no longer relate to the crisis-oriented concerns of many programs. Indeed, "Coffee and Conversation" is the name of the support group at the Age Center of Worcester, Massachusetts, where the care givers appreciate that the name does not imply that they need help or support. The real story of grandparent caregiving, and the communities that support them, is one of transcendence and empowerment. In the words of a member of the Central Illinois RAPP Program, "we have learned the power of caring, the power that voices united creates, and that we can help make a difference!" (RAPP Program Descriptions, 1997).

The tenacious creativity of the thousands of grandparent caregivers, their allies, and advocates who have developed community-based interventions demonstrates the power of local investment, institutional response, and supportive public policies. Evidence of intersectoral collaboration, volunteer commitment, lay and professional expertise, and caregiver commitment abounds in the programs across the country and the plans being laid for the future. As we close the first decade of supportive interventions for grandparents and their families, we do well to listen and learn from the field.

References

AARP (1997, summer). Parenting grandchildren, Grandparent Information Center Newsletter. Washington: AARP.

Administration on Aging. (1995, February 15). *Report on the White House Conference on Aging.* Washington, DC: Administration on Aging.

Aging Alert News. (1998, March 25). Seniors raising children get help from AARP, community organizations. *Aging Alert News.*

Boston Aging Concerns: Young and Old United, Inc. (1997, June 17). The GrandFamilies Program. Boston: Author.

Brookdale Foundation. (1996, April). *RAPP program description.* New York: Brookdale Foundation.

Brookdale Foundation. (1998, summer). *RAPP bulletin.* New York: Brookdale Foundation.

Burnette, D. (1997, September/October). Grandparents raising grandchildren in the inner city. *The Journal of Contemporary Human Services, 78,* 489–99.

Burton, L. (1992). Black grandmothers rearing children of drug-addicted parents: Stressors, outcomes and social service needs. *Research on Social Work Practice, 8,* 1–27.

Fuller-Thomson, E., Minkler, M., & Driver, D. (1997). A profile of grandparents raising grandchildren in the United States. *The Gerontologist, 37,* 406–411.

Kelley S. J., Yorker, B. C., & Whitley, D. (1998). To grandmother's house we go . . . and stay: Children raised in intergenerational families. *Journal of Geronotological Nursing, 23,* 12–20.

Minkler, M., Driver, D, & Roe, K.M. (1993). Assessing the state of the art of grandparent caregiver interventions: First year results of the Brookdale Grandparent Caregiver Information Project. *The Gerontologist, 42,* 580–585.

Minkler, M., & Roe, K. (1993). *Grandmothers as care givers: Raising children of the crack cocaine epidemic.* Newbury Park, CA: Sage.

Minkler M., & Roe, K. (1996, spring). Grandparents as surrogate parents. *Generations, 20,* 34–38.

Roe, K. M., & Minkler, M. (1998–99, winter). Grandparents raising grandchildren: Challenges and responses. *Generations, 22,* 25–32.

SECTION VI

Conclusions

Chapter 18

Conclusions

Carole B. Cox

The chapters in this book have offered a multidisciplinary perspective of the situations and issues confronting grandparents raising grandchildren. Many factors contribute to and influence their new roles as well as the ways in which these roles are enacted. Moreover, as indicated throughout the book, grandparents' abilities to fulfill the many demands associated with raising grandchildren, to a large extent, depend on policies and the availability of programs, which can further support them.

Policies provide the framework under which the grandparent-grandchild relationship is lived. Consequently, such policies as related to health care, welfare, and other benefits must be cognizant of and recognize the special situations of this group of caregivers. Such policies, as they affect the interactions of the grandparent with their adult children, their grandchildren, and social systems must contribute to the stability and security of custodial grandparents rather than undermine it. Facilitating the ability of grandparents to assume guardianship, make medical decisions, and enroll children in schools are among the areas where changes are warranted.

At the same time, grandparents must be made aware of the options available to them and what they entail. Being educated regarding the types of custodial arrangements including guardianship and foster care is critical if they are to make sound decisions regarding the care of their grandchildren. Both the legal system and child welfare agencies must assume active roles in assuring that the rights of grandparents and those in their care are recognized. Given the increasing number of grandparent caregivers, child welfare systems must begin to address their requirements for permanency planning, making them more responsive to this population's unique situations and relationships.

On a broader scale, as many custodial grandparents live on reduced incomes, assuring that they have access to public benefits including welfare, food stamps, and Medicaid is essential. Such policies must support rather than hinder the ability of grandparents to care for their grandchildren. The burdens experienced by many custodial grandparents are intensified by their worries over whether they have sufficient income with which to raise their grandchildren. Medical insurance for the grandchildren is a primary need and should be readily available to assure that their health needs, both physical and mental, are met.

Medical care is an area of particular concern as this group of grandparents is at risk of both the chronic illnesses associated with aging as well as problems precipitated by the stress of their situations. Without access to proper health care, the ability of many to raise their grandchildren may be severely compromised. Similar to their grandchildren, they require access to health insurance that can assist them in meeting their own health care needs.

Grandparents must also have suitable housing in which to raise grandchildren. In this regard, the special housing developed in Massachusetts for grandparents and grandchildren offers a compelling example of housing designed to meet the needs of these reconstituted families. Close attention should be given to this model for possible replication in other communities as it offers the promise of a stable and supportive environment which is often lacking in the community.

As policies are developed, efforts must ensure that specific groups are not being ignored. Latino and other immigrant grandparents are particularly vulnerable to being denied access to benefit programs, as they do not meet stringent eligibility criteria. These denials penalize them for accepting responsibility for caregiving and, concomitantly, increase the stress incumbent in their roles. Benefit programs should be flexible to ensure the inclusion rather than exclusion of groups of grandparents so that needs for income, food, and medical care are not ignored.

However, the effect of any policy remains limited if those it seeks to assist are not informed. Grandparents must have access to current information about policies, programs, and services pertinent to their situations. Such information must be readily available in the community and easily understood by diverse groups. Grandparents are eager for information that can assist and strengthen them, and efforts must be made to facilitate their receiving it. Such avenues stretch from resource centers to local health fairs and forums to computers and the Internet. The expansion and diversity of this population of grandparents requires that new conduits for such information be continually developed.

Creative modes of outreach to grandparents are fundamental to providing this information. Enlisting the media through public service announcements and programs as well as institutions, such as, churches and schools, can be important means for reaching large groups of grandparents. As an example, a local television broadcast in one major city about grandparents' support group resulted in myriad calls for further information by other grandparents. The national report on public radio regarding the grandparent empowerment training program resulted in calls from agencies across the country for more information on the project and ways to implement it.

The chapters throughout this book have underscored the need for services which can enhance and further enable grandparent caregivers. Support groups continue to play major roles as they address both emotional and informational needs. Various models for these groups exist and thus can be developed in congruency with the specific needs and characteristics of the grandparents. Because of the important role that these groups can have in the lives of grandparents, efforts should be made to foster their development by many sectors of the community. Libraries, schools, and health clinics are among the sites that should be encouraged to become involved in programs for custodial grandparents. Each in itself provides an important mechanism for linking them with further resources.

To help grandparents in dealing with many of the stresses they encounter, counseling programs for both themselves and their grandchildren are desperately needed. The problems involved in the new relationship, the grief and loss experienced by each generation, and the conflicts that may ensue frequently necessitate a need for professional counseling and intervention. In many families, the grandchildren come to the grandparents as a result of neglect and abuse by their own parents. Consequently, deep-rooted psychological and emotional problems further affect their ability to adapt to the new household. Access to counseling services, which can help them to deal with these issues, is fundamental for their adjustment.

In addition, grandparents often require counseling that can assist them to cope with their own emotions and grief. Feelings of loss or disappointment in their own children, worries over their ability to parent, and even resentment over their new responsibilities must be dealt with if they are to adequately cope with their new roles. Ignoring or denying these emotions can lead to further stress and barriers in the new relationships.

However, to be fully used, counseling services should not be associated with any stigma that may compromise their acceptability. Custodial grandparents, either due to cultural beliefs or a lack of familiarity with professional psychological help, may be susceptible to negatively perceiving it and thus reluctant to use services. Consequently, including these services under the rubric of other programs, such as health centers or family programs, may be necessary to encourage their use. In the same way, assuring that the titles of the services emphasize "wellness" or "well-being" rather than problems and psychological needs may also make them more acceptable to diverse groups of grandparents.

Respite programs that offer grandparents a break from caregiving can further strengthen both their physical and emotional health. Even limited hours of respite can offer grandparents an opportunity to shop or socialize and relieve the burden of constant caregiving. Organizing such programs with the assistance of other programs, such as schools or churches, is also a means of strengthening the community ties of parenting grandparents.

Professionals and service providers working with custodial grandparents must themselves be knowledgeable about the many factors that influence and affect the experiences of these grandparents. Understanding the conditions under which they assumed their grandchildren, the cultural values and norms that influence and affect their relationships, their supports, and the unique stresses they endure are critical for developing appropriate programs and interventions. Educating these professionals through in-service training, workshops, and conferences that focus on grandparents and their circumstances can help to foster their competence.

As indicated in this book, grandparents have unique strengths and abilities that must not be ignored. They can play major roles as community advocates for themselves and others. Reaching out to other grandparents in the community, taking active roles in local government, and forming coalitions with other groups are examples of the types of activities undertaken. Programs that enhance and develop innate skills and thus they empower these grandparents enable them to become important resources and educators for others. Building on the competencies of this population, rather than focusing on their limitations and problems, is empowering to the grandparents as well as to the community in which they live.

Although extensive research on custodial grandparents has occurred in the last few years, this has been largely survey based or descriptive of the circumstances of select samples of grandparents. Longitudinal studies that follow grandparent-headed families over several years are now needed to further understand the transition and the factors associated with grandparents' and grandchildrens' abilities to cope and adjust.

Research, which builds on these studies by examining the factors, that both contribute to and impede their roles, is important for the further development of interventions. Research on other populations of caregivers has documented the vital and differing roles played by informal supports as both buffers against stress and sources of assistance. Further study of the instrumental and qualitative natures of social supports, in particular the roles of friends and relatives, with diverse groups of grandparents is needed to further understand the parts they may play in the grandparent-grandchild relationship.

As noted throughout the book, many complex factors affect grandparent relationships and their ability to parent. Among these factors, income, age, marital status, health, and ethnicity appear to be particularly salient. In addition, characteristics of the grandchild, such as age, gender, previous relationship to grandparent, and circumstances leading to their placement, are also influential in the relationship. Studies, which begin to examine the interactions of these factors and their affects, can further highlight the ways in which they are associated with well-being or stress.

With the bulk of attention given to transitions into the parenting role, little, if any, attention has focused on what happens to grandparents if they are forced to relinquish their grandchildren. This transition is likely to be devastating to those who have committed themselves to the role and its success. For these grandparents, the loss of the grandchildren may be extremely stressful. Studies are needed that examine the ways that grandparents respond to these transitions and the factors that ease or hinder them.

As programs continue to expand and develop, outcome research on their effectiveness is also required. Understanding which aspects of services strengthen and enable grandparents and those that are not helpful or are perceived negatively is fundamental to service effectiveness. Studies that examine and compare interventions are necessary to assure that services are relevant to the needs of specific groups.

Qualitative research that examines the perspectives of the grandparents themselves as well as their grandchildren can further assist in developing effective services. This type of research is critical for obtaining data, which is generally not available through other large scale research designs. It is particularly important for eliciting in-depth information and insight on the types of dilemmas and problems experienced by groups of grandparents.

Focus groups may be particularly instrumental in understanding the situations of grandparents and their grandchildren. Groups of diverse populations of grandparents can highlight their specific needs and concerns. Such groups can be helpful in both the development of appropriate programs and in indicating areas for policy change.

Finally, if research on custodial grandparents is to be most helpful in both explaining and predicting responses and behaviors, it must be theory based. The new paradigm of grandparent roles and relationships provides a rich basis for both applying and testing many theories of aging. As discussed in the opening chapter, theories, such as role and developmental, may be applicable to understanding the ways in which grandparents adapt and adjust. Using these theories and others, such as social exchange, feminist, and age stratification, could contribute to both the intellectual development of social gerontology as well as provide a basis for sound policies and interventions.

Grandparents raising grandchildren are assuming major responsibilities at periods in their life when they believed that their child rearing had finished. In their efforts to fulfill their roles, to competently raise their grandchildren, and to ensure their own well-being, supportive policies and services are essential. As the population of these grandparents continues to expand, there remains a pressing urgency to ensure that supports for them and their grandchildren are in place.

Finally, policies and the services that implement them must strengthen rather than undermine custodial grandparents. Grandparents lay the foundation for future generations as well as providing links to the past. Society and its institutions must assure that these grandparents, who have accepted new roles and challenges, are given the supports they need to meet the often overwhelming demands they are their grandchildren face.

Index

Note: Italicized letters *f* and *t* following page numbers indicate figures and tables, respectively.

Kinship Advocacy Project, 291
Kinship Family Resource Center, 279
Kinship foster care, 14, 143–144
  child welfare system use of, 104
  financial need for, 31
  impact on individuals involved in,
    159–162
  as permanency option, 159
  rise in, 103
  services and interventions for abuse
    in, 98–101
Kinship Parenting Education and
  Support Program, 223–225
Kirkland, Barbara, 237
Kiwanis, tutoring programs of, 298
Knights of Columbus, tutoring
  programs of, 298

L
Language barriers, and Latino custodial
  grandparents, 225
Latinos
  children living with grandparents and
    relatives, 218–219
  custodial grandparents among, 4,
    12–14, 222–223, 308
  case vignettes of, 225–229
  and Children's Aid Society
    Community Schools, 223–229
  demographic profile of, 219–221
  social problems contributing to,
    218–219
  study of, 218–231
  elderly population among
  health of, 220
  incomes of, 219
  psychological well-being of, 220
  and familism, 13, 221–222, 227–230
  and family secrets, 227
  health status of, 39
  immigration status of, and welfare
    reform, 220
  leading cause of death among, 174
  and personalism, 227
Law enforcement, elder abuse services

in, 99
Leadership, of support groups, 239–242
Learning disability, and children under
  custodial grandparent care, 277
Legal aliens
  and Food Stamp program, 126–127
  and public benefits, 127
  and Temporary Assistance to Needy
    Families, 15, 127
Legal Assistance for Seniors program,
  291
Legal guardianship, 133, 158
Legal Services for Prisoners with
  Children program, 291
Legal status issues
  of custodial grandparents, 132–141
  among African-Americans,
    211–212
  arrangements types for, 14
  with parental planning, 133–141
  support groups based on, 243
  without parental planning, 141–146
  Grandparent Caregiver Law Center
    and, 291–292
  and pro bono legal assistance, 298
Legislation
  addressing child welfare concerns,
    152–158
  Adoption and Safe Families Act
    (1997), 156–158
  Adoption Assistance and Child
    Welfare Act (1990), 149,
    152–156
  Child Abuse Prevention and
    Treatment Act, 152–153
  consent, 137–139
  General Obligation law, 237
  Indian Child Welfare Act (1978), 153
  Older Americans Act, 98–99, 178, 180
  Personal Responsibility and Work
    Opportunities Act (1996), 15
  Ryan Whyte Comprehensive
    Resources Emergency Care Act
    (1990), 178–180
  Standby Guardianship law, 133–134

⑤ *Springer Publishing Company*

Ageism, 2nd Edition
Negative and Positive
Erdman B. Palmore, PhD

"Erdman Palmore has provided a portrait of older people in America that is both scientifically impeccable and extremely readable . . . Palmore's approach is forthright in calling attention to ways in which individual's, social groups, and social institutions undervalue older people."

—**M. Powell Lawton**, PhD, Philadelphia Geriatric Center

In this updated edition, Palmore provides a comprehensive review of many different forms of ageism-including the interesting notion of positive ageism, which projects onto the elderly a group of traditional virtues like wisdom and thrift. He discusses both the individual and social influences on attitudes towards the aged; analyzes institutional patterns of ageism; and explores ways to reduce the impact of ageism on the elderly. This book is a valuable resource for students and professionals interested in the sociology of aging in our society.

Contents: Foreword by George Maddox • Preface

- **Part I: Concepts** • Introduction and Basic Definitions • Types of Ageism • The Meaning of Age
- **Part II: Causes and Consequences** • Individual Sources • Social Influences • Cultural Sources • Consequences
- **Part III: Institutional Patterns** • The Economy • The Government • The Family • Housing and Health Care
- **Part IV:** Reducing Ageism • Changing the Person • Changing the Structure • Strategies for Change • The Future
- **Appendix :** The Facts on Aging Quizzes • Ageist Humor • Annotated Bibliography • References • Index

1999 280pp. 0-8261-7001-3 hardback 0-8261-7002-1 softback
www.springerpub.com

536 Broadway, New York, NY 10012-3955 • (212) 431-4370 • Fax (212) 941-7842

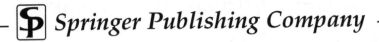 **Springer Publishing Company**

Gerontological Social Work
Theory Into Practice
Ilene L. Nathanson, DSW, BCD, Terry T. Tirrito, DSW

In this book, the authors develop a conceptual framework for task-centered social work practice with older adults. Their integrative model clearly illustrates how practitioners and students should incorporate social work practices in various settings including psychiatric, health, religious, legal, occupational, and more. Information on communication skills makes the volume more useful for students learning to work with the elderly. The authors' stimulating case studies make this an ideal text for undergraduate and graduate social work programs in gerontology.

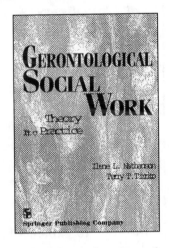

Contents: Preface
- Introduction
- Social Work Practice Revisited
- Integrative Model of Gerontological Social Work
- Special Needs of Older People: An Overview
- Gerontological Psychiatric Social Work Practice
- Formal Social Services
- Gerontological Social Work Practice in Health Services
- Social Work with the Aging in a Legal Environment
- Gerontological Social Work Practice in a Religious Environment
- Gerontological Social Work Practice in a Work Environment
- Gerontological Social Work Practice in a Political Environment
- Communication Skills for Gerontological Social Work Practice
- Epilogue

1997 176pp. 0-8261-9890-2 hardcover www.springerpub.com

536 Broadway, New York, NY 10012-3955 • (212) 431-4370 • Fax (212) 941-7842